The Science of Vitamins

Meets Optimum Health & Common Sense

DR. JOHN ZIELONKA

Wasteland Press
Shelbyville, KY USA
www.wastelandpress.net

The Science of Vitamins:
Meets Optimum Health & Common Sense
by Dr. John Zielonka

First Printing – February 2012
ISBN: 978-1-60047-681-5

The information in this book is for educational purposes only.
The taking of prescription drugs and vitamin supplements can
have both beneficial and adverse effects on your health. All
readers are strongly advised to personally consult a qualified
health care professional for conditions specific to their own health
and not to rely solely on the information in this book.

Printed in the U.S.A.

0   1   2   3   4   5

This book is dedicated to all those who choose to be healthy.

Table of Contents

INTRODUCTION

"All truth passes through three stages.
First, it is ridiculed.
Second, it is violently opposed.
Third, it is accepted as being self-evident."

-Arthur Schopenhauer,
German philosopher (1788 - 1860)

I'm sure that many of you may be familiar with the above quote, but nowhere is it more fitting than in "The Science of Vitamins". The truth is that taking essential vitamin supplementation your entire life will result in your living longer and living better.

Unfortunately, many people are still in the first stage. They don't understand or appreciate the value of health and lifelong vitamin supplementation, and they have never been properly educated on it. Their lack of knowledge or their ego's self-defence mechanism results in them ridiculing those who do value their health. This group may include many medical doctors and certainly a lot of drug reps. Unfortunately, this only results in early death and needless suffering.

There are certainly others already in the second stage. While you may not see it as "violent opposition", there is a significant and widespread lying, deceit, and purposeful misinformation perpetuated by people that you're supposed to be able to trust. Sickness and death is big business with billions upon billions of dollars at stake. Drug companies, governments, and their allies have a vested interest in ensuring that we're not all healthy at the same time.

Finally there's the third stage. I'm there already. So are many of my patients. It may take ten, twenty, or even fifty years for everyone to realize it and more importantly to act upon it, but that day will come. The day will come where we look back and wonder how we ever lived in such an insane "health care" system. While I'm looking forward to that day, I'm not waiting for it. I'm taking action now. In fact, I have been for many years. After reading this book, I hope that you will, too.

The truth is that taking essential vitamin supplementation your entire life will result in your living longer and living better

1

In the Beginning

I remember 20 years ago when I first started practice. I made the conscious decision to not carry any nutritional products in my office as I didn't want to be perceived as a salesperson pushing products on my patients or having any conflict of interest. This was despite the fact that I had advanced nutritional training as well as a Bachelor of Science in Chemistry. Instead, I made the extra effort to tell patients exactly what they should be looking for in a nutritional product and what to ask for to ensure both quality and the proper supplement.

For instance, in the case of a bone health supplement I would tell them to look for microcrystallinehydroxyapatite that had been cold processed, heavy metal assayed and verified by x-ray analysis to have a microcrystalline structure, among other things. The only problem with that approach is that the person who they would run into at the drug store or nutrition store was a salesperson whose typical response was "well I don't know what he's talking about but this is what we're promoting this month".

Needless to say, I no longer have any problems with carrying nutritional supplements in my office. I carry the absolute best products based on extensive research from the best labs that only sell to qualified health care professionals. These are the same products that my family and I take from a variety of different labs based solely on quality. Should a patient be interested, that's great, and should they have no interest, that's perfectly fine.

The reason this becomes so important is that there are millions of people out there who are trying to get healthy and millions more who would if they had the right information. Sadly, there are many millions more who are getting very poor information from health care professionals who pretend to have superior knowledge. What's worse is the hype and downright misleading marketing aimed at taking your money.

That's where this book comes in. The same advice that I've been giving my patients for years is the information that I'd like you to have. To be blunt, people are dying sooner than they were meant to because they're not getting the right information. To make matters worse, finding that right information can prove to be quite a challenge and it is also often different from commonly held beliefs.

**To be blunt,
people are dying sooner than they were meant to
because they're not getting the right information**

If you're looking for a book that tells you that vitamin A is good for your eyes and it's found in carrots, then you've come to the wrong place. There are a thousand other nutrition and vitamin books out there that will give you that information. I won't take the time and effort to write unless there's something new to say with that something being essential to your well-being.

This book is divided into 7 parts:

- The first part will confirm once and for all who really needs to take vitamins and specifically which ones are needed.
- The second part discusses the accomplishments of science as well as its significant limitations. This includes explaining how different scientific studies can come to opposite findings on whether supplementation is beneficial.
- The third part will look at the science behind how vitamins specifically play a role in preventing cancer, heart disease, high blood pressure, and diabetes, controlling cholesterol and enhancing brain function and more.
- Part 4 will explain in depth how to compare vitamin brands - other than just looking at the ingredients label - as well as the science behind the standards of the world's best labs.
- Part 5 specifically lists which vitamins and prescription drugs do not mix well as well as which vitamins are essential if you're taking prescription drugs.
- Part 6 describes the blood testing that you should have done instead of standard blood tests to accurately analyze your current health status.
- Finally, in part 7, I give you specific recommendations, including brand names, for what I feel are the very best nutritional supplements on the market today. I explain why they are the best, where to get them, and what to take for specific "health" conditions.

As I frequently tell my patients, you must not only absorb the following information, but also act upon it if you wish to achieve a lifetime of optimal health.

HEALTH – "The optimal state of physical, mental and social well being – and not merely the absence of disease or infirmity"
World Health Organization

Part One

The Need for Vitamins

2

Do I Really Need To Take Vitamins? The Question Answered Once and For All

It should be easy. Either you need vitamins or you don't. Yet while billions of dollars are spent on vitamins and nutritional supplements every year, some people firmly believe that they can get everything from their diet and even others believe that vitamins are nothing but "expensive urine".

These are, of course, all beliefs. But what if I told you that I could answer the question, once and for all? Not simply my opinion, but on a rational, logical flow chart approach to answering the question.

Do I need vitamins?

To answer this question, we need to know what a vitamin is and what it does. Do you? Most people don't.

"Vitamin" *- an organic compound that can be transformed in the body into a coenzyme that aids in specific chemical reactions in the cells and tissues.* <u>***Thus they are essential for physiological function.***</u>

So the answer is simple. You do need vitamins because they are essential for physiological function. But of course it isn't that easy because when we ask the question "Do we need vitamins?" what we are really asking is "Do we need them in a pill form?" So the real question is not do I need vitamins (you do) but rather...

Do I need vitamin supplementation?

I did say that it was a logical flow chart approach, so to answer this question I must, in fact, ask and answer another question:

Can I get everything I need from a balanced diet?

This can only be answered by asking:

What do I need?

This of course brings us to a key part of the question and a discussion of recommended daily allowances or RDAs versus optimum health. Is it your belief that RDAs are sufficient for health or do you strive for optimal health and what exactly is the difference? To begin to answer this, we must ask our next question:

What is an RDA?

Believe it or not, far too many people believe that these are numbers derived at some scientific high-level meeting held by the government with your best interests at heart that will give you all the health you need. The truth is that an RDA is:

RDA - "The amount of a vitamin necessary to prevent a disease deficiency."

What does that mean? It means that the RDA for vitamin C is how much vitamin C you need so that you don't get the disease that's caused by a lack of vitamin C. What disease is that? Scurvy! The RDA for vitamin D is how much vitamin D you need so that you don't get rickets! (Rickets is a significant "softening" of the bones.) This of course begs the real question:

Is this your health goal?

While you are free to have any goal you wish, if you really want to have a "health" goal, that goal should be based on what the word "health" actually means (previously defined on page 6). While this may seem obvious to you, most people don't know the meaning of the word (as evidenced by our so-called "health-care system") and certainly don't live their lives congruent to its true meaning.

One must also appreciate what I refer to as the "health continuum", described in detail in my previous books and most of my lectures. In a nutshell, your daily actions have the biggest influence on your health. These actions have effects, both positive and negative, and occur long before you feel them. Fortunately, you have control over these actions, thus you have incredible power over your health.

Now understanding this, if your desired level of nutrition and vitamin intake (whether through diet and/or supplementation) is simply to avoid scurvy, rickets and other deficiency diseases, then meeting RDA levels would be sufficient to accomplish such a goal. Please be aware, however, that this has nothing to do with optimum health or the health continuum and is, in fact, a major contributor to why we have so many unhealthy people on this planet.

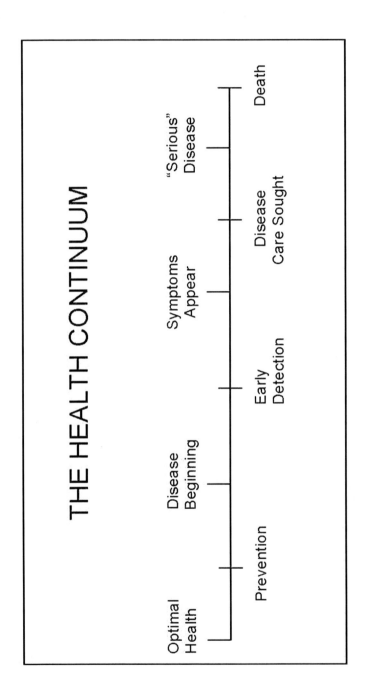

THE HEALTH CONTINUUM

Optimal Health

Prevention

Disease Beginning

Early Detection

Symptoms Appear

Disease Care Sought

"Serious" Disease

Death

Is your health goal simply to avoid scurvy?

If your health goal is optimum health, there are thousands of scientific studies (as we will discuss) that confirm the role of supplementation in helping you achieve this and how vitamin levels well above RDA levels are necessary.

It is interesting to note that there is the occasional study that is anti-vitamin and even more interesting to note that the anti-vitamin person will rely on the one negative study to justify their position while ignoring the 100 positive ones (to be discussed in greater detail later). Getting back to our flow chart of questions in discussing RDAs versus optimum health, one must now ask:

Can I get these (RDA or optimum health) levels from diet alone?

You would think the common sense thing to do would be to investigate this question, so that's exactly what I did. I went to Canada's Food Guide and took a **random sampling** to comprise my meals. For instance, if it said to have X servings of a food group and there were X number of pictures in the guide, I took one of each. I then calculated the actual nutrients I would get from those meals. The results?

A random selection of Canada's Food Guide for the following nutrients for the average adult:

Vitamin A	Vitamin C
Vitamin B1	Vitamin D
Vitamin B2	Vitamin E
Vitamin B3	Calcium
Vitamin B5	Magnesium
Vitamin B6	Iron
Vitamin B12	Zinc

Which ones achieved an "optimal health level"?

Not a single vitamin obtained an optimum level as determined by a consensus of multiple scientific studies! Hence, the answer is simple.

If your goal is to achieve optimum health and optimum levels of nutrition, you must supplement.

Please remember that the word is *supplement*, which means vitamin products *in addition* to good meals.

Eating according to Canada's Food Guide does not achieve an optimal level of health for any vitamin

But what if you're really stubborn and stuck in your old sick care paradigms?

As inadequate as RDAs are, how many people actually meet RDA levels?

Youngsters' Diets Found Inadequate
~The Associated Press~
"Hold the chips and pass the broccoli! Only 1 percent of Americans ages 2 to 19 met all government guidelines for a healthy diet, a study has found."

Of course, the next question is:

Did Canada's Food Guide meet all RDA levels?

Believe it or not, our random sampling found that following Canada's Food Guide did not even meet RDA levels for vitamins E, B5 and B12.

Please note that Canada's Food Guide also did not originate at that high-level meeting with your best interests at heart. Rather, it originated during World War II as a food rationing program. While it was updated in 2007 it is still woefully inadequate.

Hence, while it is a nice belief that you get everything you need from your meals, it's just not true 99.9 percent of the time. There are numerous factors that affect nutrient quality such as pollution, pesticides, soil quality, food contaminants, processing and cooking methods.

There are also factors that affect your vitamin requirements, such as physiological and psychological stress, infection, exercise, alcohol and poor nutrient density.

How many people fit into the above categories?

What about those who believe that God never intended us to take vitamin supplementation or that Mother Nature provides everything we need? I could simply tell you it's an unhealthy belief, but the reason I bring it up here is that you **were** right, except you were right some 10,000 years ago. As best as can be accurately determined, it is estimated that mankind did achieve optimal levels from what we ate 10,000 years ago. So God and Mother Nature did intend us to eat healthy, we just screwed it up along the way.

What about the people who think that vitamin supplementation results in "expensive urine"? They're lacking the B vitamins they need for normal brain function. That's like saying that water has no purpose since it just comes out as urine. Again, it's easier for them to believe that the vitamin-takers must be wrong and are wasting their money than it is for them to accept that they're not interested or willing to invest in their health.

Poor nutrition, or more precisely a lack of optimum nutrition, is involved in every degenerative disease known to mankind. Beyond helping to prevent disease, optimal nutrition is essential for optimal health. **Once and for all, do** you need vitamin supplementation? The answer is absolutely yes!

Finally, we must go one final step in realizing that not all vitamins are created equally. While this may sound very much like a cliché, you do get what you pay for. That doesn't mean that all expensive vitamins are good, it just simply means that most inexpensive ones, including some very well-known brand names, aren't. Different vitamins are made from different sources with different binders and fillers. Most well-known drug store brands have very poor absorption and dissolution. Paying less for a vitamin of which only 3 to 5% is absorbed by the body is not a bargain. Make the investment and buy your vitamins from health care professionals who you trust. More on this in the next chapter.

Do I need vitamins?
↓

Do I need vitamin supplementation?
↓

Can I get everything I need from a balanced diet?
↓

What do I need?
↓

RDAs or Optimal Health. What's your goal?
↓

Can I get this from my diet?
↓

Almost always, NO.

↓

Once and for all, do you need vitamin supplementation?

↓

The answer is absolutely YES!

3

WHICH VITAMINS ARE NECESSARY FOR EVERYONE?

In the previous chapter, I discussed the all-important question "Do I really need vitamins". And hopefully for the sake of your health you have come to the factual conclusion that you in fact do. If you're reading this book, you should also fully understand that everyone *needs* to be healthy, not simply that they want to be healthy.

Now of course comes the next logical question: "Which vitamins does everyone need?"

Courtesy of marketing hype, you may believe that there is no such thing as a vitamin that *everyone* needs. You would be wrong. Marketing hype, and certainly not science, has led many to the allure of the latest, greatest fad or cure for your particular condition, often with no idea of what the product actually does or with ingredients (sometimes secretive and even patented) that you may have never heard of.

You may have also been led to believe that certain blood types or certain personalities somehow have different vitamin requirements. Many people love this idea as it affirms the emotional belief that everyone is different or that we're all "individuals" or that our biochemistry is somehow unique. Unfortunately, good science does not back this up.

To answer the question "Which vitamins does everyone need?" you need to appreciate the simple fact that humans, contrary to our arrogance, are simply yet one more type of animal species[*]. You would never hear of two giraffes requiring different nutrients or taking blood tests to determine which tree they should eat from.

Now let's be clear. If you are supplementing to address a specific advanced condition that you may have in a sick care paradigm, then yes, you may be taking a different supplement.

You would never hear of two giraffes
requiring different nutrients or taking blood tests
to determine which tree they should eat from

However, if you are supplementing in a health and wellness paradigm, as everyone should, the specific vitamins that everyone needs are based on the following:

- Is the supplement necessary for optimal physiological and neurological function?
- Is it virtually impossible to obtain the required amount through normal diet?
- Is there significant and substantial scientific evidence to validate the need for and benefit of each supplement?

---

[*] This topic is discussed in detail in my DVD "Sick Care vs. The Health & Wellness Paradigm" as well as in my next book due out in the fall of 2012

Based on the above criteria, all humans require all of the following in supplement form (in addition to a good diet) if they are to achieve optimal health over the course of their lifetime:

1. A comprehensive, quality multivitamin/mineral
2. Essential fatty acids (EPA and DHA in their end form)
3. Vitamin D (specifically D3 cholecalciferol)
4. Probiotics
5. Phytonutrients

All of the above are essential for optimal health and are a requirement for all humans for proper physiological and biochemical function. This is very likely to extend the quality and quantity of your life and, the last time I checked, survival definitely qualified as a need – not simply a want.

Part Two

The Science

4

THE "SCIENCE" OF VITAMINS

When you first read the title of this book, what were your expectations? Did you expect to see the chemical structure of each vitamin? Were you hoping to see hundreds of references in scientific literature? Did you want to see a detailed chemical pathway of exactly what a vitamin does in its physiological process? Or were you simply hoping to get some rational and common-sense advice on how to choose the best nutritional supplementation without the marketing hype and differing opinions, so that you could enjoy a better quality and quantity of life?

When you think of "science", do you picture the amazing advances of performing heart surgery on a yet-to-be born baby or on creating the next six-million-dollar man? Do you picture science as one day allowing you to live to a hundred and fifty years of age with new parts? Or, is it all just grade twelve chemistry that you'd like to forget?

What many, including many scientists themselves, don't realize is that while we see "science" as the ultimate in objectivity and being completely unbiased, it does, in fact, have quite a subjective and biased component, especially depending on which health paradigm you're in and, more importantly, what question are you asking (more on this in the next chapter). This is one of the reasons why two different scientists can hold up two different studies with two completely opposite conclusions. In some cases, they may even be looking at the same study and still have completely opposite conclusions (otherwise known as "opinions").

In fact, this goes well beyond vitamins. What if I told you that the science of most aspects of healthcare is actually quite unscientific, and that the fact that it is unscientific is stated in the scientific literature?

Many people believe that healthcare, and especially medicine, must be **scientifically proven.** After all, they wouldn't experiment on us with unproven treatments and drugs, would they? But what does "scientifically proven" actually mean?

The "gold standard" for science has traditionally been something called a double-blind study or more specifically, a double-blind, randomized controlled study. What does this mean? It means that if I want to know if drug X (or vitamin X or procedure X) works to cure headaches, I can't just take it when I have a headache and consider it proven if the headache goes away. Why? Because the headache might have gone away on its own or I might have unknowingly done something else that made it go away or a host of other factors. So in a double-blind study, we would take a significant number of people with headaches and divide them into three groups. One group would get drug X, one group would get a placebo (a pill that looked just like drug X but had nothing in it or no effect to it), and one group would get nothing. Furthermore, neither the people in the study <u>nor</u> the scientist conducting the study would know who was getting what. The results would be tabulated and if, for instance, 99 percent of the people who took drug X saw headache relief whereas only 1 percent who took the placebo or took nothing experienced headache relief, then the study could conclude that drug X was effective in treating headaches for the average person. So what's the problem with that, you may ask? Many:

1. Just who is the average person? People have such varying physiological stressors and deficiencies that there is no such person as "average".
2. There are a number of health procedures that simply can't be reasonably tested using a double-blind study. For instance, a ludicrous example would be to scientifically prove that emergency surgery can repair ruptured spleens. Would we take a hundred people with ruptured spleens and repair them while leaving another hundred to bleed out just to scientifically prove that surgery is effective for ruptured spleens?
3. If everything needed to be scientifically proven before it could be done, nothing would ever happen because you couldn't perform the procedure even in the study.
4. That's great when the statistics work out as they did in our example (99 percent vs. 1 percent) but what if it's 51 percent vs. 49 percent? Yes, the mathematicians will tell you that the numbers have to be "statistically significant", but wouldn't you feel more comfortable taking drug X at 99 percent vs. 1 percent instead of 51 percent vs. 49 percent?
5. This is especially true when you consider that nowhere does the double-blind study take long-term safety into account. Think Thalidomide or Celebrex just to name two drugs that were supposedly "scientifically proven" and approved by both the U.S. FDA and Health Canada.
6. If the FDA and Health Canada are that inept, consider that most, if not all, drug trials are funded by the drug

companies. This is often the case in the handful of drug studies that have supposedly shown that a vitamin was not effective (again – more on this in the next chapter).

7. Last, but certainly not least, there is no place for anecdotal evidence. Yes, I can hear the so-called scientists shiver just hearing the word "anecdotal" as it is "unscientific", but consider the following example. One day Mary has the flu and decides to drink green Kool-Aid. The next day her flu is completely gone and she starts telling all her friends how green Kool-Aid cures the flu. Now, of course we understand that this is highly unlikely as it is simply Mary's story (her anecdote). But what if every time Mary has the flu she always drinks green Kool-Aid and her flu is always gone the next day? And what if all of Mary's friends start drinking green Kool-Aid every time they have the flu and have the same experience? Yes, it's still anecdotal. But what if everyone in Mary's entire city starts to do the exact same thing every time they have the flu and get the exact same results? Yes, it's still anecdotal, but you can be sure that they wouldn't care, and before you know it the whole country would be drinking green Kool-Aid every time they had the flu. They wouldn't wait for the "science" to confirm what they were already experiencing. This is exactly what most doctors do in their clinical practice on a daily basis.

There are many patients who I have treated successfully with widely accepted procedures that have never been "scientifically proven". Should I go back and tell all these people that they shouldn't be better?

If the "gold standard" for science has this many shortcomings, as many scientists themselves now agree, what does this have to do with healthcare and vitamins? It's relevant because many people's health beliefs insist on a standard that not only has flaws, but simply doesn't exist. Consider the following question:

What percentage of medicine has been scientifically proven?

Again, before reading the answer, please take a guess. "Why, it must be one hundred percent," you say, especially given today's technology and scientific advances. Well, according to Dr. David Eddy, M.D., Ph.D. and published in the prestigious British Medical Journal, only fifteen percent of medicine has ever been scientifically proven. That's right, eighty-five percent of medicine has never been scientifically proven. Dr. Eddy goes on to state that of the fifteen percent that has been "proven", only one percent of those studies were actually done using scientifically sound protocols.

Only 15% of medicine has ever been scientifically proven
-Dr. David Eddy, M.D., Ph.D., British Medical Journal

Now this is not to say that science does not have its place and of course continuing research and scientific advances are essential, but if your health beliefs are such that all "traditional" medicine and all FDA and Health Canada approved drugs are proven and that all vitamins, nutritional supplements and alternative healthcare is unproven (it's not alternative **medicine** unless you consider it an alternative *to* medicine) then it's time to get out of your glass house and change your beliefs. The truth is that so-called traditional medicine has only been around for two hundred years whereas alternative healthcare has been around for two thousand years. The need for essential nutrients in your body has been around since the beginning of the human race.

Having said that, please don't get the wrong idea that I'm suggesting that vitamin supplements be taken with no rhyme or reason and only on anecdotal evidence – quite to the contrary. The truth is that there exists a wealth of good scientific evidence (far more than most aspects of medicine) that clearly demonstrates both the need and effectiveness for many vitamin supplements. This will be clearly discussed in chapters to come. The purpose of this chapter was to counteract the continuing false belief that all drugs and society's "sick care" approach is traditional and scientific whereas many still believe that the jury is still out on vitamin supplementation. The next chapter will also clearly demonstrate how some have grossly skewed the "science" in an attempt to disprove the science of vitamins.

5

WHY SCIENCE ISN'T SO SCIENTIFIC

Over the past twenty years, I have treated thousands of patients, including a number of scientists and analysts. It has been my personal clinical experience, repeatedly I might add, that all of these scientists and analysts make a point of telling me that they make all of their health decisions "scientifically". Sounds reasonable, you say? I'd agree, except for the fact that it has also been my clinical experience that almost all of these same scientists and analysts end up making their health decisions anything but "scientifically". They use the same subjective opinions and sometimes false beliefs that are anything but "scientific".

They may also utilize information that they believe is from scientific sources with no idea of just how biased that so-called scientific source may be. One example would be taking the FDA and Health Canada at face value without any understanding of just how many thousands have died from "safe and approved" drugs, only for those drugs to be recalled years later. Or just how frequently it is uncovered that these two government "authorities" are found to have what many actual experts describe as incestuous ties with various drug companies. If you believe that this is some type of conspiracy theory, then come up with reasonable answers to the following questions:

1. What scientific criteria were used that found a drug safe only to discover years later that the same drug was deadly?
2. How can one scientific study prove that a vitamin is beneficial while another scientific study proves that the exact same vitamin is not beneficial? More importantly, which do you choose to believe? Isn't the whole idea of "science" to remove the need for making decisions based on beliefs?
3. If the United States believes it has the best "science" in the world and if it believes that its healthcare system is solely based on the science, then why does the United States rank 37th in the world for healthcare?

You must appreciate that double-blind randomized controlled studies have biases, and that assumes that they were conducted using sound protocols. One of the key questions that one must ask is, "Exactly what question was the study asking?".

What do I mean? Try this. How many scientific studies have proven that cholesterol-lowering drugs save lives?

The correct answer is zero. What cholesterol-lowering drug studies have shown is one thing and one thing only – that these drugs lower cholesterol. It is simply assumed that this saves lives. While this may be your belief, if it were true why would a drug company not have a single scientific study to prove it?

How many scientific studies have proven that cholesterol-lowering drugs save lives?

The correct answer is zero

The best way to understand how unreasonable a double-blind randomized controlled scientific study could be based on the question being asked is best described in this analogy from well-known wellness expert Dr. James Chestnut:

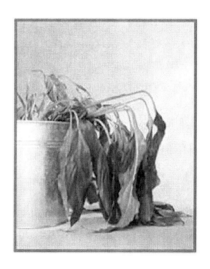

What would any reasonable person do for the above wilting plant? Water it, of course. But if I wanted to "prove" this "scientifically" in a double-blind randomized controlled study, I would need to take one hundred of these wilting plants and water them. I'd need to take another hundred wilting plants and give them a liquid that the plants thought was water but wasn't. Lastly, I would need to have another hundred wilting plants that I did nothing to. And of course the person who then assessed how the plants reacted could not know what each plant received.

So what's the problem, you ask? The problem is that you're assuming the obvious – that the wilting plants that actually received water all improved in their health. But what if in this example they didn't? You would have a scientific double-blind randomized controlled study that could officially claim that water has no health benefit in making a wilting plant no longer wilt.

This would never happen, you say? Of course it could, because what if these same plants also all had soil that was completely devoid of any nutrients? Now the logical solution to help these plants would be to add nutrients to their soil. But to prove scientifically if this was beneficial for plants, again we would need to do our double-blind randomized controlled study. In this case, we would need our control group who received nothing, a group who got water and soil nutrients, a group who got water only, a group who got soil nutrients only, and groups who got a combination of placebo water and soil nutrients.

But what if after doing all this, our water and soil nutrient plants were still wilting? Again, the drug company study would make headlines in the newspaper showing that vitamin X has been scientifically proven to have no benefit in helping disease Y. Oh, I'm sorry – we weren't talking about vitamins just yet? Alright – the newspaper headline would clearly - and accurately - I might add, state:

"New Scientific Study Shows That Water and Soil Nutrients Have No Health Benefits in Helping Wilting Plants Stop Wilting"

Couldn't happen, you say? Of course it could, because what if these same plants were all kept in a dark closet devoid of all sunlight? What many scientists and most of the general public fail to appreciate is that so-called scientific studies seek to answer a specific question and the question that is chosen can have a huge impact on just how useful the findings of that study actually are.

So what if we now do another double-blind randomized controlled study but this time with three variables, and all their placebo and control groups. Some plants received water, nutrients, and sunlight, some just water and sunlight but no nutrients, some with nutrients and sunlight but no water, etc. etc. And again, what if at the end our plants were still wilting? The newspaper headline would "accurately read" (according to the terms of the study):

"New Scientific Study Shows That Water, Nutrients, and Sunlight Have No Health Benefits in Helping Wilting Plants to Stop Wilting"

We of course know that such a finding is far from "accurate" as water, nutrients, and sunlight are essential for the health of any plant. (Try doing your own study where you stop giving these three things to your own plants and see what happens each and every time.) But according to the specific question being asked, our plants were still wilting. How is that possible, you say? Simple. All of the plants in question had gasoline poured into their soil.

While you might think that this is an extreme example, appreciate that all living creatures, including both plants and humans, will always fail to function at optimal levels if they have deficiencies that are essential for life (water, nutrients, sunlight, vitamins) and/or if they are subjected to stressors or toxins (gasoline for the plants in our example, or a whole array of human stressors and toxins).

What's the logical bottom line? A study really can't disprove that a vitamin works, especially if numerous other studies have shown that it does work. And this doesn't even begin to touch on all the other factors missed (often purposely), such as using too small a quantity of vitamins, using the wrong form of vitamin, studying the subject for too short a period of time, or not using the required co-factors to ensure that the vitamin worked effectively - not to mention conflict of interest, faulty design and media bias. This is especially prevalent in many vitamin E and beta-carotene studies that have attempted to discredit their effectiveness.

"Vitamin E Shown Not to Reduce Cardiovascular Disease" was the headline reported in the Journal of the American Medical Association (July 2005) in a study to test whether vitamin E supplementation decreased the risk of cardiovascular disease and cancer among healthy women. However, after reading the entire study it was found that for cardiovascular death there was a 24% reduction in risk! Why was the finding not heralded as a significant discovery? Because cardiovascular death was not one of the specific questions set up by the study.

In addition to asking the wrong question, there is another significant difference that is lost on most who live in the medical/drug world. As we will discuss in chapter 23, there is a huge paradigm shift between those who live in the sick-care model of "health" and those who live in the health and wellness paradigm. The idea of using the methods in the sick-care model as an accurate way of measuring the health and wellness paradigm is completely invalid and defies common-sense. As scientist and world renown supplementation expert Lyle MacWilliams states, "they're using the wrong yardstick". You cannot use a test that is designed to see if one drug has an effect on one reaction to then accurately gauge if a vitamin that works hand in hand with numerous other nutrients (not in isolation) can have the same effect on its own. As nutritional researcher Dr. Tim Wood states, "high doses of a single nutrient represent an incomplete and inappropriate approach to nutritional therapy...this would be analogous to testing the hypothesis that broccoli has cancer-preventative properties by putting people on a broccoli-only diet. It's not likely to work, and it carries the risk of creating severe nutrient imbalances, unwanted side effects, and misleading experimental artefacts."

Another way to put this into perspective would be to consider what would happen if we reversed the situation. What if we used the yardstick of the health and wellness paradigm to judge a drug from the sick-care paradigm? What would happen if we gave Lipitor or Celebrex to a healthy child over the course of their lifetime? Would the results of such an experiment show that the child enjoyed a lifetime of health? Of course not – rather we would be jailed for child endangerment.

Stop going to the sick-care experts and using their tools to judge your level of health. Your life depends on it. Stop believing that the sick care paradigm is superior as they believe they are. When it comes to health, nothing could be further from the truth.

What if we used the yardstick of the health and wellness paradigm to judge a drug from the sick-care paradigm?

What would happen if we gave Lipitor or Celebrex to a healthy child over the course of their lifetime?

Do you remember the famous vitamin E, beta-carotene cancer prevention study conducted in Finland in 1994 that many so-called experts still wrongly quote as fact in saying that beta-carotene actually caused cancer? The initial results of the study when beta-carotene was viewed in isolation led to the erroneous conclusion that high levels of beta-carotene increased the risk of cancer in male smokers. Despite objections that the study was flawed, the charge stuck and vitamin use dropped worldwide. Ten years later (July 2004), when the same data was reviewed in the American Journal of Epidemiology and total antioxidant intake was evaluated (not just beta-carotene), the findings of the original study were found to be in error. The new analysis – using the same data as the original study – came to a remarkably different conclusion: beta-carotene in combination with other antioxidants significantly reduced cancer risk in the same male smokers. Same data, different paradigms, different conclusions.

Hence, we're back to two people quoting "scientific studies" with two completely opposing *opinions*. Those who are willing to invest in their health and understand the proper use of science will see substantial benefits in vitamin supplementation. Those who don't like to make the daily effort or make the same investment or believe that someone else is supposed to pay for their health may choose to side with those who have wrongly attempted to discredit the benefit of vitamins through the misuse of science.

"Believe in gravity."
Dr. John Zielonka

People are entitled to have any belief that they choose. But as I explain to my patients, if I were to take you to the roof of my building and we both stepped off the ledge, it doesn't matter how many times you say "I don't believe in gravity" on the way down, we're still going to hit the ground.

Choose to believe in the numerous quality scientific studies listed in this book and the science of physiology and biochemistry that explains their rationale. Choose not to believe the few inaccurate "studies" that have ulterior motives or have chosen to ask the wrong question or come to the wrong conclusion. Follow this advice and you will experience a better quality and quantity of life.

**Those who are willing to invest in their health
and understand the proper use of science
will see substantial benefits in vitamin supplementation.**

**Those who don't like to make the daily effort or make
the same investment may choose to side with those
who have wrongly attempted to discredit the
benefit of vitamins through the misuse of science.**

6

Scientific References
(No – it's not the end of the book yet!)

Now that you have a much better understanding of both the benefits and limitations of science, it's time to let you know that there is a wealth of good science that strongly and repeatedly supports the role of vitamin supplementation in fighting, preventing and reversing disease as well as improving both the quantity and quality of your life.

As I have said before, while we are not even close to knowing everything there is to know about health, we know more than enough to be healthy, far healthier than we are as a whole. Contrary to those who incorrectly believe that the research on vitamins and health is limited, I have chosen to include my list of over 2,000 references and scientific studies at this point in this book simply to give you an idea of just how much scientific literature currently exists. You will now most likely fall into one of two categories: the 99% of the population that will skip these pages (that's perfectly fine and expected) or the 1% who will look up each reference trying unsuccessfully to disprove the study and the benefits of vitamin supplementation. To those who fall into the latter category: - good luck with that. While you're wasting your time defending your right to be unhealthy, the other 99% will hopefully be spending their time becoming healthy. The following chapter starts on page 145 at which point you will discover the incredible control and power you have in regards to your health.

Telomeres

Greider CW, Blackburn EH. Telomeres, telomerase and cancer. Sci Am. 1996;2:92-97.

Shay JW, Wright WE. Hayflick, his limit, and cellular ageing. Mol Cell Biol. 2000;1:72-76.

Reddel RR. The role of senescence and immortalization in carcinogenesis. Carcinogenesis. 2000;21:477-484.

Karp G. DNA replication and repair. In: Cell and Molecular Biology. 2nd ed. New York, NY: John Wiley & Sons,Inc. 1999;575-607.

Hao Y-h, Tan Z. The generation of long telomere overhangs in human cells: a model and its implication.Bioinformatics. 2002;18:666-671.

Makarov VL, Hirose Y, Langmore JP. Long G tails at both ends of human chromosomes suggest a C strand degradation mechanism for telomere shortening. Cell. 1997;88:657-666.

Griffith JD, Comeau L, Rosenfield S, et al. Mammalian telomeres end in a large duplex loop. Cell. 1999;97:503-514.

Blasco MA. Mammalian telomeres and telomerase: why they matter for cancer and aging. Eur J Cell Biol. 2003;82:441-46.

Greider CW. Telomeres do D-loop-T-loop. Cell. 1999;97:419-422.

Shay JW. At the end of the millennium, a view of the end. Nat Gen. 1999;23:382-383.

Kim S-H, Patrick K, Judith C. TIN2, a new regulator of telomere length in human cells. Nat Gen. 1999;23:405-412.

Shay JW, Zhou Y, Hiyama E, et al. Telomerase and cancer. Hum Mol Gen. 2001;10:677-685.

Enrique S, Fermin AG, Predrag S, et al. Mammalian Ku86 protein prevents telomeric fusions independently of the length of TTAGGG repeats and the G-strand overhang. EMBO Rep. 2000;11:244-252.

Bachand F, Ibtissem T, Autexier C. Human telomerase RNA-protein interactions. Nucleic Acids Res.2001;29:3385-3393.

Greider CW. Telomerase activity, cell proliferation, and cancer. Proc Natl Acad Sci U S A. 1998;95:90-92.

Haber DA. Clinical implications of basic research: telomeres, cancer and immortality. N Engl J Med.1995;332:955-956.

Belair CD, Yeager TR, Lopez PM, et al. Telomerase activity: a biomarker of cell proliferation, not malignant transformation. Proc Natl Acad Sci U S A. 1997;94:13677-13682.

Bodnar AG, Ouellette M, Frolkis M, et al. Extension of life-span by introduction of telomerase into normal human cells. Science. 1998;279:349-352.

Cong Y-S, Wright WE, Shay JW. Human telomerase and its regulation. Microbiol Mol Biol Rev. 2002;66:407-425.

Johnson FB, Sinclair DA, Guarente L. Molecular biology of aging. Cell. 1999;96:291-302.

Wright WE, Shay JW. Telomere dynamics in cancer progression and prevention: fundamental differences in human and mouse telomere biology. Nat Med. 2000;6:849-851.

Stewart SA, Hahn WC, O'Connor BF, et al. Telomerase contributes to tumorigenesis by a telomere lengthindependent mechanism. PNAS. 2002;99:12606-12611.

Judy MYW, Collins K. Telomere maintenance and disease. Lancet. 2003;362:983-988.

Simon WLC, Blackburn EH. New ways not to make ends meet: telomerase, DNA damage proteins and heterochromatin. Oncogene. 2002;21:553-563.

Herbert BS, Pitts AE, Baker SI, et al. Inhibition of human telomerase in immortal human cells leads to progressive telomere shortening and cell death. PNAS. 1999;96:14276-14281.

Halvorsen TL, Leibowitz G, Levine F. Telomerase activity is sufficient to allow transformed cells to escape from crisis. Mol Cell Biol. 1999;19:1864-1870.

Grogelny JV, McEliece MK, Broccoli D. Effects of reconstitution of telomerase activity on telomere maintenance by the alternative lengthening of telomeres (ALT) pathway. Hum Mol Gen. 2001;10:1953-1961.

Bryan TM, Englezou A, Dalla PL, et al. Evidence for an alternative mechanism for maintaining telomere length in human tumors and tumor-derived cell lines. Nat Med. 1997;3:1271-1274.

Liu JP. Studies of the molecular mechanisms in the regulation of telomerase activity. FASEB J. 1999;13:2091-2104.

Zhang XL, Mar V, Zhou W, et al. Telomere shortening and apoptosis in telomerase-inhibited human tumor cells. Gen Dev. 1999;13:2388-2399.

Hahn WC, Weinberg RA. Mechanisms of disease: rules for making human tumor cells. N Engl J Med. 2002;347:1593-1603.

Blasco MA, Lee HW, Hande MP, et al. Telomere shortening and tumor formation by mouse cells lacking telomerase RNA. Cell. 1997;91:25-34.

Blasco MA. Telomeres in cancer therapy. J Biomed Biotechnol. 2001;1:3-4.

Hodes R. Molecular targeting of cancer: telomeres as targets. Proc Natl Acad Sci U S A. 2001;98:7649-7651.

Mergny JL, Riou JF, Mailliet P, et al. Natural and pharmacological regulation of telomerase. Nucleic Acids Res.2002;30:839-865.

Herbert BS, Wright WE, Shay JW. Telomerase and breast cancer. Breast Cancer Res. 2001;3:146-149.

Blasco MA. Mouse models to study the role of telomeres in cancer, aging and DNA repair. Eur J Cancer.2002;38:2222-2228.

Cong YS, Wright WE, Shay JW. Human telomerase and its regulation. Microbiol Mol Biol Rev. 2002;66:407-425.

Meeker AK. Direct evidence of telomere shortening in the majority of human epithelial pre-cancerous lesions.

Program and abstracts of the AACR Meeting on the Role of Telomeres and Telomerases in Cancer; December 7-10, 2002; San Francisco, California.

Meeker AK, Gage WR, Hicks JL, et al. Telomere length assessment in human archival tissues: combined telomere fluorescence in situ hybridization and immunostaining. Am J Pathol. 2002;160:1259-1268.

Reddel RR. Alternative lengthening of telomeres in human cell lines and tumors. Program and abstracts of the AACR Meeting on the Role of Telomeres and Telomerases in Cancer; December 7-10, 2002; San Francisco,California.

Neumann AA, Reddel RR. Telomere maintenance and cancer -- look, no telomerase. Nat Rev Cancer. 2002;2:879-884.

DePinho RA. Crisis in the telomere checkpoint response in normal and neoplastic tissues. Program and abstracts of the AACR Meeting on the Role of Telomeres and Telomerases in Cancer; December 7-10, 2002; San Francisco, California.

Maser Rs, DePinho RA. Connecting chromosomes, crisis, and cancer. Science. 2002;297:565-569.

Chang S, Khoo CM, Naylor ML, Maser RS, DePinho RA. Telomere-based crisis: functional differences between telomerase activation and ALT in tumor progression. Genes Dev. 2003;17:88-100.

Weinberg RA. Control of replicative senescence by the telomere-associated single-strand overhang. Program and abstracts of the AACR Meeting on the Role of Telomeres and Telomerases in Cancer; December 7-10, 2002; San Francisco, California.

Stewart SA, Hahn WC, O'Connor BF, et al. Telomerase contributes to tumorigenesis by a telomere lengthindependent mechanism. Proc Natl Acad Sci U S A. 2002;99:12606-12611.

Harley CB. Status and issues for therapeutics based on telomere biology. Program and abstracts of the AACR Meeting on the Role of Telomeres and Telomerases in Cancer; December 7-10, 2002; San Francisco,California.

Chin AC. Treatment with GRN163 (novel telomerase template antagonist) selectively inhibits growth of myeloma and lymphoma cell lines and tumor xenografts by inducing proliferative arrest and apoptosis inmalignant cells with short telomeres. Program and abstracts of the AACR Meeting on the Role of Telomeres and Telomerases in Cancer; December 7-10, 2002; San Francisco, California.

Irving J. An oncolytic adenovirus controlled by the human telomerase promoter provides broad-spectrum antitumor activity. Program and abstracts of the AACR Meeting on the Role of Telomeres and Telomerases inCancer; December 7-10, 2002; San Francisco, California.

Novak KD. Telomeres and telmoerase in cancer: Highlights From an AACR Special Conference; December 7-11, 2002; San Francisco, California.

Medscape General Medicine 5(1), 2003. © 2003 Medscape Posted 01/23/200

Telomere Length in Different Tissues of Elderly Patients. Friedrich U, Griese E, Schwab M, Fritz P, Thon K, Klotz Uech Ageing Dev. 2000;15:89-99

Proc Natl Acad Sci USA 2004. www.pnas.org/cgi/doi/10.1073/pnas.040716210

Free Radicals and Antioxidants

Meyers DG, Maloley PA, Weeks D. Safety of antioxidant vitamins. *Arch Intern Med.* 1996;156:925-35.

Sun Y. Free radicals, antioxidant enzymes, and carcinogenesis. *Free Radic Biol Med.* 1990;8:583-99.

Loudon GM. *Organic Chemistry.* Menlo Park, Calif: Benjamin/Cummings Publishing Company Inc; 1988.

Winkler BS, Boulton ME, Gottsch JD, Sternberg P. Oxidative damage and age-related macular degeneration. *Mole Vis.* 1999;5:32.

Bulger EM, Helton WS. Nutrient antioxidants in gastrointestinal diseases. *Gastroenterol Clin North Am.*1998;27:403-19

Machlin LJ, Bendich A: Free radical tissue damage: protective role of antioxidant nutrients. FASEB J 1987;1:441-445

Ames BN, Shigenaga MK, Hagen TM: Oxidants, antioxidants, and the degenerative diseases of aging. Proc Natl Acad Sci U S A 1993; 90:7915-7922

Barja G The flux of free radical attack through mitochondrial DNA is related to aging rate. Aging (Milano) 2000 Oct;12(5):342-55

Bonnefoy M; Drai J; Kostka T Antioxidants to slow aging, facts and perspectives] Presse Med 2002 Jul 27;31(25):1174-84

Bonnefoy M; Drai J; Kostka T Oxidative stress, aging and longevity in Drosophila melanogaster. FEBS Lett 2001 Jun 8;498(2-3):183-6

Reiter R. Melatonin. Bantom Books. 1995: 15-44

Klatz R and Goldman R. The New Anti-Aging Revolution. Basic Health Publications, Inc. 2003: 19-38

Halliwell B and Gutteridge J. Free Radicals in Biology and Medicine (second edition) 1991: 1-20; 416-508

Antioxidants and Cancer

Cancer In General

Ames Bruce N, et al. Oxidants, Antioxidants, and the Degenerative Diseases of Aging; Proceedings of the National Academy of Science 1993 Sep;90:7915-22

Block G. Vitamin C and cancer prevention: the epidemiologic evidence. Am J Clin Nutr. 1991;53(1):270-282

Block G, et al. Fruits, Vegetables and Cancer Prevention: A Review of the Epidemiologic Evidence; Nutrition and Cancer 1992;187:1029

Gutteridge John M. Antioxidants, Nutritional Supplements, and Life-Threatening Diseases; British Journal of Biomedical Science 1994;31:288-95

Weisburger J. Nutriitonal Approach to Cancer Prevention with Emphasis on Vitamins, Antioxidants, and Carotenoids; American journal of Clinical Nutrition 1991;53:2265-2375

Zeigler, R. Vegetables, Fruits, and Carotenoids and the Risk of Cancer; American Journal of Clinical Nutrition 1991;53:2515-2595

Colon Cancer

Blot WJ, et al. The Linxian trails: mortality rates by vitamin-mineral intervention group. AM J Clin Nutr.;1995;62:14245-65

Bostick R.M, et al. Reduced risk of colon cancer with high intake of vitamin E:the Iowa Women's Health Study. Cancer Res 1993;53:4230-7

Bussey HJR, DeCosse JJ, Deschner EE, et al. A randomized trial of ascorbic acid in polyposis coli. Cancer 1982;50:1434–9.

Clark L, Cantor K, Allaway W. Selenium in forage crops and cancer mortality in US counties. Arch Environ Health 1991;46:37-42

Clark L, Combs GF, Turnbull BW, Slate EH, Chalker DK, et al. Effects of selenium supplementation for cancer prevention in patients with carcinoma of the skin. JAMA 1996;276: 1957-1964

Clark L, Hixson L, Combs G, Reid M, Turnbull B, et al. Plasma selenium concentration predicts the prevalence of colorectal adenomatous polyps. Cancer Epidemiol Biomarkters Prev 1993;2:41-45

DeCosse JJ, Miller HH, Lesser ML. Effect of wheat fiber and vitamins C and E on rectal polyps in patients with familial adenomatous polyposis. J Natl Cancer Inst 1989;81:1290–7

Dion PW, et al. The effect of dietary ascorbic acid and alpha-tocopherol on fecal mutagencity.Mutat Res.1982;102:27-37

Fiala E, Joseph C, Sohn O, El-Bayoumy K, and Reddy B. Mechanism of benzylselenocyanate inhibition of azoxymethane-induced colon carinogenesis in F344 rats. Cancer Res 1991;51:2826-2830

Greenberg ER, et al. A clinical trial of antioxidant vitamins to prevent colorectal adenoma. Ployp Provention Study Group. N Engl J Med 1994;331:141-7

Greenburg ER, Baron JA, Tosteson TD, et al. A clinical trial of antioxidant vitamins to prevent colorectal adenoma. N Engl J Med 1994;331:141–7

Jacobs M. Selenium inhibition of 1,2-dimethylhydralyzine-induced colon carcinogenesis." Cancer Res1983;43:1646-1649

Kiremidjian-Schumacher L, et al. Supplementation with selenium and human immune cell functions; II, effect on cytotoxic lymphocytes and natural killer cells. Bio Trace Elem Res 1994;41:103-114

Lanfear J, Fleming J, Wu L, Webster G, Harrison PR The selenium metabolite selenodiglutathione induces p53 and apoptosis." Carcinogenesis 1994;15:1378-1392

Langnecker MP, et al. Serum alpha-tocopherol concentration in relation to subsequent colorectal cancer; pooled data from five cohorts.J Natl Cancer Inst 1992;84:430-5

Lavender OA, et al. Bioavailability of selenium to Finnish men as assessed by platelet glutathione peroxidase activity and other blood parameters. AM J Clin Med 1983;37:887-897

McKeown-Eyssen G, et al. A randomized trial of vitamin C and E in the prevention of recurrence of colorectal polyps. Cancer Res 1988;48:4701-5

McKeown-Eyssen G, Holloway C, Jazmaji V, et al. A randomized trial of vitamins C and E in the prevention of recurrence of colorectal polyps. Cancer Res 1988;48:4701–5

Mutanen M, Bioavailability of selenium. Annals Clin Res 1986;18:48-54

Paganelli GM, et al. Effect of vitamin A, C and E. Supplementation on rectal cell proliferation in patients with colorectal adenomas. J Natl Cancer Inst. 1992;84:47-51

Ponz de Leon M, Roncucci L. Chemoprevention of colorectal tumors: role of lactulose and of other agents. Scand J Gastroenterol Suppl 1997;222:72–5

Reddy B, Rivenson A, Kulkarni N, Upadhyaya P, El-Bayoumy K. Chemoprevention of colon carcinogenesis by the synthetic organoselenium compound 1,4phenylenebis (methylene) selenocyanate. Cancer Res 1992;52:5635-5640

Reddy B, Tanaka T, El-Bayoumy K. Inhibitory effect of dietary p-methoxybenzeneselenol on azoxymethaneinduced colon and kidney carcinogenesis in female 344 rats.: JNCI 1985;74:1325-1328

Russo MW, et al. Plasma selenium levels and the risk of colorectal adenomas:, Nutrition and Cancer1997;28(2):125-129

Salonen, J, Alfthan G, Huttunen J, Puska P. Association between serum selenium and the risk of cancer. Am J Epidemiol 1984;120:342-349

Soullier B, Wilson P, Nigro, N Effect of selenium on azoxymethane-induced intestinal cancer in rats fed a high fat diet Cancer Lett 198;12:343-348

Stone, W.L. and Papas, A.M. Tocopherols and the Etiology of Colon Cancer.J Natl Cancer Inst. 1997;14(89):1006-1014

The effect of vitamin E and beta-carotene on the incidence of lung cancer and other cancers in male smokers. The Alpha-Tocopherol, Beta-carotene Cancer prevention Study Group. N Engl J med 1994;330:1029-35

Thompson CD, et al. Effect of prolonged supplementation with daily supplements of selenomethionine and sodium selenite on glutathione peroxidase activity in blood of New Zealand residents. AM J Clin Nutr 1982;36:24-31

Virtamo, J, Valkeila, E, Alfthan, G, Punsar, S, Huttunen, J, et al.: "Serum selenium and risk of cancer: a prospective follow-up of nine years." Cancer 1987;60:145-148

Willett WC, Polk PF, Morris JS, Stampfer MJ, Pressel S, et al.: "Prediagnostic serum selenium and risk of cancer." Lancet 1983;2:130-134

Prostate Cancer

Grovannucci et al. Intake of carotenoids and retinol in relation to risk of prostate cancer. J Natl Cancer Inst 1995; 87; 23:1767-76

Heinonen OP, et al. Prostate cancer and supplementation with Alpha-Tocopheral and Beta-Carotene : Incidence and mortality in a controlled trial. J Natl Cancer Inst 1998; 90; 6:440-446

Liehr JG. Androgen – Induced redox changes in prostate cancer cells: what are causes and effects? J Natl Cancer Inst 1997;1:3-6

Linehan WM. Inhibition of prostate cancer metastasis: a critical challenge ahead. J Natl Cancer Inst 1995; 87; 5: 331-32

Olson KB, et al. Vitamins A and E: Further clues for prostate cancer prevention. J Natl Cancer Inst 1998; 90(6):414-415

Rao VA, et al. Serum and tissue lycopene and biomarkers of oxidation in prostate cancer patients: A casecontrol study.
Nutr and Cancer, 1999; 33(2):159-164

Sigounas G, et al. DL-alpha-tocopherol induces apoptosis in erythroleukemia, prostate and breast cancer cells., Nutrition and Cancer 1997;28(1):30-35

Breast Cancer

Fleischauer A, et al. Antioxidant supplements and risk of breast cancer recurrence and breast cancer-related mortality among postmenopausal women. Nutrition and Cancer, 2003;46(1):15-22

Lockwood K, et al. Apparent partial remission of breast cancer in 'high risk' patients supplemented with nutritional antioxidants, essential fatty acids and coenzyme Q10. Mol Aspects Med. 1994;15 Suppl:s231-40

Sung L, et al. Vitamin E: The evidence for multiple roles in cancer. Nutrition and Cancer, 2003; 46(1):1-14

Cervical Cancer

B-carotene on the regression and progression of cervical dysplasia: a clinical experiment. J Clin Epidemiol 1991;44:273-293

Brock KE, Berry G, Mock PA, MacLennan R, Truswell AS et al. Nutrients in diet and plasma and risk of in situ cervical cancer. JNCI 1988;80:580-585

Buckley DI, McPherson S, North CQ, Becker TM. Dietary micronutrients and cervical dysplasia in southwestern American Indian women. Nutr Cancer 1992;17:179-185

Cuzik J, Stavola BL, Russell MJ, Thomas BS. Vitamin A, vitamin E and the risk of cervical intraepithelial
neoplasia. Br J Cancer 1990;62:651-652

De Vet HCW, Knipschild PG, Willebrand D, Schouten HJA, Sturmans F. The effect of intraepithelial and invasive cervical neoplasia. Gynegol Oncol 1988;30:187-195

De Vet, HCW, Knipschild PG, Grol MEC, Schouten HJA, Sturmans F. The role of B-carotene and other dietary factors in the aetiology of cervical dysplasia: results of a case-control study. Int J Epidemiol 1991;20:603-610

Di Masio P, Kaiser S, Sies H. Lycopene as the most efficient biological carotenoid singlet quencher. Arch Biochem Biophys 1989;274:532-538

Harris RWC, Forman D, Doll R, Vessey MP, Wald NJ. Cancer of the cervix uteri and vitamin A. Br J Cancer 1986;53:653-659

Knekt P. Serum vitamin E level and risk of female cancer. Int L Epidemiol 1988;17:281-286

La Vecchia C, Decarli A, Fasoli M, Parazzini F, Franceschi S et all Dietary vitamin A and tho rick of Liu T, Soong S, Wilson NP, Craig CR, Cole P, et al. A case control study of nutritional factors and cervical dysplasia. Cancer Epidemiol Biomarkers Prev 1993;2:525-530

Slattery ML, Abbott TM, Overall JC, Jr., Robinson LM, French TK et al. Dietary vitamins A, C, and E and selenium as risk factors for cervical cancer. Epidemiology 1990;1:8-15

Van Eenwyk J., Davis FG, Bowen PE. Dietary and serum carotenoids and cervical intraepithelial neoplasia. Int J Cancer 1991;48:34-38

Wylie-Rosett, JA, Romney SL, Slagle NS, Wassertheil-Smoller S, Miller GL et al. Influence of vitamin A on cervical dysplasia and carcinoma in situ.
Nurt Cancer 6, 49-57, 1984.

Ziegler RG, Jones CJ, Briton LA, Norman SA, Mallin K, et al. Diet and the risk of in situ cervical cancer among white women in the United States,Cancer Causes Control 1991;2:17-29

Stomach Cancer

Block G. Vitamin C and cancer prevention: the epidemiologic evidence. Am J Clin Nutr 1991 Jan;53(1):270S-282S

Kyrtopoulos SA. Ascorbic acid and the formation of N-nitroso compounds:possible role of ascorbic acid in cancer prevention. Am J Clin Nutr 1987May;45(5):1344-50

Tannenbaum SR, Wishnok JS, Leaf CD. Inhibition of nitrosamine formatin by ascorbic acid. Am J Clin Nutr 1991Jan;53(1):247S-250S

Selenium and Colon Cancer

Spallholz, J.E., et al. Dimethyldiselenide and methylseleninic Acid Generate Superoxide in an In Vitro Chemiluminescence Assay in the presence of Glutathione: Implications for the Anticarcinogenic Activity of l- Selenomethionine and L-Se-Methylselenocysteine. Nutrition and Cancer : 40 (1); 34-41

Woo Youn, B., et al. Mechanisms of Organoselenium Compounds in Chemoprevention: Effects on Transcription Factor-DNA Binding. Nutrition and Cancer: 40 (1); 28-33

El-Bayoumy, Karam, et al. Multiorgan Sensitivity to Anticarcinogenesis by the Organoselenium 1, 4- Phenylenebis (Methylene) Selenocyanate. Nutrition and Cancer: 40 (1); 18-27

Fleming, J, et al. Molecular Mechanisms of Cancer Prevention by Selenium Compounds. Nutrition and Cancer: 40 (1); 42-49

Kim, Y.S., Milner, J. Molecular Targets for Selenium in Cancer Prevention. Nutrition and Cancer: 40 (1); 50-54

Combs, Jr., Gerald F. Impact of Selenium and Cancer-Prevention Findings on the Nutrition-Health Paradigm. Nutrition and Cancer: 40 (1); 6-11

Doll R., Peto R. The Causes of Cancer. Oxford, Oxford University Press; 1981

Mendeloff A. Dietary fiber and gastrointestinal disease. American Journal of Clinical Nutrition; 45:1267-70, 1987

Doll R., Peto R. The Causes of Cancer: Quantitative estimates of avoidable risks of cancer in the United States today.
J Natl Cancer Instit 66:1191-1308, 1981

Burkitt, DP: "Epidemiology of Cancer of the Colon and Rectum." Cancer 28,3-13, 1971

Potter, JD, and McMichael, AJ: "Diet and Cancer of Colon and Rectum: A Case-Control Study." J Natl Cancer Instit 76,.557-569, 1986

Wattenberg, LW: "Inhibition of Neoplasia by Minor Dietary Constituents." Cancer Res 43, 2448s –2453s-2453s,1983

Shekelle, RB, Lepper, M, Liu, S, Maliza, C, Raynor, et al.: "Dietary Vitamin A and Risk of Cancer in the Western Electric Study *Lancet* 28, 1185-1191, 1981

Narbonne, JF, Cassand, P, Decoudu, S, and Leveque, F: "Effect of Fat Soluble Vitamins on Chemical Carcinogenesis in Rat Liver. " *Int J Viam Nutr Res* 60, 188, 1990

Silverman, J, Katayama, S, Zelenakas, K, Lauber, J, Musser, et al.: "Effect of Retinoids on the Induction of Colon Cancer in F344 Rats by N-Methyl-N-Nitrosourea or by 1,2-Dimethylhydrazine.: *Carcinogenesis* 2, 1167-1172, 1981

Alabaster, O, Tang, ZC, Frost, A, and Shivapurkar, N: "Effect of Beta-Carotene and Wheat Bran Fiber on Colonic Aberrant Crypt and Tumor Formation in Rats Exposed to Azoxymethane and High Dietary Fat." *Carcinogenesis* 16, 127-132, 1995

Soullier, B, Wilson, P, and Nigro, N: "Effect of selenium on azoxymethane-induced intestinal cancer in rats fed a high fat diet." *Cancer Lett* 12, 343-348, 1981

Jacobs, M: "Selenium inhibition of 1,2-dimethylhydralyzine-induced colon carcinogenesis." *Cancer Res* 43,1646-1649, 1983

Fiala, E, Joseph, C, Sohn, O, El-Bayoumy, K, and Reddy, B: "Mechanism of benzylselenocyanate inhibition of azoxymethane-induced colon carcinogenesis in F344 rats." *Cancer Res* 51, 2826-2830, 1991

Reddy, B, Tanaka, T, and El-Bayoumy, K: "Inhibitory effect of dietary p-methoxybenzeneselenol on azoxymethane-induced colon and kidney carcinogenesis in female 344 rats: *J Natl Cancer Instit* 74, 1325-1328,1985

Clark, L, Cantor, K, and Allaway, W: "Selenium in forage crops and cancer mortality in US counties." *Arch Environ Health* 46, 37-42, 1991

Virtamo, J, Valkeila, E, Alfthan, G, Punsar, S, Huttunen, Jet al.: "Serum selenium and risk of cancer: a prospective follow-up of nine years." *Cancer* 60, 145-148, 1987

Clark, L, Hixson, L, Combs, G, Jr, Reid, M, Turnbull, B, et al.: "Plasma selenium concentration predicts the prevalence of colorectal adenomatous polyps." Cancer Epidemiol Biomarkers Prev 2, 41-45, 1993

Clark, L., Combs, G.F., Jr, Turnbull, B.W., Slate, E.H., Chalker, D.K., et al.: "Effects of selenium supplementation for cancer prevention in patients with carcinoma of the skin." *JAMA* 276, 1957-1964, 1996

Russo MW et al: "Plasma selenium levels and the risk of colorectal adenomas:, *Nutrition and Cancer* 28(2),125-129, 1997

Reddy, B, Rivenson, A, Kulkarni, N, Upadhyaya, P, and El-Bayoumy, K: "Chemoprevention of colon carcinogenesis by the synthetic organoselenium compound 1,4-phenylenebis(methylene)selenocyanate." *Cancer Res* 52, 5635-5640, 1992

Lanfear, J, Fleming, J, Wu, L, Webster, G, and Harrison, PR: "The selenium metabolite selenodiglutathione induces p53 and apoptosis." *Carcinogenesis* 15, 1378-1392, 1994

Willett, WC, Polk, PF, Morris, JS, Stampfer, MJ, Pressel, S, et al.: "Prediagnostic serum selenium and risk of cancer." *Lancet* 2, 130-134, 1983

Salonen, J, Alfthan, G, Huttunen, J, and Puska, P: "Association between serum selenium and the risk of cancer." *Am J Epidemiol* 120, 342-349, 1984

Hendler, S,. The Doctor's Vitamin and Mineral Encyclopedia. Simon and Schuster, 1990

Thompson CD, et al., Effect of prolonged supplementation with daily supplements of selenomethionine and sodium selenite on glutathione peroxidase activity in blood of New Zealand residents. *AM J Clin Nutr* 36, 24-31,1982

Lavender OA, et al., Bioavailability of selenium to Finnish men as assessed by platelet glutathione peroxidase activity and other blood parameters. *AM J Clin Med* 37, 887-897, 1983

Mutanen M, Bioavailability of selenium. *Annals Clin Res* 18, 48-54, 1986

Murray, M. Encyclopedia of Nutritional Supplements. Prima Publishing, 1996

National Research Council, Diet and Health. Implications for Reducing Chronic Disease Risk. National Academy Press; Washington, D.C.:1989, pp. 376-379

Clark, L. The Epidemiology of Selenium and Cancer. 1985, Fed Proc; 44: 2584-2589

Clot, W.J., et al. The Linxian trials: mortality rates by vitamin-mineral intervention group. *Am J Clin Nutr.*1995, 62 (suppl): 14245-14265

Kiremidjian-Schumacher, L., et al. Supplementation with selenium and human immune cell functions, II, effect on cytotoxic lymphocytes and natural killer cells. 1994, Bio Trace Elem Res 41; 103-114

Tarp, U., et al. Selenium treatment in rheumatoid arthritis. *Scard J Rheumatol*, 1985, 14: 364-368

Salomen, J.R. Association between cardiovascular death and myocardial infarction and serum selenium in a matched-pair longitudinal study. *Lancet*, 1982; 2: 175-179

Multivitamins, Vitamin E and Colon Cancer

White E, Shannon JS, Patterson RE. Relationship between vitamin and calcium supplement use and colon cancer. Cancer Epidemiology, Biomarkers & Prevention. Oct1997;6(10):769-774

Colon Cancer and Folic Acid

Giovannucci et al: Folate, methionine, and alcohol intake and risk of colorectal adenoma. J. Natl Cancer Inst. 1993; 85; 11: 875-83

Doll R, Peto R: The causes of cancer: Quantitative estimates of avoidable risks of cancer in the United States today. JNCI 66:1191-1308, 1981

Willet W: The search for the causes of breast and colon cancer. Nature 338:398, 394, 1989

Haenszel W, Kurihara M: Studies of Japanese migrants. I. Mortality from cancer and other diseases among Japanese in the United States. J Natl Cancer Inst 40:43-68, 1968

McKeown-Eyssen GE, Bright-See E: Dietary factors in colon cancer: International relationships, Nutr Cancer 6:160-170, 1984

Potter JD, McMichael AJ: Diet and cancer of the colon and rectum: A case-control study. JNCI 76:557-569,1986

Graham S, Dayal H, Swanson M, et al: Diet in the epidemiology of cancer of the colon and rectum. J Natl Cancer Inst 55:15-18, 1978

La Vecchia C, Negri E, Decarli A, et al: A case-control study of diet and colo-rectal cancer in northern Italy, Int J Cancer 41:492-498, 1988

Nyce J, Weinhouse S, Magee PN: 5-Methylcytosine depletion during tumor development: An extension of the miscoding concept, Br J Cancer 48:463-475, 1983

Hoffman RM: Altered methionine metabolism, DNA methylation and oncogene expression in carcinogenesis. Biochim Biophys Acta 738:49-87, 1984

Shivapurkar N. Poirer LA: Tissue levels of S-adenosylmethionine and S-adenosylhomocysteine in rats fed methyl-deficient diets for one to five weeks. Carcinogenesis 4:1052-1057, 1983

Wainfan E, Dizik M, Stender M, et al: Rapid appearance of hypomethylated DNA in livers of rats fed cancerpromoting, methyl-deficient diets. Cancer Res 49:4094-4097, 1989

Wainfan E, Poirier LA: Methyl groups in carcinogenesis: Effects of DNA methylation and gene expression. Cancer Res 52:2071s-2077s, 1992

Cravo ML, Mason JB, Dayal Y, et al: Folate deficiency enhances the development of colonic neoplasia in dimethylhydrazine-treated rats. Cancer Res 52:5002-5006, 1992

Feinberg AP, Vogelstein B: Hypomethylation distinguishes genes of some human cancers from their normal counterparts. Nature 301:89-92, 1983

Goelez SE, Vogelstein B, Hamilton SR, et al: Hypomethylation of DNA from benign and malignant human colon neoplasms. Science 228:187-190, 1985

Feinberg AP, Gehrke CW, Kuo KC, et al: Reduced genomic 5-methylcytosine content in human colonic neoplasia. Cancer Res 48:1159-1161, 1988

Freudenheim JL, Graham S, Marshall JR, et al: Folate intake and carcinogenesis of the colon and rectum, IntJ Epidemiol 20:368-374, 1991

Lashner BA, Heidenreich PA, Su GL, et al: Effect of folate supplementation on the incidence of dysplasia and cancer in chronic ulcerative colitis. A case-control study, Gastroenteral 97:255-259, 1989

MRC Vitamin Study Research Group: Prevention of neural tube defects: results of the medical research council vitamin study. Lancet 338:131-137, 1991

Sauberlich HE: Evaluation of folate nutrition in population groups. In: Folic Acid Metabolism in Health and Disease

(Picciano MF, Stokstad ELR, Gregory JF, eds). New York: Wiley-Liss, 1990, pp211-235

Essential Fatty Acids

Calder PC. Dietary modification of inflammation with lipids. Proc Nutr Soc. 2002 Aug;61(3):345-58

Dietary Supplement Information bureau (Dietary Supplement Education Alliance, U.S.A.) www.supplementinfo.org/omega-6 fatty acids, omega-3 acidsDiGiacoma RA, Kremer JM, Shah DM. Fish-oil dietary supplementation in patients with Raynaud's phenomenon: a double-blind, controlled, prospective study. Am J Med 1989;86:158–64

Galland L. Increased Requirements for Essential Fatty Acids in Atopic Individuals: A Review with Clinical Descriptions. J Am Coll Nutr. 1986;5(2):213-28

Garg ML, et al. Alpha-linolenic Acid and Metabolism of Cholesterol and Long-chain Fatty Acids. Nutrition. Jun1992;8(3):208-10

Geusens P, et al. Long-term Effect of Omega-3 Fatty Acid Supplementation in Active Rheumatoid Arthritis. A 12-month, Double-blind, Controlled Study. Arthritis Rheum. Jun1994;37(6):824-29

Gibson RA, Neumann MA, Makrides M. Effect of dietary docosahexaenoic acid on brain composition and neural function in term infants. Lipids 1996;31:177S–81S

Harris WS, Park Y, Isley WL. Cardiovascular disease and long-chain omega-3 fatty acids. Curr Opin Lipidol. 2003 Feb;14(1):9-14

Health Notes. www.puritan.com/Health Notes/Supp/EPA

Holland PA, et al. Drug Therapy of Mastalgia. What are the Options? Drugs. Nov1994;48(5):709-16

Horrobin DF, Manku M, Brush M, et al. Abnormalities in plasma essential fatty acid levels in women with premenstrual syndrome and with non-malignant breast disease. J Nutr Med 1991;2:259–64

Horrobin DF. Essential fatty acids in clinical dermatology. J Am Acad Dermatol 1989;20:1045–53

Horrobin DF. The importance of gamma-linolenic acid and prostaglandin E1 in human nutrition and medicine. J Holistic Med 1981;3:118–39

Isseroff RR. Fish Again for Dinner! The Role of Fish and other Dietary Oils in the Therapy of Skin Disease. J Am Acad Dermatol. Dec1988;19(6):1073-80

Joe LA, Hart LL. Evening primrose oil in rheumatoid arthritis. Ann Pharmacother 1993;27:1475–7 [review]

Keen H, Payan J, Allawi J, et al. Treatment of diabetic neuropathy with gamma-linolenic acid. Diabetes Care 1993;16:8–15

Kinsella JE, et al. Dietary n-3 Polyunsaturated Fatty Acids and Amelioration of Cardiovascular Disease: Possible Mechanisms. Am J Clin Nutr. Jul1990;52(1):1-28

Knapp HR, et al. The Antihypertensive Effects of Fish Oil. A Controlled Study of Polyunsaturated Fatty Acid Supplements in Essential Hypertension. N Engl J Med. Apr1989;320(16):1037-43

Kremer JM, Lawrence DA, Petrillow GF, et al. Effects of highdose fish oil on rheumatoid arthritis after stopping nonsteroidal antiinflammatory drugs. Arthritis Rheum 1995;38:1107–14.

Leventhal LJ, et al. Treatment of Rheumatoid Arthritis with Gammalinolenic Acid. Ann Intern Med. Nov1993;119(9):867-73

Maes M, Christophe A, Bosmans E, et al. In humans, serum polyunsaturated fatty acid levels predict the response of proinflammatory cytokines to psychological stress. Biol Psychiatry 2000;47:910–20

Makrides M, Neumann MA, Gibson RA. Is dietary docosahexaenoic acid essential for term infants? Lipids1996;31:115–9

Manku MS, Horrobin, DF, Morse NL, et al. Essential fatty acids in the plasma phospholipids of patients with atopic eczema. Br J Derm 1984;110:643

Masuev KA. The Effect of Polyunsaturated Fatty Acids of the Omega-3 Class on the Late Phase of the Allergic Reaction in Bronchial Asthma Patients. Ter Arkh. 1997;69(3):31-33

Mate J, Castanos R, Garcia-Samaniego J, Pajares JM. Does dietary fish oil maintain the remission of Crohn's disease: a case control study. Gastroenterology 1991;100:A228 [abstract].

Murray M. Encyclopedia of Nutritional Supplements. (Prima publishing, 1996):239-278

Pye JK, et al. Clinical Experience of Drug Treatments for Mastalgia. Lancet. Aug1985;2(8451):373-77

Stevens L, Zentall SS, Deck JL. Essential fatty acid metabolism in boys with attention-deficit hyperactivity disorder. Am J Clin Nutr. 1995;62:761-7681.

Nesbitt PD, et al. Human metabolism of mammalian lignan precursors in raw and processed flaxseed. *Am J Clin Nutr* 1995;69(3):549-555

Hutchins AM, et al. Flaxseed influences urinary lignan excretion in a dose-dependent manner in postmenopausal women.
Cancer Epidemiol Biomarkers Prev 2000;9(10):1113-1118

Tham DM, et al. Clinical Review 97: Potential health benefits of dietary phytoestrogens: a review of the clinical, epidemiological, and mechanistic evidence. *J Clin Endocrinol Metab* 1998;83(7):2223-2235

Zeigler J. Just the Flax, Ma'am: Researchers Testing Linseed. *J Natl Cancer Instit* 1994;86(23):1746-1748

Cunnane SC, et al. Nutritional attributes of traditional flaxseed in healthy young adults. *Am J Clin Nutr* 1995;61(1):62-68

Prasad K, et al. Reduction in hypercholesterolemia atherosclerosis by CDC-flaxseed with very low alphalinolenic acid. *Atherosclerosis* 1998;136(2):367-375

Kitts DD, et al. Antioxidant activity of the flaxseed lignan secoisolariciresinol diglycoside and its mammalian lignan metabolites enterodiol and enterolactone *Mol Cell Biochem* 1999;202(1-2):91-1008.

Kurzer MS, et al. Dietary Phytoestrogens. *Annu Rev Nutr* 1997;17:353-381

Richard SE, et al. Plasma insulin-like growth factor-1 levels in rats are reduced by dietary supplementation
of flaxseed or lignan secoisolariciresinol diglycoside. *Cancer Lett* (Ireland) 2000;161(1):47-55

Li D, et al. Dietary supplementation with secolariciresinol diglycoside (SDG) reduces experimental metastasis of melanoma cells in mice. *Cancer Lett* 1999;142(1):91-96

Brzezinksi A, Debi A. Phytoestrogens: the natural selective estrogen receptor modulators? *Eur J Obstet Gynecol Reprod Biol* 1999;85(1):47-51

Tou JC, Thompson LU. Exposure to flaxseed as its lignan component during different developmental stages influences rat mammary gland structures. *Carcinogenesis* 1999;20(9):1831-1835

Haggans CJ, et al. Effect of flaxseed consumption on urinary estrogen metabolites in postmenopausal women. *Nutr Cancer* 1999;33(2):188-195

Haggans CJ, et al. The effect of flaxseed and wheat bran consumption on urinary estrogen metabolites in premenopausal women. *Cancer Epidemiol Biomarkers Prev* 2000;9(7):719-725

Thompson LU, et al. Anti-tumorigenic effect of mammalian lignan precursor from flaxseed. *Nutr Cancer* 1996;26:159-165

Gross PE, et al. Effect of dietary flaxseed in women with cyclical mastalgia. Program and abstract of the 23rd Annual San Antonio Breast Cancer Symposium. Dec 6-9, 2000; San Antonio Texas. Abstract 153.
Breast Cancer Res Treat 2000;64:p49

Arjmandi BH, et al. Whole flaxseed consumption lowers serum LDL-cholesterol and lipoprotein (a) concentrations in postmenopausal women. *Nutr Res* 1998;18:1203-1214

Jenkins DJP, et al. Health aspects of partially defatted flaxseed, including effects on serum lipids, oxidative measures, and ex vivo androgen and progestin activity: a controlled crossover trial. *Am J Clin Nutr* 1999;69(3):395-402

Flaxseed Lowers Cholesterol. *Nutr. Science News* 1998;3(11):575

Velasquez M, et al. Dietary Phytoestrogens: a Possible role in renal disease protection. *Am J Kidney Dis* 2001;37(5):1056-1068

Clark WF, et al. A novel treatment for lupus nephritis: lignan precursor derived from flaxseed. *Lupus* 2000;9(6):429-436

Denis L, et al. Diet and its preventive role in prostate disease. *Eur Urol* 1999;35(5-6):377-387

Chen, WJL, et al. Hypocholesterolemic effects of soluble fibers. In Kritchevsky D , Yahouny, GD, eds.*Dietary Fiber: Basic and Clinical Aspects.* New York:Plenum Press 1986:275-289

Sanghui A, et al. Inhibition of rat liver cholesterol 7-alpha hydroxylase and acyl C-A: cholesterol acyl transferase activities by enterodiol and enterolactone. In Kritchovsky D, ed. *Proceedings of the Symposium on Drugs Affecting Lipid Metabolism.* New York:Plenum Press, 1984:311-322

Flaxseed and Breast Cancer

Ziegler J. Just the flax, Ma'am: Researchers testing linseed. J Natl Cancer Inst 1994; 86; 23: 1746-48

Cunnane SC. et al. Nutritional attributes of traditional flaxseed in healthy young adults. Am J Clin Nutr. 1995;61; 62-8

Thompson LU, Robb P, Serraino M, Cheung F, Mammalian lignan production from various foods. Nutr Cancer 1991; 16:43-52

Chan JK, McDonald BE, Gerrard JM, Bruce VM, Weaver BJ, Holub BJ. Effect of dietary a-linolenic acid and its ratio to linoleic acid on platelet and plasma fatty acids and thrombogenesis. Lipids 1993;28:811-7

Cunnane SC, Ganguli S, Menard C, et al. High alpha-linolenic acid flaxseed (Linum usitatissimum): some nutritional properties in humans. Br J Nutr 1993;69:443-53

Setchell KDR, Adlercreutz H. Mammalian lignans and phytoestrogens; recent studies in the formation, metabolism and biological role in health and disease. In: Rowland I, ed. Role of the gut flora in toxicity and cancer. London: Academic Press, 1988:315-45.

Adlecreutz H, Mousavi Y, Hockerstedt K. Diet and breast cancer. Acta Oncologia 1992;31:175-81

Serraino M. Thompson LU. The effect of flaxseed supplementation on the initiation and promotional stages of mammary tumorigenesis. Nutr Cancer 1991;17:153-9

Serraino M, Thompson LU. The effect of flaxseed supplementation on early risk markers for mammary carciogenesis. Cancer Lett 1991;60:135-42

Serraino M, Thompson LU. Flaxseed supplementation and early markers of colon carcinogenesis. Cancer Lett 1992;63:159-65

Axelson M, Sjovall J, Gustafsson BE, Setchell KDR. Origin of lignans in mammals and identification of a precursor from plants. Nature 1982;2298:659-60

Shultz TD, Bonorden WR, Seaman WR. Effect of short term flaxseed consumption on lignan and sex hormone metabolism in men. Nutr Res 1991;11:1089-100

Lampe JW, Martini MC, Kurzer MS, Adlercreutz H, Slavin Jl. Urinary lignan and isoflavonoid in premenopausal women consuming flaxseed powder. Am J Clin Nutr 1994;60:122-8

Thompson LU, Potential health benefits and problems associated with antinutrients in foods. Food Res Int 1993;26:131-49

Adlercreutz H, Mousavi Y, Clark H, et al. Dietary phytoestrogens and cancer: in vitro and in vivo studies. J Steroid Biochem Mol Biol 1992;41:331-7

Mousavi Y, Adlercreutz H. Enterolactone and estradiol inhibit each others proliferative effect on MCF-7 breast cancer cells in culture. J Steroid Mol Biol 1992;41:615-9

Fotsis T, Pepper M, Adlercreutz H, et al. Genistein, a dietary-derived inhibitor of in vitro angiogenesis. Proc Natl Acad Sci USA 1993;90:22690-4

Gamma-Linolenic Acid *(GLA)*

1. Murray M. Encyclopedia of Nutritional Supplements. Rocklin, CA: Prima Publishing; 1996. p. 252-68.
2. Joe LA, Hart LL. Evening primrose oil in rheumatoid arthritis. Ann Pharmacother 1993;27:1475-7[review].
3. Horrobin DF. The importance of gamma-linolenic acid and prostaglandin E1 in human nutrition and medicine. J Holistic Med 1981;3:118-39.
4. Horrobin DF, Manku M, Brush M, et al. Abnormalities in plasma essential fatty acid levels in women with pre-menstrual syndrome and with non-malignant breast disease. J Nutr Med 1991;2:259-64.
5. Keen H, Payan J, Allawi J, et al. Treatment of diabetic neuropathy with gamma-linolenic acid. Diabetes Care 1993;16:8-15[reviews].
6. Horrobin DF. Essential fatty acid metabolism in diseases of connective tissue with special reference to scleroderma and to Sjogren's syndrome.Med Hypoth 1984;14:233-47.
7. Horrobin DF, Campbell A. Sjogren's syndrome and the sicca syndrome: the role of prostaglandin E1 deficiency. Treatment with essential fatty acids and vitamin C. Med Hypoth 1980;6:225-32.
8. Vaddadi KS, Gilleard CJ. Essential fatty acids, tardive dyskinesia, and schizophrenia. In: Horrobin DF, editor. Omega-6 Essential Fatty Acids: Pathophysiology and Roles in Clinical Medicine. New York, NY: Alan R Liss; 1990. p. 333–43.
9. Manku MS, Horrobin, DF, Morse NL, et al. Essential fatty acids in the plasma phospholipids of patients with atopic eczema. Br J Derm 1984;110:643.

10. Horrobin DF. Essential fatty acids in clinical dermatology. J Am Acad Dermatol 1989;20:1045-53.

11. Mansel RE, Pye JK, Hughes LE. Effects of essential fatty acids on cyclical mastalgia and noncyclical breast disorders. In: Omega-6 Essential Fatty Acids: Pathophysiology and Roles in Clinical Medicine. Horrobin DF, editor. New York, NY: Alan R Liss, 1990. p. 557-66.

12. Keen H, Payan J, Allawi J, Walker J, Jamal GA, Weir AI, et al. Treatment of diabetic neuropathy with gamma-linolenic acid. Diabetes Care 1993;16:8-15.

13. Horribin DF. Essential fatty acid metabolism in diseases of connective tissue with special reference to scleroderma and to Sjogren's syndrome. Med Hypoth 1984;14:233-47.

14. Vaddadi KS, Gilleard CJ. Essential fatty acids, tardive dyskinesia, and schizophrenia. In: Horrobin DF, editor. Omega-6 Essential Fatty Acids: Pathophysiology and Roles in Clinical Medicine. New York, NY: Alan R Liss; 1990. p. 333-43.

15. Schalin-Karrila M, Mattila L, Jansen CT, Uotila P. Evening primrose oil in the treatment of atopic eczema: effect on clinical status, plasma phospholipid fatty acids and circulating blood prostaglandins. Brit J Dermatol 1987;117:11-9.

16. Janti J. Evening primrose oil in rheumatoid arthritis: changes in serum lipids and fatty acids. Annals Rheumatol Dis 1989;48:124-7.

17. Keen H, Payan J, Allawi J, Walker J, Jamal GA, Weir AI, et al. Treatment of diabetic neuropathy with gamma-linolenic acid. The Gamma-Linolenic Acid Multicenter Trial Group. Diabetic Care 1993;16:8-15.

18. Zurier RB, Rossetti RG, Jacobson EW, et al. Gamma-linolenic acid treatment of rheumatoid arthritis. A randomized, placebo-controlled trial. Arthritis Rheum 1996;11:1808-17.

19. Leventhal LJ, Boyce EG, Zurier Rb. Treatment of rheumatoid arthritis with black currant seed oil. Br J Rheumatol 1994;9:847-52.

20. Jantti J, Nikkari T, Solakivi T, Vapaatalo H, et al. Evening primrose oil in rheumatoid arthritis. Changes in serum lipids and fatty acids. Annals Rheum Dis 1989;48:124-7.

21. Andreassi M, Forleo P, Di Lorio Z, Masci S, Abate G, Amerio P. Efficacy of gamma-linolenic acid in the treatment of patients with atopic dermatitis. J Int Med Res 1997;5:266-74.

22. Borrek S, Hildebrandt A, Forster J. Gamma-linolenic acid-rich borage seed oil capsules in children with atopic dermatitis. A placebo-controlled double-blind study. Klin Padiatr 1997;3:100-4.

23. Hederos C, Berg, A. Epogam evening primrose oil treatment on atopic dermatitis and asthma. Arch Dis Child 1996;6:494-7.

24. Collier PM, Ursell A, Zaremba K, Payne CM, Staughton RC, Sanders T. Effect of regular consumption of oily fish compared with white fish on chronic plaque psoriasis. Ew J Clin Nutr 1993;4:251-4.

25. Vaddadl KS. The use of gamma-linolenic acid and linolenic acid to differentiate between temporal lobe epilepsy and schizophrenia. Prostaglandins Med 1981;6:375-9.

26. Holman CP, Bell AFJ. A trial of evening primrose oil in the treatment of chronic schizophrenia. J Orthomol Psychiatr 1983;12:302-4.

27. Miller LG. Selected clinical considerations focusing on known or potential drug-herb interactions. Arch Intern Med 1998;158:2200-11.

Flaxseed Oil and Alpha-Linolenic Acid

1. Nordstrom DCE, Honkanen VEA, Nasu Y, Antila E, Friman C, Konttinen YT. Alpha-linolenic acid in the treatment of rheumatoid arthritis. A double-blind placebo-controlled and randomized study: flaxseed vs safflower oil. Rheumatol Int 1995;14:231-4.

2. Von Schacky C, Angerer P, Kothny W, Theisen K, Mudra H. The effect of dietary omega-3 fatty acids on coronary atherosclerosis. A randomized, double-blind, placebo-controlled trial. Ann Intern Med 1999;130:554-62.

3. Mate J, Castanos R, Garcia-Samaniego J, Pajares JM. Does dietary fish oil maintain the remission of Crohn's disease: a case control study. Gastroenterology 1991;100:A228[abstract]

4. Gonzalez MJ. Fish oil, lipid peroxidation and mammary tumor growth. J Am Coll Nutr 1995;14:325.

5. Schlomo Y, et al. Modulating the learning pain thresholds, and thermoregulation in the rat by preparations of free purified alpha-linolenic and linolenic acids: Determination of the optimal w3-to w6 ratio. Proc Nat Acad Sci 1993;90:10345-7.

6. Murray M. Encyclopedia of Nutritional Supplements. Rocklin, CA: Prima Publishing; 1996. p. 249-78

7. Lee TH, Hoover RL, Williams JD, Sperling RI, Ravalese J, Spur BW, et al. Effect of dietary enrichment with eicosapentaenoic and docosahexanoic acids on in vitro neutrophil and monocyte leukotriene generation and neutrophil generation. New Eng J Med 1985;312:1217-24.

8. Strasser T, Fischer S, Weber P. Leukotrien B5 is formed in human neutrophils after dietary supplementation with eicosapentaenoic acid. Proc Natl Acad Sci 1985;82:1540-3.

9. Bjerve KS, et al. Clinical studies with alpha-linolenic acid and long n-3 fatty acids. Nutrition 1992;8:130-2.

10. Mantzioris E, James MJ, Gibson RA, Cleland LG. Dietary substitution with alpha-linolenic acid-rich vegetable oil increases EPA concentrations in tissues. Am J Clin Nutr 1994;59:1304-9.

11. Kelly DS. Alpha-linolenic acid and immune response. Nutrition 1992;8:215-7.

12. Erasmus U. Fats and oils. Vancouver, BC: Alive Books; 1986. p. 273.

13. Lockwood K, Moesgaard S, Folkers K. Partial and complete regression of breast cancer in patients in relation to dosage of coenzyme Q10. Biochem Biophys Res Comm 1994;199:1504-8.

14. Chan JK, Bruce VM, McDonald BE. Dietary alpha-linolenic acid is as effective as oleic acid and linoleic acid in lowering blood cholesterol in normolipidemic men. Am J Clin Nutr 1991;53:1230-4.

15. Singer P, Jaeger W, Berger I, et al. Effects of dietary oleic, linoleic and alpha-linolenic acids on blood pressure, serum lipids, lipoproteins and the formation of eicosanoid precursors in patients with mild essential hypertension. J Human Hypertansion 1990;4:227-233.

16. Healthnotes online. 2000 Healthnotes Inc: Flaxseed Oil.

Eicosapentaenoic Acid

1. Von Schacky C, Angerer P, Kothny W, Theisen K, Mudra H. The effect of dietary omega-3 fatty acids on coronary atherosclerosis. A randomized, double-blind, placebo-controlled trial. Ann Intern Med 1999;130:554-62.

2. Mate J, Castanos R, Garcia-Samaniego J, Pajares JM. Does dietary fish oil maintain the remission of Crohn's disease: a case study. Gastroenterology 1991;100:A228[abstract].

3. Lee TH, Hoover RL, Williams JD. Effect of dietary enrichment with eicosapentaenoic and docosahexanoic acids on in vitro neutraphil and monocyte leudotriene generation and neutrophil generation. New Eng J Med 1985,312:1217-24.

4. Strasser T, Fischer S, Weber P. Leukotriene B5 is formed in human neutrophils after dietary supplementation with EPA. Proc Nat Acad Sci 1985;82:1540-3.

5. Kinsella JE, Lokesh B, Stone RA. Dietary n-3 polyunsaturated fatty acids and amelioration of cardiovascular disease: possible mechanisms. Am J Clin Nutr 1990;52:1-28.

6. Murray M. Encyclopedia of Nutritional Supplements. Rocklin, CA: Prima Publishing; 1996. p. 249-78.

7. Cobiac L, Clifton PM, Abbey M, et al. Lipid, lipoprotein, and hemostatic effects of fish vs fish oil w-3 fatty acids in mildly hyperlipidemic males. Am J Clin Nutr 1991;53:1210-6.

8. Schmidt EB, Dyerberg J. Omega-3 fatty acids: Current status in cardiovascular medicine. Drugs 1994;47:405-24.

9. Appel LJ, Miller ER, Seidler AJ, Whelton PK. Dose supplementation of diet with "fish oil" reduce blood pressure? A meta-analysis of controlled clinical trials. Arch Intern Med 1993;153:1429-38.

10. Singer P. Alpha-linolenic acid vs long-chain fatty acids in hypertension and hyperlipidemia. Nutrition 1992;8:133-5.

11. Swank RL. Multiple sclerosis: fat-oil relationship. Nutrition 1991;7:368–76.

12. Swank RL, et al. The Multiple Sclerosis Diet Book. Garden City, NY: Doubleday; 1977.

13. Belluzzi, A, Boschi, S, Brignola, C, Munarini, A, Cariani, G, Miglio F. Polyunsaturated fatty acids and inflammatory bowel disease. Am J Clin Nutr 2000;71(Suppl):339S-42S.

14. DiGiacoma RA, Kremer JM, Shah DM. Fish-oil dietary supplementation in patients with Raynaud's phenomenon: A double-blind, controlled prospective study. Am J Med 1989;86:158-64.

15. Piche LA, Draper HH, Cole PD. Malondialdehyde excretion by subjects consuming cod liver oil vs a concentrate of n-3 fatty acids. Lipids 1988;23:370-1.

16. Clarke JTR, Cullen-Dean G, Reglink E, et al. Increased incidence of epistaxis in adolescents with familial hypercholesterolemia treated with fish oil. J Pediats 1990;116:139-41.

17. Pederson HS, et al. n-3 fatty acids as a risk factor for hemorrhagic stroke. Lancet 1999;353:812-3.

18. Schectman G, Kaul S, Kassebah AH. Effect of fish oil concentrate on lipoprotein composition in NIDDM. Diabetes 1988;37:1567-73.

19. Axelrod L, Camuso J, Williams E, Kleinman K, Briones E, Schoenfeld D. Effects of a small quantity of omega-3 fatty acids on cardiovascular risk factors in NIDDM: a randomized, prospective, double-blind, controlled study. Diabetes Care 1994;17:37-44.

Docosahexaenoic Acid

1. Davidson MH, Maki KC, Kalkowski J, Schaefer EJ, Torri SA, Drennan KB. Effects of docosahexaenoic acid on serum lipoproteins in patients with combined hyperlipidemia: A randomized, double-blind, placebcontrolled trial. J Am coll Nutr 1997:16,3:236-43.

2. Conquer JA, Holub BJ. Supplementation with an algae source of DHA increases (n-3) fatty acid status and alters selected risk factors for heart disease in vegetarian subjects. J Nutr 1996;126:3032-9.

3. Nelson GJ, et al. The effect of dietary DHA on platelet function, platelet fatty acid composition, and blood coagulation in humans. Lipids 1997;32:1129-36.

4. Gibson RA, Neumann MA, Makrides M. Effect of dietary DHA on brain composition and neural function in term infants. Lipids 1996;31 (Suppl):1775S-81S.

5. Makrides M, Neumann MA, Gibson RA. Is dietary DHA essential for term infants? Lipids 1996;31:115-9.

6. Werkman SH, Carlson SE. A randomized trial of visual attention of preterm infants fed DHA until nine months. Lipids 1996:31:91-7.

7. Soyland E, et al. Dietary supplementation with very long-chain n-3 fatty acids in patients with atopic dermatitis: a double-blind, multi-centre study. Br J Dermatol 1994;130:757-64.
8. Arm JP, et al. The effects of dietary supplementation with fish oil lipids on the airway response to inhaled allergen in bronchial asthma. Am Rev Respiratory Dis 1989;139:1395-400.
9. Dry J, et al. Effect of a fish oil diet on asthma: Results of a 1-year double-blind study. Int Arch Allergy Apply Immunol 1991;95:156-7.
10. Broughton KS, Johnson CS, Pace BK, Liebman M, Kleppinger KM. Reduced asthma symptoms with n-3 fatty acid ingestion are related to 5-series leukotriene production. Am J Clin Nutr 1997;65:1011–7.
11. Burgess JR, Stevens L, Zhang W, Peck L. Long-chain polyunsaturated fatty acids in children with attention-deficit hyperactivity disorder. Am J Clin Nutr 2000;71,7(Suppl):327S-30S.
12. Schectman G, Kaul S, Kassebah AH. Effect of fish oil concentrate on lipoprotein composition in NIDDM. Diabetes 1988;37:1567-73.
13. Axelrod L. Effects of a small quantity of omega-3 fatty acids on cardiovascular risk factor in non-insulin dependent diabetics(NIDD). Diabetes Care 1994;17:37-45.
14. Healthnotes Online. Healthnotes Inc 2000:DHA.
15. Martinez M. Resortin the DHA levels in the brains of Zellweger patients. J Mol Neurosci 2001;85(6):966-74.
16. Dietary Supplementation Information Bureau. www.content.intramedicine.com:DHA.

Non-Pharmacological Prevention of Cardiovascular Disease

1. Carleton R A . Dwyer J., Finberg I, et al. Report of the Expert Panel on Population Strategies for Blood Cholesterol Reduction: A statement from the National Cholesterol Education Program, National Heart, Lung and Blood Institute, National Institutes of Health Circulation 1991; 83(6)2154-232.
2. Kingsley C M, Gupta, S C. How to Reduce the Risk of Coronary Artery Disease. Post Graduate Medicine Vol. 91, No.4, March 1992:147-160.
3. Lipid Research Clinics Program. The Lipid Research Clinics Coronary Primary Prevention Trial Results. II. The relationship of reduction in incidence of coronary heart disease to cholesterol lowering. JAMA 1984; 251(3):365-74,
4. Frick M H, Elo 0, Haapa K, et al. Helsinki Heart Study: primary-prevention trial with gemfibrozil in middleaged men with dyslipidemia. Safety of treatment, changes In risk factors, and incidence of coronary heart disease. N Engl J Med 1983;317(20):1237-45.
5. Manninen V, Elo M O, Frick N H, et al. Lipid alterations and decline in the Incidence of coronary heart disease in the Helsinki Heart study. JANA 1988;260(5): 641-51.
6. Gordon D J., Probstfield J L., Rubenstein C , et al. Coronary risk factors and exercise test performance in asymptomatic hypercholesterolemic men; application of proportional hazards analysis. AM J Epidemiol 1984;120(2):21-24
7. Gofman J W ., Yound W., Tandy R. Ischemic heart disease, atherosclerosis and longevity. Circulation 1966; 34(4): 679-97
8. Castelli , W P Garrison, R J Wilson, P W et al. Incidence of coronary heart disease and lipoprotein cholesterol levels: the Framingham study. JAMA 1986; 256(20) 2835-8.
9. Anderson J W , Gustafson N J Hypocholesterolemic effect of oat and bean products. AM J Clinical Nutrition I988; 48: 749-53.
10. Paffenbarger, R S, Hyde R T , Wing A L, Hsieh, C. Physical activity, all-cause mortality and longevity of college alumni. N Engl J Med 314:605-613,1986.

11. Pekkanen J, Marti B, Nissinen A, Tuomilehto J, Punsar S, Karvonen M J, Reduction of premature mortality by high physical activity: a 20 year follow-up of middle-aged Finnish men. Lancet 1:1473-1477, 1987.
12. Powell, K E, Thompson P D, Caspersen C J, Kendrick J S. Physical activity and the incidence of coronary heart disease. Annu Rev Public Health 8:253-287, 1987.
13. Quinn, T.J., Sprague H A, Van Huss W D, Olson H W. Caloric expenditure, life status, and disease in former male athletes and non-athletes Med Sci Sports Exerc 22:742-750, 1990,
14. Tsevat J, Weinstein M C, Williams L W, Tosteson, A N A, Goldman, L. Expected gains in life expectancy from various coronary heart disease risk factor modifications. Circulation 83:1194-1201, 1991.
15. Rotevatn S, Akseln L A, Bjelke, E. Lifestyle and mortality among Norwegian man. Prev Med 18:433-443, 1989.
16. Butler R N, Goldberg, L. Exercise and prevention of coronary heart disease. Prim Care 1989;16(1):99-114.
17. Enstrom J E, Kanin, L E, Klein, M A, 1992. Vitamin C intake and mortality among a sample of the U.S. Population. Epidemiology 2:194-202.
18. Gey, K F, Brubacher G B and Stehelin, H B, 1987. Plasma levels of anti-oxidant vitamins in relation to ischemic heart disease and cancer. American Journal of Clinical Nutrition 45:1368-1377.
19. Salonen J T, et al. 1987. Serum fatty acids, apolipoproteins, selenium and vitamins in relation to ischemic heart disease and cancer. American Journal of Clinical Nutrition 45:1368-1377.
20. Lavie, C J, et al. High-density lipoprotein cholesterol. Post Graduate Medicine vol. 87 (7): 36-51, May, 1990.
21. Castelli, W P, Griffin G C, 1988. Cutting back on saturated fat and cholesterol. Post Graduate medicine vol. 84 (3): 44-56
22. Keys A, Seven Countries: a multivariate analysis of death and coronary artery disease.. Cambridge, MA; Harvard University Press, 1980.

Antioxidants That Reduce Heart Disease Risk

Boscoboinik D, Szewczyk A, Hensey C, Azzi A. Inhibition of cell proliferation by a-tocopherol: role of protein kinase C. J Biol Chem 1991;266;6188-94

DeMaio SJ, King SB, Lembo NJ, et al. Vitamin E supplementation, plasma lipids and incidence of restenosis after percutaneous transluminal coronary angioplasty (PTCA). J Am Coll Nutr 1992;11:68-73

Enstrom J E, Kanin L E, Klein M A. Vitamin C intake and mortality among a sample of the U.S. Population. Epidemiology 1992;2:194-202

Frei B. Ascorbic acid protects lipids in human plasma and low-density lipoprotein against oxidative damage. Am J Clin Nutr 1991;54 (suppl):1113s-8s

Gey K F, Brubacher G B, Stehelin HB. Plasma levels of anti-oxidant vitamins in relation to ischemic heart disease and cancer. American Journal of Clinical Nutrition 1987;45:1368-1377

Gey KF, Brubacher GB, Stahelin HB. Plasma levels of antioxidant vitamins in relation to ischemic heart disease and cancer. AM J Clin Nutr 1987;45(suppl):1368-77

Gey KF, et al. Inverse correlation between plasma Vitamin E and mortality from ischemic heart disease in cross-cultural epidemiology. Am J Clin Nutr 1991; 53:326s-34s

Gey KF, Moser UK, Jordan P, Stahelin HB, Eichholzer M, Ludin E. Increased risk of cardiovascular disease at sub-optimal plasma concentrations of essential antioxidants: an epidemiological update with special attention to carotene and vitamin C. Am J Clin Nutr 1993;57(suppl):787S-97S

Gillilan RE, Mondell B, Warbasse JR. Quantitative evaluation of vitamin E in the treatment of angina pectoris. AM Heart J 1977;93:444-9

Ginter E, et al. The effect of ascorbic acid on cholesterolemia in healthy subjects with seasonal deficit of vitamin C. Nutr Metab 1970;12:76-86

Harats D, et al. Citrus fruit supplementation reduces lipoprotein oxidation in young men ingesting a diet high in saturated fat: presumptive evidence for an interaction between vitamin C and E in vivo.Am J Clin Nutr 1998Feb; 67:240-245

Hodis HN, Mack WJ, LaBree L, et al. Serial angioghaphic evidence that antioxidant vitamin intake reduces progression of coronary artery atherosclerosis. JAMA 1995;273:1849-54

Knekt P, et al. Antioxidant vitamin intake and coronary mortality in a longitudinal population study. Am J Epidemiol 1994;139:1180-9

Knekt P, Reunanen A, Järvinen R Seppänen R, Heliövaara M Aromaa A. Antioxidant vitamin intake and coronary mortality in a longitudinal population study. AM J Epidemiol 1994;139:1180-9

Kok FJ, de Bruijn AM, Vermeeren R, et al. Serum selenium, vitamin antioxidants, and cardiovascular mortality: a 9 y follow-up study in the Netherlands.AM J Clin Nutr 1987;45:462-8

Paolisso G, et al. Metabolic benefits deriving from chronic vitamin C supplementation in aged non-insulin dependent diabetics. J Am Coll.Nutr.1995;14:387-92

Princen HMG, von Poppel G, Vogelezang C, Buytenhek R, Kok FJ. Supplementation with Vitamin E but not bcarotene in vivo protects low density lipoprotein from lipid peroxidation in vitro: effect of cigarette smoking. Arterioscler Thromb 1992;12:554-62

Puurunen M, Manttari M, Mannienen V, et al. Antibody against oxidized low-density lipoprotein predicting myocardial infraction. Arch Intern Med 1994; 154:2605-9

Riemersma RA, Wood DA, Macintyre CCA, Elton RA, Gey KF, Oliver MF. Risk of angina pectoris and plasma concentrations of vitamins A, C and E and carotene. Lancet 1991;337:1-5

Rimm EB, Stampfer MJ, Ascherio A, Giovannucci E, Colditz GA, Willett WC. Vitamin E consumption and risk of coronary heart disease among men. N Engl J Med 1993;328:1450-6.

Salonen JT, et al. Serum fatty acids, apolipoproteins, selenium and vitamins in relation to ischemic heart disease and cancer. American Journal of Clinical Nutrition 1987;45:1368-1377

Salonen R, Nyyssönen K, Porkkala E, et al. Low vitamin E status is associated with increased risk of myocardial infarction only if vitamin C status is low: a population study in men in Eastern Finland. Circulation 1995;91:933(abstr)

Stamfer MJ, Rimm EB, Epidemiologic evidence for vitamin E in prevention of cardiovascular disease. Am J Clin.Nut 1995;62;1365s-1369s

Stampfer MJ and Rimm EB Epidemiologic evidence for vitamin E in prevention of cardiovascular disease. AM J Clin Nutr 1995;62(suppl):1365S-9S

Stampfer MJ, Hennekens CH, Manson JE, Colditz GA, Rosner B, Willet WC. A prospective study of vitamin E consumption and risk of coronary disease in women. N Engl J Med 1993;328:1444-9

Stampfer MJ, Rimm EB. A review of the epidemiology of dietary antioxidants and risk of coronary heart disease. Can J Cardiol 1993;9:14B-8B

Steinberg D. Antioxidants and artherosclerosis. A current assessment. Circulation 1991;84:1420-5 (editorial)

Steiner M, Glantz M, Lekos A. Randomized, double-blind study of vitamin D plus aspirin compared with aspirin alone for the prevention of recurrent strokes and transient ischemic attacks. Am J Clin Nutr 1995;62(suppl):1381S-4S

Street DA, Comstock GW, Salkeld RM, Schuep W, Klag M. Serum antioxidants and myocardial infarction: are low levels of carotenoids and a-tocopherol risk factors for myocardial infarction? Circulation 1990;90:1154-61

Williams HTG, Fenna D, Macbeth RA. Alpha-tocopherol in the treatment of intermittent claudication. Surg Gynecol Obstet 19971;132:662-6

Vitamin E In Prevention of Heart Attack and Stroke

Stamfer M.J., Rimm E.B., Epidemiologic evidence for vitamin E in prevention of cardiovascular disease. 1995. Am J Clin. Nut. 62 (suppl); 1365s-1369s.

Steinberg D. Antioxidants and artherosclerosis. A current assessment. Circulation 1991;84:1420-5 (editorial).

Puurunen M, Manttari M, Mannienen V, et al. Antibody against oxidized low-density lipoprotein predicting myocardial infraction. Arch Intern Med 1994; 154:2605-9.

Princen HMG, von Poppel G, Vogelezang C, Buytenhek R, Kok FJ. Supplementation with Vitamin E but not bcarotene in vivo protects low density lipoprotein from lipid peroxidation in vitro: effect of cigarette smoking. Arterioscler Thromb 1992;12:554-62.

Boscoboinik D, Szewczyk A, Hensey C, Azzi A. Inhibition of cell proliferation by a-tocopherol: role of protein kinase C. J Biol Chem 91;266;6188-94.

Steiner M, Glantz M, Lekos A. Randomized, double-blind study of vitamin D plus aspirin compared with aspirin alone for the prevention of recurrent strokes and transient ischemic attacks. Am J Clin Nutr 1995;62(suppl):1381S-4S.

Stampfer MJ, Rimm EB. A review of the epidemiology of dietary antioxidants and risk of coronary heart disease. Can J Cardiol 1993;9:14B-8B.

Vitamin E – Heart Disease, Cancer, All-Cause Mortality

Losonczy KG, Harris TB, Havlik RJ. Vitamin E and Vitamin C supplement use and risk of all-cause and coronary heart disease mortality in older persons: The Established Populations for Epidemiologic Studies of the Elderly. The American Journal Clinical Nutrition, 1996; 64; 2:190-196.

Wang Y, Huang DS, Eskelson CD, Watson RR. Long-term dietary vitamin E retards development of retrovirusinduced disregulation in cytokine production. Clin Immunol Immunopathol 1994; 72:70-5.

Omach EH, Kidao S, Sanders BG, Kline K. Effects of RRR-a-tocopherol succinate on IL-1 and PGE2 production macrophages. Nutr Cancer 1993:20:205-14.

Bendich A. Physiological role of antioxidants in the immune system. J Dairy Sci 1993;76:2789-94.

Meydani SN, Hayek M, Coleman L. Influence of vitamins E and B6 on immune response. Ann N Y Acad Sci 1992;669:125-39 (discussion 139-40).

Roebothan BV, Chandra RK. Relationship between nutritional status and immune function of elderly people. Age Ageing 1994;23:49-53.

Kelleher J. Vitamin E and the immune response. Proc Nutr Soc 1991;50:245-9.

Penn ND, Purkins L, Kelleher J, et al. The effect of dietary supplementation with vitamins A, C and E on cellmediated immune function in elderly long-stay patients: a randomized controlled trial. Age Ageing 1991;20:169-74.

Hodis HN, Mack WJ, LaBree L, et al. Serial coronary angiographic evidence that antioxidant vitamin intake reduces progression of coronary artery atherosclerosis. JAMA 1995;273:1849-54.

Meyers DG, Maloley PA. The antioxidant vitamins: impact on atherosclerosis. Pharmacotherapy 1993;13:574-82.

Manson JE, Gaziano JM, Jonas MA, Hennekens CH. Antioxidants and cardiovascular disease: a review. J AM Coll Nutr 1993; 12:426-32.

Donnan PT, Thomson M, Fowkes FGR, Prescott RJ, Housely E. Diet as a risk factor for peripheral arterial disease in the general population: The Edinburgh Artery Study. Am J Clin Nutr 1993;57:917-21.

Maxwell Sr. Can antioxidants prevent ischaemic heart disease? J Clin Pharm Ther 1993;18:85-95.

Gey KF, Brubacher GB, Stahelin HB. Plasma levels of antioxidant vitamins in relation to ischemic heart disease and cancer. Am J Clin Nutr 1987;45:1368-77.

Riemersma RA, Wood DA, Macintyre CC, et al. Risk of angina pectoris and plasma concentrations of vitamins A, C, and E and carotene. Lancet 1991;337:1-5.

Gey KF, Puska P, Jordon P, Moser UK. Inverse correlation between plasma vitamin E and mortality from ischemic heart disease in cross-cultural epidemiology. Am J Clin Nutr 1991;53:326S-34S.

Hennekens CH. Antioxidant vitamins and cancer. Am J Med 1994;97(suppl):2S-4S(discussion 22S-8S).

Kirkpatrick CS, White E, Lee JA. Case-control study of malignant melanoma in Washington State. II. Diet alcohol and obesity. Am J Epidemiol 1994;139:869-80.

Taylor Pr, Li B, Dawsey SM, et al. Prevention of esophageal cancer: the nutrition intervention trials in Linxian, China. Cancer Res 1994; 54 (suppl 7):2029S-31S.

Li JY, Li B, Blot WJ, Taylor PR. Preliminary report on the results of nutrition prevention trials of cancer and other common diseases among residents in Linxian, China. Chung Hua Chung Liu Tsa Chih 1993;15:165-81.

Gridley G, McLaughlin JK, Block G, et al. Vitamin supplement use and reduced risk of oral and pharyngeal cancer. Am J Epidemiol 1992;135:1083-92.

Knekt P, Reunanen A, Jarvinen R, et al. Antioxidant vitamin intake and coronary mortality in a longitudinal population study. Am J Epidemiol 1994;139:1180-9.

Bolton-Smith C, Woodward M, Tunstall-Pedoe H. The Scottish Heart Health Study. Dietary intake by food frequency questionnaire and odds ratios for coronary heart disease risk. II. The antioxidant vitamins and fibre. Eur J Clin Nutr 1992;45:85-93.

Rimm EB, Stampfer MJ, Ascherio A, et al. Vitamin E consumption and the risk of coronary heart disease in men. N Engl J Med 1993;328:1450-6.

Stampfer MJ, Hennekens CH, Manson JE, et al. Vitamin E consumption and the risk of coronary disease in women. N Engl J Med 1993;328:1444-9.

Ginter E. Decline in coronary mortality in United States and vitamins C. Am J Clin Nutr 1979;32:511-2(letter)

Vitamin C, Heart Attack and Stroke

Harats, D. et al. Citrus fruit supplementation reduces lipoprotein oxidation in young men ingesting a diet high in saturated fat: presumptive evidence for an interaction between vitamin C and E in vivo.Am J Clin Nutr. Feb 1998; 67:240-245

Gey, K.F. et al. Inverse correlation between plasma Vitamin E and mortality from ischemic heart disease in cross-cultural epidemiology. Am J Clin Nutr.1991; 53 (suppl):326s-34s.

Frei, B. Ascorbic acid protects lipids in human plasma and low-density lipoprotein against oxidative damage. Am J Clin Nutr. 1991;54 (suppl):1113s-8s.

Knekt, P. et al. Antioxidant vitamin intake and coronary mortality in a longitudinal population study. Am J Epidemiol 1994;139:1180-9

Ginter, E. et al. The effect of ascorbic acid on cholesterolemia in healthy subjects with seasonal deficit of vitamin C. Nutr Metab 1970;12:76-86

Paolisso, G. et al. Metabolic benefits deriving from chronic vitamin C supplementation in aged non-insulin dependent diabetics. J Am Coll.Nutr.1995;14:387-92.

Vitamin E, Insulin Action, Heart Disease in Elderly

Paolisso et al. Chronic intake of pharmacological doses of vitamin E might be useful in the therapy of elderly patients with coronary heart disease.Am J Clin Nutr 1995; 61:848-52.

De Fronzo RA, Ferrannini E. Insulin resistance. A multifaceted syndrome responsible for NIDDM, obesity, hypertension, dyslipidemia and atherosclerotic cardiovascular disease. Diabetes Care 1991; 14:173-94.

Young MH, Jeng CY, Sheu WHH et al. Insulin resistance, glucose intolerance, hyperinsulinemia and dyslipidemia in patients with angiographically demonstrated coronary artery disease. Am J Cardiol 1993; 72:458-60.

Paolisso G, Gambardella A, Galzerano D et al. Metabolic features of patients with and without coronary artery disease but with a superimposable cluster of cardiovascular factors. Coronary Artery Disease 1993; 4:1085-91.

Gey FK, Puska P, Jordan P, Moser UK. Inverse correlation between plasma vitamin E and mortality from ischemic heart disease in cross-cultural epidemiology. Am J Clin Nutr 1991; 53(suppl):326S-34S.

Stampfer MJ, Hennekens CH, Manson JAE, Colditz GA, Rosuer B, Willet WC. Vitamin E consumption and the risk of coronary heart disease in women. N Engl J Med 1993;328:1444-9.

Rimm EB, Stampfer MJ, Ascherio A, Giovanucci E, Colditz GA, Willet WC. Vitamin E consumption and the risk of coronary heart disease in men. N Engl J Med 1993;328:1450-6.

Paolisso G, D'Amore A, Guigliano D, Cereillo A, Varricchio M, D'Onofrio F. Pharmacological doses of vitamin E improve insulin action in healthy subjects and non-insulin-dependent diabetic patients. Am J Clin Nutr 1993;57:650-6.

Paolisso G, Di Maro G, Galzerano D, Cacciapuotti F, Varricchio M, O'Onofrio F. Pharmacological doses of vitamin E and insulin action in elderly subjects.Am J Clin Nutr 1994;59:1291-6.

Paolisso G, D'Amore A, Galzerano D et al. Daily vitamin E supplements improve metabolic control but not insulin secretion in elderly type II diabetic patients. Diabetes Care 1993;16:1433-7.

Paolisso G, Di Maro M, Pizza G et al. Plasma GHS/GSSG affects glucose homeostasis in healthy subjects and non-insulin dependent diabetes mellitus.Am J Physiol 1992;263:E435-40.

Reaven GM. The role of insulin resistance and hyperinsulinemia in coronary heart disease. Metabolism 1992; 41(suppl 1):16-9.

Kaardinal AFM, Kok FJ, Ringstad J et al. Antioxidants in adipose tissue and the risk of myocardial infarction: the EURAMIC study. Lancet 1993;342:1379-84.

Douglas CE, Chan AC, Chay PC. Vitamin E inhibits platelet phospholipase A2. Biochem Biophys Acta 1986; 876:639-45.

Tengerdy RP. The effect of vitamin E on immunoresponse and disease-resistance. Ann N Y Acad Sci 1989;570:335-44.

Jandank JM, Steiner M, Richardson PD. Reduction of platelet adhesiveness by vitamin E supplementation in humans. Thromb Res 1988; 49:393-404.

Castelli WP, Wilson PWF, Levy D, Anderson K. Cardiovascular risk factors in the elderly. Am J Cardiol 1989;63(suppl):12H-9H.

Paolisso G, D'Amore A, Balbi V et al. Plasma vitamin C effects glucose homeostasis in healthy subjects and in non-insulin-dependent diabetics. Am J Physiol 1994; 266:E261-8.

Heart Disease in Women, Folic Acid, Homocysteine

Rimm E.B. et al. Folate and vitamin B6 from diet and supplements in relation to risk of coronary heart disease among women. JAMA 1998;279;5:359-64

McCull KS. Vascular pathology of homocysteinemia; implications for pathogenesis of arteriosclerosis. Am J Pathol, 1969;56:111-128

Mudd SH, FinkelsteinJD, Irreverre F, Laster L. Homocysteinuria: an enzymatic defect. Science. 1964;143:1443-1445.

Brattstrom L, Israelsson B, Norrving B, et al. Impaired homocysteine metabolism in early-onset cerebral and peripheral occlusive arterial disease: effects of pyridoxine and folic acid treatment. Atherosclerosis. 1990;81:51-60

Morrison HI, Schaubel D, Desmeules M, Wigle DT. Serus folate and risk of fatal coronary heart disease. JAMA.1996;275:1983-1896

Chasan-Taber L, Selhub J, Roseberg IH, et al. A prospective study of folate and vitamin B6 and risk of myocardial infarction in US physicians. J Coll Nutr. 1996;15:136-143

Giovannucci E, Stampfer MJ, Colditz GA, et al. Folate, methionine, and alcohol intake and risk of colorectal adenoma J Natl Cancer Inst. 1993;85:875-884

Selhub J, Jacques PF, Wilson PWF, Rush D, Roseberg IH. Vitamin status and intake as primary determinanats of homocysteinemia in an elderly population. JAMA, 1993;270:2693-2698

Nygard O, Nordrehaug JE, Refsum H, Ueland PM, Farstad M, Vollset SE. Plasma homocysteine levels and mortality in patients with coronary artery disease. N Engl J Med. 1997;337:230-236

Rimm EB, Stampfer MJ, Ascherio A, Giovannucci E, Willett WC. Dietary folate, vitamin B6, and vitamin B12 intake and risk of CHD among a large population of men. Circulation. 1996;93:625.

Abstract Tsai JC, Perrella MA, Yoshizumi M, et al. Promotion of vascular smooth muscle cell growth by homocysteine: a link to atherosclerosis. Proc Natl Acad Sci USA. 1994;91:6369-6373

Stamler JS, Osborne JA, Jaraki O, et al. Adverse vascular effects of homocysteine are modulated by endothelium-derived relaxing factor and related oxides of nitrogen. J Clin Invest. 1993;91:308-318

Tawakol A, Omland T, Gerhard M, Wu JT, Creager MA. Hyper homocysteinemia is associated with impaired endothelium-dependent vasodilation in humans. Circulation. 1997;95:1119-1121

Pancharuniti N, Lewis CA, Sauberlich HE, et al. Plasma homocysteine, folate, and vitamin B12 concentrations and risk for early-onset coronary artery disease. Am J Clin Nutr. 1994;59:940-948

Bendich A. Folic and prevention of neural tube birth defects: critical assessment of FDA proposals to increase folic acid intakes. J Nutr Educ. 1994; 26:294-299

Higher Folic Acid Intake, Reduced Risk of Stroke

Bazzano L.A et al, Dietary intake of folate and risk of stroke in US men and women: NHANES I Epidemiologic follow-up study. Stroke. 2002; 33, 5: 1183

B-Vitamins and Heart Disease

Rimm E.B. et al. Folate and vitamin B6 from diet and supplements in relation to risk of coronary heart disease among women. JAMA 1998;279;5:359-64

McCull KS. Vascular pathology of homocysteinemia; implications for pathogenesis of arteriosclerosis. Am J Pathol, 1969;56:111-128

Mudd SH, FinkelsteinJD, Irreverre F, Laster L. Homocysteinuria: an enzymatic defect. Science. 1964;143:1443-1445.

Brattstrom L, Israelsson B, Norrving B, et al. Impaired homocysteine metabolism in early-onset cerebral and peripheral occlusive arterial disease: effects of pyridoxine and folic acid treatment. Atherosclerosis. 1990;81:51-60

Morrison HI, Schaubel D, Desmeules M, Wigle DT. Serus folate and risk of fatal coronary heart disease. JAMA. 1996;275:1983-1896

Chasan-Taber L, Selhub J, Roseberg IH, et al. A prospective study of folate and vitamin B6 and risk of myocardial infarction in US physicians. J Coll Nutr. 1996;15:136-143

Giovannucci E, Stampfer MJ, Colditz GA, et al. Folate, methionine, and alcohol intake and risk of colorectal adenoma J Natl Cancer Inst. 1993;85:875-884

Selhub J, Jacques PF, Wilson PWF, Rush D, Roseberg IH. Vitamin status and intake as primary determinanats of homocysteinemia in an elderly population. JAMA, 1993;270:2693-2698

Nygard O, Nordrehaug JE, Refsum H, Ueland PM, Farstad M, Vollset SE. Plasma homocysteine levels and mortality in patients with coronary artery disease. N Engl J Med. 1997;337:230-236

Rimm EB, Stampfer MJ, Ascherio A, Giovannucci E, Willett WC. Dietary folate, vitamin B6, and vitamin B12 intake and risk of CHD among a large population of men. Circulation. 1996;93:625.

Abstract Tsai JC, Perrella MA, Yoshizumi M, et al. Promotion of vascular smooth muscle cell growth by homocysteine: a link to atherosclerosis. Proc Natl Acad Sci USA. 1994;91:6369-6373

Stamler JS, Osborne JA, Jaraki O, et al. Adverse vascular effects of homocysteine are modulated by endothelium-derived relaxing factor and related oxides of nitrogen. J Clin Invest. 1993;91:308-318

Tawakol A, Omland T, Gerhard M, Wu JT, Creager MA. Hyper homocysteinemia is associated with impaired endothelium-dependent vasodilation in humans. Circulation. 1997;95:1119-1121

Pancharuniti N, Lewis CA, Sauberlich HE, et al. Plasma homocysteine, folate, and vitamin B12 concentrations and risk for early-onset coronary artery disease. Am J Clin Nutr. 1994;59:940-948

Bendich A. Folic and prevention of neural tube birth defects: critical assessment of FDA proposals to increase folic acid intakes. J Nutr Educ. 1994; 26:294-299

Reducing High Blood Pressure, Natural Therapies

1. Quick Reference to Clinical Nutrition, Halpern, S. (ed.); Nutrition and Cardiovascular Disease; J.B. Lippincott Company, Philadelphia, 1987: 139-153

2. Canadian Guidelines for Cardiac Rehabilitation and Cardiovascular Disease Prevention (Canadian Assoc. of Cardiac Rehab.) 1st edition, 1999; 94-104

3. Fowler, F.E. Myocardial infarction in the 1990's; Postgraduate Medicine, May 1995; 97, 5: 135-146

4. Complete Guide to Prescription and Non-Prescription Drugs (1999 edition) Griffith H.W. The Body Press,1998: 168-169, 194-195, 54-55

5. Murray, C.J.L.M., et al. Evidence-based health policy – lessons from the global burden of disease study. Science 1996; 274: 740-743

6. Joffres, M.R., et al. Awareness, treatment, and control of hypertension in Canada. Am J Hypertens. 1997; 10, (Pt-1): 1097-1102

7. 2000 Canadian hypertension recommendations (summary of recommendations affecting family physicians) – the Canadian Hypertension Recommendations Working Group. Canadian Family Physician. April 2001; 47: 793-794

8. Modern Nutrition in Health and Disease (sixth edition) Goodhart, R., and Shils, M. Lea and Febiger: 733

9. McCarron, D., et al. Body weight and blood pressure regulation. Am J Clin Nutr. 1996; 63 (suppl): 423-425

10. Pate, R.R., et al. Physical Activity and Public Health. JAMA. Feb. 1, 1995; 272, 5: 402-407

11. McCarron, D. Role of adequate dietary calcium intake in the prevention and management of salt-sensitive hypertension. Am J Clin Nutr. 1997; 62: 2 (suppl): 712-716

12. Cappuccio, F., et al. Double-blind randomized trial of modest salt restriction in older people. Lancet, 1997; 350; 9081: 850-854.

13. Graudal, N. et al. Effects of sodium restriction on blood pressure, rennin, aldosterone, catecholamines, cholesterols, and triglycerides. JAMA, 1998; 279: 1383-1391

14. Meese, R.B., et al. The inconsistent effects of calcium supplements upon blood pressure in primary hypertension. Am J Med Sci. 1987; 29: 4219-4224

15. Motoyama, T., et al. Oral magnesium supplementation in patients with essential hypertension. Hypertension, 1989; 13: 227-232

16. Murray, M., and Pizzorno, J. Encyclopedia of Natural Medicine (2nd edit.) Prima Publishing, 1997; 425-535

17. Foushee, D.B., et al. Garlic as a natural agent for the treatment of hypertension. A preliminary report. Cytobios. 1982; 34: 145-162

18. Digiesi, V., et al. Mechanism of action of Coenzyme Q10 in essential hypertension. Curr Ther Res. 1992; Res 51: 668-672

19. Langsjoen, P., et al. Treatment of essential hypertension with Coenzyme Q10. Mol Aspects Med. 1994; Med 15 (suppl): 265-272

20. Digiesi, V., et al. Coenzyme Q10 in essential hypertension. Mol Aspects Med. 1994; Med 15 (suppl): 257-263

21. McCarty, M.F. Coenzyme Q versus hypertension: does CoQ decrease endothelial superoxide generation? Med Hypotheses. 1999; 53, 4: 300-304

22. Singh, R.B., et al. Effect of hydrosoluble Coenzyme Q10 on blood pressure and insulin resistance in hypertensive patients with coronary artery disease. J Hum Hypertens. 1999; 13, 3: 203-208

23. Yamagami, T., et al. Bioenergetics in Clinical Medicine. Studies on Coenzyme Q10 and Essential Hypertension. Research Comm. in Chem. Path and Pharmacol 1975; 11, 2: 273-288

24. Yamagami, T., et al. Bioenergetics in Clinical Medicien, VIII. Administration of Coenzyme Q10 to patients with essential hypertension. Research Comm in Chem Path and Pharmacol. 1976; 14, 4: 721-727

25. Encyclopedia of Nutritional Supplements. Murray, M., PRIMA publishing, 1996: 300-301

26. Nutritional Influences on Illness. Werbach, M.R. Third Line Press., Inc. 1987: 227-240

27. Encyclopedia of Natural Medicine (2nd edit) Murray, M. and Pizzorno, J. Prima Publishing 1997: 524-535

28. Petrella, R.J. Lifestyle approaches to managing high blood pressure. Can Family Phys. 1999; 45: 1750-1755

29. Elmer, J.P., et al. Lifestyle intervention: results of the Treatment of Mild Hypertension Study. (TOHMS). Prev Med 1995; 24: 378-388

30. Stamler, R., et al. Nutritional therapy for high blood pressure. Final report of a four-year randomized controlled trial – the hypertension control program. JAMA. 1987; 257: 1484-1491

31. Iso, H., et al. Community-based education classes for hypertension control: a 1.5-year randomized controlled trial. Hypertension. 1996; 27: 968-974

32. Appel, L.J., et al. A clinical trial of the effects of dietary patterns on blood pressure (DASH-study) N Engl J Med 1997; 336: 1117-1124

34. Shariff, S., et al. Herbal Fervor and Vitamin Vigor: Herbs and vitamins for cardiac disease. Perspective in Cardiology. 2000; 16, 1: 21-29

35. McCarron, D., et al. Blood pressure response to oral calcium in persons with mild to moderate hypertension. A randomized, double-blind, placebo-controlled, crossover trial. Ann Intern Med, 1985; 103,6: 825-831

Natural Supplements, Cholesterol, Triglycerides, Gugulipid

1. Murray MT, The Healing Power of Herbs (2nd edition), Prima Publishing, 1995.

2. Satyavati GV, A Primising Hypolipidaemic Agent from Gum Guggul (Commiphora Wightii), Econ Med Plant Res 5, 1991, 47-82.

3. Nityand S and Kapoor NK, Hypocholesterolemic Effect of Commiphora Mukul Resin, Indian J Exp Biol 9, 1971, 376-377.

4. Kuppurajan K, et.al., Effect of Gugglu on Serum Lipids in Obese Hypercholesterolemic and Hyperlipidemic Cases, J Assoc Physicians India 26, 1978, 367-371.

5. Malhotra SC, Ahuja MMS, and Sundaram KR, Long Term Clinical Studies on the Hypolipidaemic Effect of Commiphora Mukul (Guggulu) and Clofibrate, Indian J Med Res 65, 1977, 390-395.

6. Verna SK and Bordia A, Effect of Commiphora Mukul (Gum Guggulu) in Patients of Hyperlipidemia with Special Reference to HDL –cholesterol, Indian J Med Res 87, 1988, 356-360.

7. Agarwal RC, et.al., Clinical Trial of Gugulipid a New Hypolipidemicagent of Plant Origin in Primary Hyperlipidemia, Indian J Med Res 84, 1986, 626-634.

8. Nityanand S, Srivastava JS, and Asthana OP. Clinical Trials with Gugulipid, a New Hypolipidaemic Agent, J Assoc Physicians India 37, 1989, 321-328.

9. Singh V, et.al., Stimulation of Low Density Lipoprotein Receptor Activity in Liver Membrane of Guggulsterone Treated Rats, Pharmocol Res 22, 1990, 37-44.

10. Sharma JN and Sharma JN, Commparison of the Anti-inflammatory Activity of Commiphora Mukul (an indigenous drug) with those Pfhenylbutazone and Ibuprofen in Experimental Arthritis Induced by Mycobacterial Adjuvant, Arzneimittel-Forsch 27, 1977, 1455-1457.

11. Dietary Supplement Information Bureau. www.content.intramedicine.com: Guggul.

12. Natural Health Products Encyclopedia. www.consumerslab.com: Guggul.

13. Healthnotes, Inc.200.www.healthnotes.com: Guggul

14. Satyavati GV. Gum guggul (Commiphora mukul) – The success of an ancient insight leading to a modern discovery. Indian J Med 1988;87:327-35

15. Singh RB, Niaz MA, Ghosh S. Hypolipidemic and antioxidant effects of Commiphora mukul as an adjunct to dietary therapy in patients with hypercholesterolemia. Cardiovasc Drugs Ther 1994;8:659-64

16. Singh K, Chander R, Kapoor NK. Guggulsterone, a potent hypolipidaemic, prevents oxidation of low density lipoprotein. Phytother Res 1997;11:291-4

17. Mester L, Mester M, Nityanand S. Inhibition of platelet aggregration by guggulu steroids. Planta Med 1979;37:367-9
18. Thappoa DM, Dogra J. Nodulocystic acne: oral gugulipid versus tetracycline. J Dermatol 1994;21:729-31
19. Satyavati GV et al. Experimental studies on the hypocholesterolemic effect of commiphora mukul. Indian J Med Res 1969;57(10):1950-62
20. Nityanand S et al. Clinical trials with gugulipid. A new hypolipidaemic agent. J Assoc Physicians India 1989;37(5):323-8
21. Satyavati GV et al. Guggulipid: a promising Hypolipidemic agent from gum guggul (Commiphora Wightii). Econ Med Plant Res 1991;5:48-82
22. Tripathi YB et al. Thyroid stimulatory action of (Z)-Guggulsterone: mechanism of action. Planta Med 1988;54(4):271-7
23. Panda S, Kar A. Gugulu (Commiphora mukul) induces triiodothyronine production: possible involvement of lipid peroxidation. Life Sci 1999;65(12):PL137-41
24. Dalvi SS et al. Effects of gugulipid on bioavailability of diltiazem and propranolol. J Assoc Physicians India 1994;42(6):454-5

Policicosanol

1. Gouni-Berthold I, Berthold HK. Policosanol: Clinical pharmacology and therapeutic significance of a new lipid-lowering agent. Am Heart J 2002Feb;143(2):356-65
2. Torres O, Agramonte AJ, Illnait J, Más Ferreiro R, Fernández L, Fernández JC. Treatment of hypercholesterolemia in NIDDM with policosanol. Diabetes Care 1995Mar;18(3):393-7
3. Castaño G, Más R, Roca J, Fernández L, Illnait J, Fernández JC, Selman E. A double-blind, placebocontrolled studyof the effects of policosanol in patients with intermittent claudication. Angiology 1999Feb;50(2):123-30
4. A Natural Anti-Cholesterol Dietary Supplement: Policosanol. Life Extension Jun2001;7(6):24
5. Prat H, et al. Comparative effects of policosanol and two HMG-CoA Reductase inhibitors on type II hypercholesterolemia. Rev Med Chil Mar 1999;127(3):286-94
6. Menéndez R, Amor AM, Rodeiro I, González RM, González PC, Alfonso JL, et al. Policosanol modulates HMG-CoA Reductase activity in cultured fibroblasts. Arch med Res 2001Jan-Feb;32(1):8-12
7. Canetti M, Moreira M, Más R, Illnait J, Fernández L, Fernández, JC, et al. A two-year study on the efficacyand tolerability of policosanol in patients with type II hyperlipoproteinaemia. Int J Clin Pharmacol Res1995;15(4):159-65
8. Stusser R, et al. Long-term therapy with policosnol improves treadmill exercise-ECG testing performance of coronary heart disease patients. Int J Clin Pharmacol Ther 1998;36:469-73
9. Mirkin A, Más R, Martinto M, Boccanera R, Robertis A, Poudes R, et al. Efficacy and tolerability of policosanol in hypercholesterolemic postmenopausal women. Int J Clin Pharmacol Res 2001;21(1):31-41
10. Más R, Castaño G, Illnait J, Fernández L, Fernández J, Alemán C, et al. Effects of policosanol in patients with type II hypercholesterolemia and additional coronary risk factors. Clin Pharmacol Ther 1999Apr;65(4):439-47
11. Castaño G, Más R, Fernández JC, Illnait J, Fernández L, Alvarez E. Effects of policosanol in older patients with type II hypercholesterolemia and high coronary risk. J Gerontol A Biol Sci med Sci 2001Mar;56(3):186-92

12. Castaño G, Más R, Arruzazabala ML, Noa M, Illnait J, Fernández JC, et al. Effects of policosanol and pravastatin on lipid profile, platelet aggregation and endothelemia in older hypercholesterolemic patients. Int J Clin Pharmacol Res 1999;19(4):105-16

13. Prat H, Román O, Pino E. Comparative effects of policosanol and two HMG-CoA Reductase inhibitors on type II hypercholesterolemia. Rev Med Chil 1999Mar;127(3):286-94

14. Marcello S, Gladstein J, Tesone P, Más R. Current Therapeutic Research 2000Jun;61(6):346-57

15. Castaño G, et al. A double-blind placebo-controlled study of the effects of policosanol in patients with intermittent claudication. Angiology. Feb 1999; 50(2):123-30

16. Stüsser R, Batista J, Padrón R, Sosa F, Pereztol O. Long-term therapy with policosanol imporves treadmill exercise-ECG testing performance of coronary heart disease patients. Int J Clin Pharmacol Ther 1998Sep;36(9):469-73

17. Batista J, Stüsser R, Saéz F, Peréz B. Effect of policosanol on hyperlipidemia dn coronary heart diseases in middle-aged patients.A 14-month pilot study. Int J Clin Pharmacol Ther Mar1996;34(3):134-7

18. Torres O, et al. Treatment of hypercholesterolemia in NIDDM with policosanol. Diabetes Care. Mar1995;18(3):393-7

19. Arruzazabala ML, et al. Effect of policosanol successive dose increases on platelet aggregation in healthy volunteers. Pharmacol Res Nov 1996;34(5-6):181-5

20. Arruzazabala ML, et al. Comparative study of policosanol, aspirin and the combination therapy policosanol-aspirin on platelet aggreagation in healthy volunteers. Pharmacol Res Oct1997;36(4):293-7

21. Carbajal D, et al. Effect of policosanol on platelet aggregation and serum levels of arachidonic acid metabolites in healthy volunteers. Prostaglandins Leukot Essent Fatty Acids Jan1998;58(1):61-4

22. Mesa AR, Mas R, Noa M et al. Toxicity of policosanol in beagle dogs: one-year study. Toxicol Lett 1994;73:81-90

23. Aleman CL, Mas R, Hernandez C et al. A 12-month study of policosanol oral toxicity in Sprague Dawley rats. Toxicol Lett 1994;70:77-87

24. Mas R, et al. Effects of policosanol in patients with type II hypercholesterolemia dn additional coronary risk factors. Clin Pharmacol Ther Apr1999;65(4):439-47

25. Carbajal D, Arruzazabala ML, Valdes S, Mas R. Effect of policosanol on platelet aggreagation and serum levels of arachidonic acid metabolites in healthy volunteers. Prostaglandins Leukot Essent Fatty Acids Jan1998;58(1):61-4

26. Arruzazabala ML, et al. Comparative study of policosanol, aspirin and the combination therapy policosanol-aspirin on platelet aggregation in healthy volunteers. Pharmacol Res Oct1997;36(4):293-7

27. Stusser R, Batista J, Padron R, et al. Long-term therapy with policosanol improves treadmill exercise-ECG testing performance of coronary heart disease patients. Int J Clin Pharmacol Ther Sep1998;36(9):469-73

28. Carbajal D, et al. Interaction policosanol-warfarin on bleeding time and thrombosis in rats. Pharmacol Res Aug1998;38(2):89-91

29. Molina Cuevas V, et al. Effect of policosanol on arterial blood pressure in rats. Study of the pharmacological interaction with nifedipine and propranolol. Arch Med Res Mar1998;29(1):21-4

30. Griffith W, MD. Complete Guide to Prescription and Nonprescription Drugs. The Body Press 1999;MHGCoA Reductase inhibitors:418-419

CoEnzyme Q10: An Essential Anti-Aging Nutrient

General Anti-Aging/DiseasePrevention

Alleva R, Scararmucci A, Mantero F, et al. The protective role of ubiquinol-10 against formation of lipid hydroperoxides in human seminal fluid. Mol Aspects Med. 1997;18(Suppl):S221-8

Bargossi AM, Grossi G, Fiorella PL, et al. Exogenous CoQ10 supplementation prevents plasma ubiquinone reduction induced by HMG-CoA reductase inhibitors. Mol Aspects Med. 1994;15(suppl):S187-S193

Carper J. Stop Aging Now. HarperCollins Publishers, Inc 1995;The Amazing New Age Terminator: Coenzyme Q10:138-147

Folkers K, Langsjoen P,Willis R, et al. Lovastatin decreases Coenzyme Q10 levels in humans. Proc Natl Acad Sci USA. 1990; 87;8931-8934

Ghirlanda G, Oradei A, Manto A, et al. Evidence of plasma CoQ10-lowering effect by HMG-CoA reductase inhibitors: a double-blind, placebo-controlled study. J Clin Pharmacol. 1993;33:226-229

Kishi H, Kishi T, Folkers K. Bioenergetics in clinical medicine. III. Inhibition of Coenzyme Q10-enzymes by clinically used anti-hypertensive drugs.Res Commun Chem Pathol Pharmacol. 1975;12:533-540

Kishi T, Kishi H, Watanabe T, et al. Bioenergetics in clinical medicine. XI. Studies on Coenzyme Q10 and diabetes mellitus. J Med. 1976;7:307-321

Kishi T, Makino K, Ochi T, et al. Inhibition of myocardial respiration by spychotherapeutic drugs and prevention by coenzyme Q. Biomed Clin Aspects Coenzyme Q. 1980;4:139-157

Kishi T, Watanabe T, Folkers K. Bioenergetics in clinical medicine XV. Inhibition of Coenzyme Q10-enzymes by clinically used adrenergic blockers of beta-receptors. Res Commun Chem Pathol Pharmacol. 1977;17:157-164

Lewin A, Lavon H. The effect of Coenzyme Q10 on sperm motility and function. Mol Aspects Med. 1997;18(Suppl):S213-9

Mortensen SA, Leth A, Agner E, et al. Dose-related decrease of serum Coenzyme Q10 during treatment with HMG-CoA reductase inhibitors. Mol Aspects Med. 1997;18(suppl):S137-S144

Murray M and Pizzorno J. Encyclopedia of Natural Medicine (revised 2nd edition) Prima Health 1998; Heart Disease:500-506

Murray M. The Encyclopedia of Nutritional Supplements. Prima Publishing 1996; Chapter 35: Coenzyme Q10:296-308

Murray M. The Healing Power Of Herbs (2nd edition). Prima Publishing 1995; Hawthorn:203-209

Reavley N. The New Encyclopedia of Vitamins, Minerals, Supplements & Herbs. M. Evans and Company, Inc 1998;Coenzyme Q10: 353-361

Weber C, Jacobsen TS, Mortensen SA, et al. Antioxidative effect of dietary coenzyme Q10 in human blood plasma. Int J Vitam Nutr Res 1994; 64:311-5

Burke BE, Neuenschwander R, Olson RD. Randomized, double-blind, placebo-controlled trial of Coenzyme Q10 in isolated systolic hypertension. South Med J. 2001;94:1112-1117

Digiesi V, Cantini F, Brodbeck B. Effect of coenzyme Q10 on essential arterial hypertension. Curr Ther Res. 1990;47:841-845

Digiesi V, Cantini F, Oradei A, et al. Coenzyme Q10 in essential hypertension. Mol Aspects Med. 1994;15(suppl):S257-S263

Hofman-Bang C, Rehnquist N, Swedberg K, et al. Coenzyme Q10 as adjunctive treatment of congestive heart failure. J Am Coll Cardiol. 1992;19:216A

Hofman-Bang C, Rehnquist N, Swedberg K, et al. Coenzyme Q10 as an adjunctive treatment of congestive heart failure. J Am Coll Cardiol. 1992;19:216A

Kamikawa T, Kobayashi A, Yamashita T, et al. Effects of coenzyme Q10 on exercise tolerance in chronic stable angina pectoris. AM J Cardiol 1985;56:247

Khatta M, Alexander BS, Krichten CM, et al. The effect of coenzyme Q10 in patients with congestive heart failure. Ann Intern Med. 2000;132:636-640

Lampertico M, Comis S. Italian muticenter study on the efficacy and safety of Coenzyme Q10 as adjuvant therapy in heart failure. Clin Investig. 1993;71(8 suppl):S129-S133

Langsjoen H, Langsjoen P, Langsjoen P, et al. Usefulness of coenzyme Q10 in clinicl cardiology: a long-term study. Mol Aspects Med. 1994;15(suppl):S165-S175

Langsjoen P, Langsjoen P, Willis R, et al. Treatment of essential hypertension with Coenzyme Q10. Mol Aspects Med. 1994;15(suppl):S265-S272

Langsjoen PH, Vadhanavikit S, Folkers. Response of patients in classes III and IV of cardiomyopathy to therapy in a blind and crossover trial with Coenzyme Q10. Proc Natl Acad Sci USA. 1985;82:4240-4244

Morisco C, Trimarco B, Condorelli M. Effect of coenzyme Q10 therapy in patients with congestive heart failure: a long-term multicenter randomized study. Clin Investig. 1993; 71(8 suppl): S134-S136

Munkholm H, Hansen HH, Ramussen K. Coenzyme Q10 treatment in serious heart failure. Biofactors.1999;9:285-289

Pogessi L, Galanti G, Comeglio M, et al. Effect of Coenzyme Q10 on left ventricular function in patients with dilative cardiomyopathy. Curr Ther Res. 1991;49:878-886

Singh RB, Niaz MA, Rastogi SS, et al. Effect of hydrosoluble coenzyme Q10 on blood pressures and insulin resistance in hypertensive patients with coronary artery disease. J Human Hypertens. 1999;13:203-208

Tanaka J, Tominaga R, Yoshitoshi M, et al. Coenzyme Q10: the prophylactic effect on low cardiac output following cardiac valve replacement. Ann Thorac Surg 1982;33:145-51

Thomas SR, Neuzil J, Stocker R. Inhibition of LDL oxidation by ubiquinol-10. A protective mechanism for coenzyme Q in atherogenesis? Mol Aspects Med 1997; 18:S85-103

Watson PS, Scalia GM, Galbraith A, et al. Lack of effect of Coenzyme Q10 on left ventricular function in patients with congestive heart failure. J Am Coll Cardiol. 1999;33:1549-1552

Brain Function

Albano CB, Muralikrishnan D, Ebadi M. Distribution of coenzyme Q homologues in brain. Neurochemical Research. 2002 May; 27 (5), pp. 359-68

Baker SK, Tarnopolsky MA. Targeting cellular energy production in neurological disorders. Expert opinion on investigational drug. 2003 Oct; 12(10):1 655-79

Huntington Study Group. A randomized, placebo-controlled trial of Coenzyme Q10 and remacemide in Huntington's disease Neurology 2001;57:397-40

Imagawa M, Naruse S, Tsuji S, et al. Coenzyme Q10, iron, and vitamin B6 in genetically-confirmed Alzheimer's disease. Lancet 1992;340:671 (letter)

Matthews RT, Yang L, Browne S, et al. Coenzyme Q10 administration increases brain mitochondrial concentrations and exerts neuroprotective effects. Proc Natl Acad Sci USA. 1998;95:8892-8897

Naini A, Lewis VJ, Hirano M, DiMaura S. Primary Coenzyme Q deficiency and the brain. Biofactors. 2003; Vol. 18 Issue ¼, p145, 8P

Baker SK. Targeting cellular energy production in neurological disorders. Expert Opin Investig Drugs 2003 Oct; Vol. 12 (10), pp. 1655-79; PMID:

14519086 Beal M. Coenzyme Q10 administration and its potential for treatment of neurodegenerative diseases. Flint Biofactors, 1999;Vol.9Issue2-4,p261,6p; (An 2135916)

Beal MF. Coenzyme Q10 as a possible treatment for neurodegenerative diseases. Free Radic Res, 2002 Apr; Vol. 36 (4), pp. 455-60; PMID: 12069110

Beal MF. Coenzyme Q10 attenuates the 1-methyl-4-pheyl-1,2,3, tetrahydropyridine (MPTP) induced loss of striatal dopamine and dopaminergic axon in aged mice. Brain Res, 1998 Feb 2; Vol. 783 (1), pp. 109-14; PMID: 9479058

Beal MF. Mitochondria, oxidative damage, and inflammation in Parkinson's disease. Ann N Y Acad Sci, 2003 Jun; Vol. 991 120-31; PMID:12846981

Ebadi M. Ubiquinone (coenzyme Q10) and complex I in mitochondrial oxidative disorder of Parkinson's disease. Proc West Pharmacol Soc, 2000;Vol.43,pp.55-63;PMID: 11056957

Ebadi M. Ubiquinone (coenzyme q10) and mitochondria in oxidative stress of parkinson's disease. Biol Signals Recept, 2001 May-Aug; Vol. 10(3-4) pp. 224-53; PMID: 11351130

Frankish H. Coenzyme Q10 could slow functional decline in Parkinson's disease. Lancet 10/19/2002;Vol.360 Issue 9341, p1227, 1p; (AN 7557063)

Jiménez-Jiménez FJ. Serum levels of coenzyme Q10 in patients with Parkinson's disease. J Neural Transm, 2000; Vol 107 (2), pp. 177-81; PMID:10847558

Kidd PM. Parkinson's disease as multifactorial oxidative neurodegeneration: implications for integrative management. Altern Med Rev, 200 Dec; Vol. 5 (6), pp. 502-29; PMID: 11134975

Müller T. Coenzyme Q10 supplementation provides mild symptomatic benefit in patiens with Parkinson's disease. Neurosci Let, 2003 May 8;Vol.341(3);201-4; PMID: 12697283

Ogawa O. Mitochondrial abnormalities and oxidative imbalance in neurodegenerative disease. Sci Aging Knowledge Environ. 2002 Oct 16; Vol. 2002 (41), pp. pe16; PMID: 14603007

Shults CW, Haas RH. A possible role of coenzyme Q10 in the etiology and treatment of Parkinson's disease. Biofactors, 1999, Vol. 9 Issue 2-4, p267,6p, 1 chart, 1 graph; (AN 2135917)

Shults CW. Absorption, tolerability, and effects on mitochondrial activity of oral coenzyme Q10 in parkinsonian patients. Neurology, 1998 Mar; Vol. 50 (3), pp. 793-5; PMID: 9521279

Shults CW. Coenzyme Q10 in neurodegenerative diseases. Med Chem, 2003 Oct; Vol. 10 (19), pp. 1917-21; PMID: 12871093

Shults CW. Coenzyme Q10 levels correlate with the activities of complexes I and II/III in mitochondria from parkinsonian and non parkinsonian subjects.Ann Neurol, 1997 Aug; Vol. 42 (2), pp. 261-4: PMID: 9266740

Strijks E. Q10 Therapy in patients with idiopathic Parkinson's disease. Mol Aspects Med, 1997; Vol. 18 Suppl, pp. S237-40; PMID: 9266528

Immune Function and Cancer Treatment Support

Folkers K, Shizukuishi S, Takemura K, et al. Increase in levels of IgG in serum of patients treated with Coenzyme Q10. Res Commun Pathol Pharmacol 1982

Judy WV. Nutritional Intervention in cancer prevention and treatment. American College for Advancement in Medicine Spring Conference, Ft.Lauderdale, FL. May 3, 1998

Lockwood K, et al. Apparent partial remission of breast cancer in "high risk" patients supplemented with nutritional antioxidants, essential fatty acids and coenzyme Q10. Mol Aspects Med, 1994;15 Suppl:s231-40

Lockwood K, et al. Progress on therapy of Breast Cancer with Vitamin Q10 and the Regression of Metastases. Biochem Biophys Res Commun. Jul 1995;212(1):172-77

Hawthorn

Degenring FH, Suter A, Weber M, Saller R. A randomized double-blind placebo controlled clinical trial of a standardized extract of fresh Crataegus berries (Crataegisan) in the treatment of patients with congestive heart failure NYHA II. Phytomedicine. 2003;10(5):363-9

Leuchtgens H. Crataegus Special Extract WS 1442 in NYHA II heart failure. A placebo controlled randomized double-blind study. Forschr Med 111,352-354, 1993

Murray M. The Healing Power Of Herbs (2nd edition). Prima Publishing 1995; Hawthorn:203-209

O'Conolly VM, et al. Treatment of cardiac performance (NYHA stage I to II) in advanced age with standardized crataegus extract. Forschr Med 104,805-808, 1986

Petkov E, et al. Inhibitory Effect of Some Flavonoids and Flavonoid Mixtures on Cyclic AMP Phosphodiesterase Activity of Rat Heart. Planta Medica. 1981;43:183-86

Tauchert M, Ploch M, Huebner WD. Effectiveness of Hawthorn Extract LI132 Compared with the ACE Inhibitor Captopril: Muticenter double-blind study with 132 NYHA Stage II. Muench Med Wochenschr. 1994;136(supp):S27-S33

Hawthorn

1. Petkov V, Plants with Hypotensive, Antiatheromatous and Coronarodilating Action, Am J Clin Med 7, 1979,197-236.

2. Wagner H, Bladt S, and Zgainski EM, Plant Drug Analysis, Springer-Verlag, New York, 1984, 166 & 178-179.

3. Ammon HPT, Handel M, Crataegus, Toxicology and Pharmacology, I Toxicity, Planta Medica 43, 1981, 105-120, II Pharmacodynamics, Planta Medica 43, 1981, 209-239, III Pharmacodynamics and Pharmacokinetics, Planta Medica 43(4), 1981, 313-322.

4. Mavers VWH, and Hensel H, Changes in Local Myocardial Blood Flow Following Oral Administration of a Crataegus Extract to Non-anesthetized Dogs, Arzneimittel-Forsch 24, 1974, 783-785.

5. Roddewig VC, and Hensel H, Reaction of Local Myocardial Blood Flow in Non-anaesthetic Dogs and Anesthetized Cats to Oral and Parental Application of Crataegus Fraction (Ologomer Procyanidins), Arzneimittel-Forsch 27, 1977, 1407-1410.

6. Rewerski VW, et.al., Some Pharmacological Properties of Oligometric Procyanidin Isolated from Hawthorn (Crataegus Oxyacantha), Arzneimittel-Forsch 17, 1967, 490-491.

7. Uchida S, et.al., Inhibitory Effects of Condensed Tannins on Angiotensin Converting Enzyme, Jpn J Pharmacol 43, 1987, 242-245.

8. Blesken R, Crataegus in Cardiology, Forschr Med 110, 1992, 290-292.

9. O'Connoly VM, et.al., Treatment of Cardiac Performance (NYHA Stages I to II) in Advanced Age with Standardized Crataegus Special Extract, Forschr Med 104, 1986, 805-808.

10. Leuchrgens H, Crataegus Special Extract WS 1442 in NYHA II heart failure. A Placebo Controlled Randomized Double-blind Study, Forschr Med 111,1993, 352-354.

11. Murray MT, The Healing Power of Herbs (2nd edition), Prima Publishing, 1995.

12. Dietary Supplement Information Bureau.www. content.intramedicine.com: Hawthorn

13. Natural Products Encyclopedia. www.consumereslab.com: Hawthorn

14. Healthnotes, Inc. 2001. www.healthnotes.com: Hawthorn

15. Principles and Practice of Phytotherapy. Mills M and Bone K. Churchill Livingstone.2000: 444-445

16. Wagner H et al. Cardioactive Drugs IV. Cardiotonic amines from crataegus oxyacantha. Planta Medica 1982;45:99-101

17. Weihmayr T, Ernst E. Therapeutic effectiveness of crataegus. Forschr Med 1996;114:27-9

18. Tauchert M. Efficacy and safety of crataegus extract WS 1442 in comparison with placebo in patients with chronic stable New York heart Association class-III heart failure. Am Heart J 2002;143(5):910-5

19. Tauchert M, Siegel G, Schulz V. Hawthorn extract as plant medication for the heart; a new evaluation of it therapeutic effectivenss [translated from German]. MMW Munch Med Wochenschr. 1994;136(suppl 1):S3-S5

20. Popping S, Rose H, Ionescu I et al. Effect of a hawthorn extract on contraction and energy turnover of isolated rat cardiomyocytes. Arzneimittelforschung 1995;45:1157-61

21. Joseph G, Zhao Y, Klaus W. Pharmacolgic action profile of crataegus extract in comparison to epinephrine, amirinone, milrinone and digoxin in the isolated perfused guinea pig heart [in German; English abstract]. Arzneimittelforschung 1995;45:1261-5

22. Schulz V, Hansel R, Tyler VE. Rational Phytotherapy: A Physician's Guide to Herbal medicine. 3rd ed. Berlin, Germany, Springer-Verlag 1998:91-4

23. Murray M, Pizzonro J. Encylopedia of Natural Medicine (2nd ed) Prima Publishing 1997:524-35

24. Petkov V. Plants and hypotensive, Antiatheromatous and coronarodilatating action. Am J Chinese Med 1979;7:197-236

25. Wagner H et al. Cardioactive Drugs IV. Cadiotonic amines from crataegus oxyacantha. Planta Medica 1982;45:99-101

26. Uchida S et al. Inhibitory effects of condensed tannins on agiotensin converting enzyme. Jap J Pharmacol 1987;43(2):242-6

27. Taskov M. On the coronary and cardiotonic action of crataemon. Acta Physiol Pharmacol Bulg 1977;3(4):53-7

Carnitine

1. Bermer J. Carnitine-metabolism and function. Physiol Rev 1983;63:1420-80.

2. Bamji MS. Nutritional and health implications of lysine carnitine relationship. Wld Rev Nutr Diet 1984;44:185-211.

3. Engel AG, Angelini C. Carnitine deficiency of human skeletal muscle with associated lipid storage myopathy: A new syndrome. Science 1973;179:899-902.

4. Murray M. Encyclopedia of Nutritional Supplements. Rocklin, CA: Prima Publishing; 1996. ch.34.

5. Bazzato G, Mezzina C, Ciman et al. Myasthenia-like syndrome associated with carnitine in patients on long term dialysis. Lancet 1979;I:1041-2.

6. Paulson DJ, Shug AL. Tissue specific depletion of L-carnitine in rat heart and skeletal muscle by Dcarnitine. Life Sci 1981;28:2931-8.

7. Watanable S, et al. Effects of L- and DL-carnitine on patients with impaired exercise tolerance. Jap Heart J 1995;36:319-31.

8. Bowman B. Acetyl-carnitine and Alzheimer's disease. Nutrition Reviews 1992;50:142-4.

9. Carta A, et al. Acetyl-L-carnitine and Alzheimer's disease. Pharmacological considerations beyond the cholinergic sphere. Ann NY Acad Sci 1993;49:1137-41.

10. Goa KL, Brogden RN. L-carnitine – a preliminary review of its pharmacokinetics, and its therapeutic use in ischemic cardiac disease and primary and secondary carnitine deficiencies in relationship to its role in fatty acid metabolism. Drugs 1987;34:1-24.

11. Silverman Na, Schmitt G, Vishwanath M, et al. Effect of carnitine on myocardial function and metabolism following global ischemia. Ann Thor Surg 1985;40:30-5.

12. Cherchi A, Lai C, Angelino F, Trucco G, Caponnetto S, Mereto PE, et al. Effects of L-carnitine on exercise tolerance in chronic stable angina: a multicenter, double-blind,

randomized, placebo controlled crossover study. Int H Clin Pharm Ther Tox 1985;23:569-72.

13. Orlando G, Rusconi C. Oral L-carnitine in the treatment of chronic cardiac ischemia in elderly patients. Clin Trials 1986;23:338-44.

14. Kamikawa T, Suzuki Y, Kobayashi A, Hayashi H, Masumura Y, Nishihara K, et al. Effects of L-carnitine on exercise tolerance in patients with stable angina pectoris. Jap Heart J 1984:25:587-97.

15. Kosolcharoen P, et al. Improved exercise tolerance after administration of carnitine. Curr Ther Res 1981;30:753-64.

16. Pola P, Savi L, Serricchio M, et al. Use of physiological substance, acetyl-carnitine, in the treatment of angiospastic syndromes. Drugs Exp Clin Res 1984;X:213-7.

17. Lagioia R, Scrutinio D, Mangini SG, et al. Propionyl-L-carnitine: a new compound in the metabolic approach to the treatment of effort angina. Int J Cardiol 1992;34:167-72.

18. Bartels GL, Remme WJ, Pillay M, Schonfeld DH, Kruijssen DA. Effects of L-propionylcarnitine on ischemia-induced myocardial dysfunction in men with angina pectoris. Am J Cardiol 1994;74:125-30.

19. Cacciatore L, Cerio R, Ciarimboli M, Cocozza M, Coto V, D'Alessandro A, et al. The therapeutic effect of L-carnitine in patients with exercise-induced stable angina: a controlled study. Drugs Exp Clin Res 1991;17:225-35.

20. Davini P, Bigalli A, Lamanna F, Boem A. Controlled study on L-carnitine therapeutic efficacy in postinfarction. Drugs Exp Clin Res 1992;18:355-65.

21. Iliceto S, Scrutinio D, Bruzzi P, D'Ambrosio G, Boni L, Di Biase M, et al. Effects of L-carnitine administration on left ventricular remodelling after acute anterior myocardial infarction: the L-Carnitine Ecocardiografia Digitalizzata Infarto Miocardico (CEDIM) trial. J Am Coll Cardiol 1995;26:380-7.

22. Mancini M, Rengo F, Lingetti M, Sorrentino GP, Nolfe G. Controlled study on the therapeutic efficacy of propionyl-L-carnitine in patients with congestive heart failure. Arzneim Forsch 1992;42:1101-4.

23. Pucciarelli G, Mastursi M, Latte S, Sacra C, et al. The clinical and hemodyanamic effects of propionyl-Lcarnitine in the treatment of congestive heart failure. Clin Ther 1992;141:379-84.

24. Brevetti G, Perna S, Sabba C, et al. Comparison between the effect of L-propionylcarnitine, L-carnitine in improving walking capacity in patients with peripheral vascular disease: an acute, intravenous, doubleblind, cross-over study. Eur Heart J 1992;13:251-5.

25. Sabba C, Berardi E, Antonica G, Ferraioli G, Buonamico P, Godi L, et al. Comparison between the effect of L-propionylcarnitine, L-acetylcarnitine and nitroglycerin in chronic peripheral arterial disease: a haemodynamic double blind echo-Doppler study. Eur Heart J 1994;15:1348-52.

26. Brevetti G, Chiariello M, Ferulano G, Policicchio A, Nevola E, Rossini A, et al. Increases in walking distance in patients with peripheral vascular disease treated with L-carnitine: a double-blind, cross-over study. Circulation 1988;77:767-73.

27. Calvani M, Carta A, Caruso G, Bendetti N, Iannuccelli M. Action of acetyl-L-carnitine in neurodegeneration and Alzheimer's disease. Ann NY Acad Sci 1993;663:483-6.

28. Pettegrew JW, Klunk WE, Panchalingam K, Kanfer JN, McClure RJ. Clinical and neurochemical effects of acetyl-L-carnitine in Alzheimer's disease. Neurobiol Agin 1995;16:1-4.

29. Sano M, Bell K, Cote L, Dooneief G, Lawton A, Legler L, et al. Double-blind parallel design pilot study of acetyl levocarnitine in patients with Alzheimer's disease. Arch Neurol 1995;49:1137-41.

30. Spagnoli A, Lucca U, Menasce G, Bandera L, Cizza G, Forloni G, et al. Long-term acetyl-L-carnitine treatment in Alzheimer's disease. Neurology 1991;41:1726-32.

31. Vecchi GP, Chiari G, Cipolli C, et al. Acetyl-L-carnitine treatment of mental impairment in the elderly: evidence from a multicenter study. Arch Gerontol Geriatr 1991;2(Suppl):159S-68S.

32. Savioli G, Neri M. L-acetylcarnitine treatment of mental decline in the elderly. Drugs Exp Clin Res 1994;20:169-76.

33. Cipolli C, Chiari G. Effects of L-acetylcarnitine on mental deterioration in the aged: initial results. Clin Ther 1990;132:479-510.

34. Garzya G, Corallo D, Fiore A, Lecciso G, Tetrelli G, Zotti C. Evaluation of the effects of the Lacetylcarnitine on senile patients suffering from depression. Drugs Exp Clin Res 1990;16(2):101-6.

35. Tempesta E, Casella L, Pirrongelli C, Janiri L, Calvani M, Ancona L. L-acetylcarnitine in depressed elderly subjects. A cross-over study vs. placebo. Drugs Exp Clin Res 1987;8:417-23.

36. Bornman MS, et al. Seminal carnitine, epididymal function and spermatozoal motility. S Afr Med J 1989;75:20,21.

37. Mechini Fabris GF, et al. Free L-carnitine in human semen: its variability in different andologic pathologies. Feril Steril 1984;42:263-7.

38. Costa M, Canale D, Filicori M, D'Lddio S, Lenzi A. L-carnitine in idiopathic asthenozoospermia: a multicenter study. Andrologia 1994;26:155-9.

39. Dragan AM, Vasiliu D, Eremia NM, Georgescu E. Studies concerning some acute biological changes after exogenous administration of 1 g L-carnitine in elite athletes. Physiologie 1987;24:231-4.

40. Dragan GI, Vasiliu A, Georgescu E, Dumas I. Studies concerning acute and chronic effects of L-carnitine on some biological parameters.Physiologie 1987;24:23-8.

41. Dragan DI, Wagner W, Ploesteaunu E. Studies concerning the ergogenic value of protein supply and Lcarnitine in elite junior cyclists. Physiologie 1988;25:129-32.

42. Furitano G, et al. Polygraphic evaluation of effects of carnitine in patients on Adriamycin treatment. Drugs Exp Clin Res 1984;10:107-11.

43. Murray M, editor. Encyclopedia of Nutritional Supplements. Rocklin, CA: Prima Publishing 1996. p. 294-5.

44. Van Wouwe JP. Carnitine deficiency during valporic acid treatment. Int J Vitamin Nutr Res 1995;65(3):211-4.

45. Dalakas MC, Leon-Monzon ME, Bernardini I, Gahl WA. Zidovudine-induced mitochondrial myopathy is associated with muscle carnitine deficiency and lipid storage. Ann Neurol 1994;35(4):482-7.

46. Bertelli A, Ronca F, Ronca G, Palmieri L, Zucchi R. L-carnitine and coenzyme Q10 protective action against ischaemia and reperfusion of working rat heart. Drugs Exp Xlin Res 1992;18:431-6.

47. Daily JW III, Sachan DS. Choline supplementation alters carnitine homeostasis in humans and guinea pigs. J Nutr 1995;125:1938-44.

Taurine

1. Hendler S. The Doctor's Vitamin and Mineral Encyclopedia. Simon and Schuster 1990;224-5

2. Gonzalez-Qevedo A, Obregon F, Santiesteban Freixas R, et al. Amino acids as biochemical markers in epidemic and endemic optic neuropathies.Rev Cubana med Trop 1998;50(Suppl):241-4

3. Thompson GN. Excessive fecal taurine loss predisposes to taurine deficiencyin cystic fibrosis. J Pediatr Gastroenterol Nutr Mar1988;7(2):214-9

4. Smith LJ, Lacaille F, Lepage G, et al. Taurine decreses fecal faty acid and sterol excretion in cystic fibrosis. A randomized double-blind trial. Am j Dis Child Dec1991;145(12):1401-4

5. Dietary Suplement Information Bureau, USA: Taurine (Dietary Supplementation Education Alliance, copyright 2001)

6. Azuma J, et al. Therapeutic Effect of taurine in congestive heart failure: a double-blind crossover trial. Clin Cardiol May 1985;8(5):276-82

7. Azuma J, et al. Therapy of congestive heart failure with orally administered taurine. Clin Ther 1983;5(4):398-408

8. Franconi F et al. Plasma and platelet taurine are reduced in subjects iwith insulin-dependent diabetes mellitus: effects of taurine supplementation. Am J Clin Nutr May1995;61(5):1115-9

9. Hwang DF, Wang LC. Effect of taurine on toxicity of cadmium in rats. Toxicology Oct2001;167(3):173-80

10. Waters E, Wang JH, Redmond HP, et al. Role of taurine in preventing acetaminophen-induced hepatic injury in the rat. Am J Physiol Gastrointest Liver Physiol Jun2001;280(6):G1274-9

11. Wu C, Kennedy DO, Yano Y, et al. Thiols and polyamines in the cytoprotective effect of taurine on carbon tetrachloride-induced heptotoxicity. J Biochem Mol Toxicol 1999;13(2):71-6

12. Drugs.com

13. Barbeau A. Zinc, taurine and epilepsy. Archives of Neurology 1974:30-52

14. Barbeau A, et al. The neuropharmacology of taurine. Life Sciences 1975;17:669-78

15. Takahashi R, Nakane Y. Clinical trial of taurine in epilepsy. In:Barbeau A and Huxtable RJ (eds.), Taurine and Neurological Disorders, New York. Raven Press 1978:p375

16. Desai TK, Maliakkal J, Kinzie JL, et al. Taurine deficiency after intensive chemotherapy and/or radiation. Am J Clin Nutr 1992;55:708-11

Glucosamine Sulfate

1. Bland, J.H., and Cooper, S.M. Osteoarthritis: A review of the cell biology involved and evidence for reversibility. Management rationally related to known genesis and pathophysiology. *Sem Arthr Rheum* 14:106-33, 1984.

2. Murray, Michael, T. Glucosamine sulfate: nature's arthritis cure. Excerpt from *The Chiropractic Journal* – March 1998

3. Williams & Wilkins. *Basic Medical Biochemistry: A Clinical Approach.* 1996: 452-453.

4. Glucosamine Sulfate. *Altern Med Rev* 1999 Jun; 4(3): 193-5 (ISSN: 1089-5159)

5. Vidal, Y., and Plana, R.R., et al. Articular cartilage pharmacology. In vitro studies on glucosamine and non-steroidal anti-inflammatory drugs. *Pharmacol Res Comm* 10, 557-569, 1978.

6. Deal, C.L., Moskowitz, R.W. Nutraceuticals as therapeutic agents in osteoarthritis. The role of glucosamine, chondroitin sulfate, and collagen hydrolysate. *Rheum Dis Clin North Am,* 1000 May; 25 (2): 379-95 (ISSN: 0889-857X)

7. Setnikar, I., et al: Pharmacokinetics of glucosamine in the dog and man. *Arzneim Forsch,* 43: (10) 1109-13, 1993.

8. Setnikar, I, et al: Pharmacokinetics of glucosamine in the dog and man. *Arzneim Forsch,* 36 (4) 729- 35, 1986.

9. Baici, A., et al. Analysis of glycosaminoglycans in human sera after oral administration of chondroitin sulfate. *Rheumatol Int* 12:81-8, 1992.

10. Conte, A., et al. Biochemical and pharmacokinetic aspects of oral treatment with chondroitin sulfate. *Arzneim Forsch* 45:918-25, 1995.

11. Baici, A. and Wagenhauser, F.J.: Bioavailability of oral chondroitin sulfate. *Rheumatology Int.* 13:41- 43, 1993.

12. Peperno, M., Reboul, P., Hellio Le Graverand, M.P., Peschard, J.J., Annefeld, M., Richard, M., Vignon, E. Glucosamine sulfate modulates dysregulated activities of human osteoarthritic chondrocytes in vitro. *Osteoarthritis Cartilage*, 2000 May; 8 (3): 207-12 (ISSN: 1063-4584)

13. Kelly, G.S. The role of glucosamine sulfate and chondroitin sulfates in the treatment of degenerative joint disease. *Altern Med Rev* 1998 Feb.; 3 (1): 27-29 (ISSN: 1089-5159)

14. Gottlieb, Marc S. Conservative Management of Spinal Osteoarthritis with Glucosamine Sulfate and Chiropractic Treatment. *Journal of Manipulative and Physiological Therapeutics*, Volume 20, (6) July/August, 1997.

15. Sullivan, M.S. and Hess, W.C. Cysteine content of fingernails in arthritis. *J Bone Joint Surg* 16: 185-8, 1935.

16. Senturia, B.D., "Results of treatment of chronic arthritis and rheumatoid conditions with colloidal sulphur." *J Bone Joint Surg* 16: 119-25, 1934.

17. Lawrence, R.M. Methylsulfonylmethane (MSM): A double-blind study of its use in Degenerative Arthritis. Int J Anti-Aging Med., 1998; 1, 1:50

18. Challem, J., Sulfur Power. *Natural Way For Better Health* (magazine). 1999 (02/28): 34-35

19. Methylsulfonylmethane (MSM). *Herbal Advisor*. www.herbaladvisor.com, Samtech Research, 2001

20. Noack, W., et al. Glucosamine sulfate in osteoarthritis of the knee. *Osteoarthritis Cartilage* 2: 51-9, 1994.

21. Vaz, A.L. Double-blind clinical evaluation of the relative efficacy of ibuprofen and glucosamine sulfate in the management of osteoarthrosis of the knee in outpatients. *Curr Med Res Opn* 8. 145-9, 1982.

22. Muller-Fassbender, H. et al. Glucosamine sulfate compared to ibuprofen in osteoarthritis of the knee. *Osteoarthritis Cartilage* 2: 61-9, 1994.

23. Rovati, L.C., et al. A large randomized placebo-controlled, double-blind study of glucosamine sulfate vs. piroxicam and vs. their association on the kinetics of the symptomatic effect in knee osteoarthritis. Osteoarthritis Cartilage 2 (suppl 1): 56, 1994.

24. Tapadinhas, M.J., et al. Oral glucosamine sulfate in the management of arthrosis: report on a multicentre open investigation in Portugal. Pharmatherapeutica 3: 157-68, 1982.

25. Qiu, G.X., Gao, S.N., Giacovelli, G., Rovati, L., Setnikar, I. Efficacy and safety of glucosamine sulfate versus ibuprofen in patient with knee osteoarthritis. Arzneimittelforschung. 1998 May; 48 (5): 469-74 (ISSN: 0004-4172)

26. Barclay, T.S., Tsourounis, C., McCart, G.M. Glucosamine. *Ann Pharmacother* 1998 May; 32 (5): 574-9 (ISSN: 1060-0280)

27. Reginster, Y.J., Deroisy, R., Paul, I., et al. Glucosamine sulfate significantly reduces progression of knee OA over 3 years: a large randomized, placebo-controlled, double-blind prospective trial. *ArthritisRheum*. 1999; 42 (suppl).

28. Reginster, J.Y., Deroisy, R., Rovati, L.C., Lee, R.L. , Lejeune, E., Bruyere, O., Giacovelli, G., Henrotin, Y., Dacre, J.E., Gossett, C. Long-term effects of glucosamine sulphate on osteoarthritis progression: a randomized, placebo-controlled clinical trial. *Lancet* 2001, Jan. 27; 357 (9252):251-6 (ISSN: 0140-6736)

29. McCarty, M.F. Glucosamine for Wound Healing. *Medical Hypotheses*, 1996. 47; 273-275.

30. Shankland, W.E. The effects of glucosamine and chondroitin sulfate on osteoarthritis of the TMJ: a preliminary report of 50 patients. *Cranio* 1998 Oct.; 16 (4): 230-5 (ISSN: 0886-9634)

31. McCarty, Mark F. Vascular Heparan Sulfates May limit the Ability of Leukocytes to Penetrate the Endothelial Barrier – Implications for Use of Glucosamine in Inflammatory Disorders.

32. Vlodavsky, I., Fuks, Z., Bar-Ner, M., et al. Lymphoma-cell-mediated degradation of sulfated proteoglycans in the subendothelial extracellular matrix: Relationship to tumor cell metastasis. *Cancer Res* 1983; 43: 2704-2711.

33. Nakajima, M., Irimura, T., Di Ferrante, D., et al. Heapran sulfate degradation: Relation to tumor invasion and metastatic properties of mouse B16 melanoma sublines. *Science* 983; 220: 611-612

34. Ricoveri, W., Cappelletti, R. Heparan sulfate endoglycosidase and metastatic potential in murine fibrosarcoma and melanoma. *Cancer Res* 1986; 45: 3855-3861.

35. Nakajima, M., Irimura, T., Nicolson, G.L. Heparanase and tumor metastasis. *J Cell Biochem* 1988; 36: 157-167.

36. Vlodavsky, I., Eldor, A., Bar-Ner, M., et al. Heparan sulfate degradation in tumor cell invasion and angiogenesis. *Adv Exp Med Biol* 1988; 233: 201-210.

37. Vlodavsky, I., Korner, G., Ishai-Michaeli, R., et al. Extracellular-matrix-resident growth factors and enzymes: Possible involvement in tumor metastasis and angiogenesis. *Cancer Metastasis Rev* 1990; 9: 203-226.

38. Russell, A.L. Glucosamine in osteoarthritis and gastrointestinal disorders: an example of the need for a paradigm shift. *Med Hypotheses* 1998 Oct.; 51 (4): 347-9 (ISSN: 0306-9877)

39. Monauni, T., Zenti, M.G., Cretti, A., et al. Effects of glucosamine infusion on insulin secretion and insulin action in humans. *Diabetes* 2000 Jun;49 (6): 926-35 (ISSN: 0012-1797)

40. McAlindon, T.E., La Valley, M.P., Gulin, J.P., Felson, D.T. Glucosamine and chondroitin for treatment of osteoarthritis: a systematic quality assessment and meta-analysis. *JAMA* 2000 Mar. 15; 283 (11): 1469-75 (ISSN: 0098-7484)

41. McAlindon, T., Glucosamine for osteoarthritis: dawn of a new era? Lancet, 2001; 357, 9252: 247-248.

42. Nutrition News Focus, February 13, 2001.

Chondroitin Sulfate

1. Conte A, Volpi N, Palmieri L, Bahous I, Ronca G. Biochemical and pharmacokinetic aspects of oral treatment with chondroitin sulfate. Arzneum Forsch/Drug Res 1994;45(8):918-25.

2. Setnikar I, Palumbo R, Canali S, Zanolo G. Pharmacokinetics of glucosamine in man. Arzneum Forsch/Drug Res 1993;43,10:1109-13.

3. Murray M. Encyclopedia of Nutritional Supplements. Rocklin, CA: Prima Publishing; 1996.

4. Baici A, Horler D, Moser B, et al. Analysis of glycosaminoglycans in human sera after oral administration of chondroitin sulfate. Rheumatol Int 1992;12:81-8.

5. Vaz AL. Double-blind clinical evaluation of the relative efficacy of ibuprofen and glucosamine sulfate in the management of osteoarthrosis of the knee in out patients. Curr Med Res Opin 1982;8:145-9.

6. Baici A, Wagenhauser FJ. Bioavailability of oral chondroitin sulfate. Rheumatology Int 1993;13:41-3.

7. Pipitone VR. Chondroprotection with chondroitin sulfate. Drugs Exptl Clin Res 1991;18:3-7.

8. Hirondel JL. Double-blind clinical study with oral administration of chondroitin sulfate versus placebo in tibiofemoral gonarthrosis. Litera Rheumatologica 1992;14:77-82.

9. Conrozier T, Vignon E. The effect of chondroitin sulfate treatment in coxarthritis. Litera Rheumatologica 1992;14:69-75.

10. Morreale P, Manopulo R, Galati M, Boccanera L, Saponati G, Bocchi L. Comparison of the anti-inflammatory efficacy of chondroitin sulfate and diclofenac sodium in patients with knee osteoarthritis. J Rheumatol 1996;23:1385-91.

11. Reginster JY, Deroisy R, Rovati LC, Lee RL, Lejeune E, Bruyere O, et al. Long-term effects of glucosamine sulfate on osteoarthritis progression: a randomized, placebo-controlled clinical trial.Lancet 2001;357:251-6.

12. Healthnotes 2000, Healthnotes, Inc (www.healthnotes.com): chondroitin sulfate.

MSM

1. Lovelock, J.E. Atmospheric dimethyl sulphide and the natural sulphur cycle. Nature 237, 453-453, 1972

2. Hucker, H.B., et al. Studies on the absorption, excretion and metabolism of dimethyl sulfoxide (DMSO) in man. J Pharmacol Exp Ther 155(2):309-317, 1967

3. Herschler, R.J. MSM: The Scientific Rationale For Nutritional Sulfur – A summary of writings and conversations with R.J. Herschler

4. Williams, K.I.H., et al. Dimethyl sulfone: isolation from cows' milk. Proc Soc Exp Biol Med 122: 865, 1966

5. Pearson, T.W. Natural occurring levels of dimethyl sulfoxide in selected fruits, vegetables, grains, and beverages. J Agr Food Chem 29: 1089, 1981

6. Williams, K.I.H. Dimethyl sulfone: Isolation from human urine. Arch Biochem Biophys 113: 251-252,1966

7. Herschler, R.J. 1986. MSM: A nutrient for the horse. Equ. Vet. Data 7:268-269

8. Herschler, R. Use of Methylsulfonylmethane to enhance the diet of an animal. 1991, United States Patent 5,071,878

9. Metcalf, J. MSM – A dietary derivative of DMSO. Equine Vet Data 3(5): 174-175, 1983

10. Cronin, J.R. Methylsulfonylmethane. Nutraceutical of the Century. Alternative and Complementary Therapies, December 1999, pp: 386-389

11. Rubin, L.F. Barnett, K.C. Ocular effects of oral and dermal application of dimethyl sulfoxide in animals. Ann NY Acad Sci 141: 333-345, 1967

12. National Academy of Sciences Research Council. Dimethyl sulfoxide as a therapeutic agent: Report of the ad hoc committee on dimethyl sulfoxide.New York: National Academy of Sciences, 1973.

13. Challem, J. Sulfur Power, Natural Way Publications, 1998; 02/28

14. Richmond, V.L. Incorporation of methylsulfonylmethane sulfur into guinea pig serum proteins. Life Sci 1986; 39: 263-8

15. Richmond, V.A. Incorporation of methylsulfonylmethane sulfur into methionine and cysteine of guinea pig serum protein. Am J Clin Nutrition, 43(6): Abs 42

16. Richmond, V.A. Incorporation of methylsulfonylmethane sulfur into guinea pig serum proteins. Life Sciences, 39: 263-268, 1986

17. Hanson, R.R. DVM, DACVS. Will medicine keep your horse sound? 1996, The Horse, April issue, p.38-40

18. Teigland, M.B., Saurino, V.R. Clinical evaluation of dimethyl sulfoxide in equine applications. Ann N.Y. Acad. Sci., 1975; 243: 471-477

19. Jacob, S.W., Lawrence, R.M., Zucker, M. The Miracle of MDM: The Natural Solution for Pain. New York. G.P. Putman's Sons, 1999.
20. Lawrence, R.M. Methylsulfonylmethane (MSM): A double-blind study of its use in Degenerative Arthritis. Int J Anti-Aging Medicine, 1998; 1, 1:50
21. MSM Herbal Advisor, www.herbaladvisor.com, 2001
22. Jacob, S.W., Herschler, R. Introductory Remarks: Dimethyl sulfoxide after twenty years. 1983, Ann NY Acad Sci. 411: xiii-xvii
23. Metcalf, J.W. 1986 MSM status report, Eq. Vet. Data 7: 332-334
24. Deichman, W.B. Gerards, H.W. (eds.) Toxicology of Drugs and Chemicals. (the ed.) New York: Academic Press, 1969
25. Challem, Jack. The Power of MSM: Let's Live (magazine) January, 2001
26. 2000 Healthnotes, Inc.; Sulfur. www.healthnotes.com
27. Moore, R.D., Morton, J.I. Diminished inflammatory joint disease in MRL/1pr mice ingesting dimethyl sulfoxide (DMSO) or dimethylsulfone (MSM). Federation of American Societies for Experimental Biology, 69th Annual Meeting, April 1985, p.692
28. Layman, D. Growth inhibitory effects of dimethyl sulfoxide and dimethyl sulfone on vascular smooth muscle and endothelial cells in vitro. In Vitro Cell Develop Biol 23(6): 422-428, 1987
29. Richmond, V.I. Incorporation of methylsulfonylmethane sulfur into guinea pig serum proteins. Life Sci 39: 263-268, 1986
30. Morton, J.I., Siegel, B.V. Effects of oral dimethyl sulfoxide and dimethyl sulfone on marine autoimmune lymphoproliferative disease. Proc Soc Exp Biol med 183: 227-230, 1986

Clinical Use of Anti-Inflammatory Herbs

1. Gottlieb M S. Conservative management of spinal osteoarthritis with glucosamine sulfate and chiropractic treatments. J. Manipulative Physiol Ther.1997 July-Aug; 20 (6): 400-414 (JPMT)
2. Murray M. The Healing Power of Herbs. Prima Publishing, 1995. Rocklin, CA.
3. Hayliyar J et al. Gastro protection and nonsteroidal anti-inflammatory drugs. Drug Safety, 7, 86; 86- 105, 1992.
4. Ament P W et al. Prophylaxis and treatment of NSAID-induced gastropathy. Am Fam Phys 1997. 1997;4:1323-6.
5. Silverstein F E et al. Gastrointestinal toxicity with celecoxib vs nonsteroidal anti-inflammatory drugs for osteoarthritis and rheumatoid arthritis. JAMA, 284 (10): 1247-1255, 2000.
6. Simon L S. Osteoarthritis: A Review Clinical Cornerstone. 2 (2):26-34, 1999.
7. Dobrilla G et al. The epidemiology of the gastroduodenal damage induced by aspirin and other nonsteroidal anti-inflammatory drugs. Recenti Pog Med 1997, May; 88 (5): 202-11.
8. Boon H and Smith M. Health Care Professional Training Program in Complementary Medicine. Instit. Of Applied Complementary Med., 1997.
9. Borenstein O. Osteoarthritis: Clinical Update. Am College of Rheumatology. 1999 Annual Scientific Meeting. Medscape, 1999.
10. Deadhar 50 et al. Preliminary studies on anti rheumatic activity of curcumin. Ind J Med Res 1980; 71:632-34.
11. Satoskar R R et al. Evaluation of anti-inflammatory property of curcumin in patients with postoperative inflammation. Int J Clin Pharmacal Ther Toxical 1986; 24:651-54.
12. Murray M T. The Healing Power of Herbs. Prima Publishing, Rocklin CA; 1995: 327-35.

13. Arora R B et al. Anti-inflammatory studies on curcuma longa (turmeric). Ind J Med, Res 1971; 50: 1289-95.

14. Heck A. et al. Potential interactions between alternative therapies and warfarin. Am J Health – Syst Phar, 2000; 57, 13: 1221-1227.

15. Schweizer S et al. Workup-dependent formation of 5-lipoxygenase inhibitory boswellic acids analogues. J Nat Prod 2000, Aug; 63 (8): 1058-1061.

16. Etzel R. Special extract of boswellia serrata (H15) in the treatment of rheumatoid arthritis. Phytomed 1996; 3: 91-94.

17. Bradley P R et al. British Herbal Compendium, Vol 1, Bournemouth, Dorset, UK: British Herbal Med Assoc., 1992, 224-26.

18. Mills S Y et al. Effects of a proprietary herbal medicine on the relief of chronic arthritic pain: A double-blind study. Br J Rheum 1996; 35: 874-78.

19. Chrubasik S et al. Treatment of low back pain exacerbations with willow bark extract: a randomized double – blind study. Am J Med 2000 July; 109 (1):9-14.

20. Srivastava K C et al. Ginger in rheumatism and musculoskeletal disorders. Medical Hypotheses 1992; 39:342-8.

21. Bliddal H et al. A randomized placebo – controlled, cross-over study of ginger extracts and ibuprofen in osteoarthritis, osteoarthritis cartilage 2000, Jan; 8 (1): 9-12.

22. Klein G et al. Short-term treatment of painful osteoarthritis of the knee with oral enzymes. Clin Drug Invest 19 (1): 15-23, 2000.

23. Cohen A et al. Bromelain therapy in rheumatoid arthritis. Pennsyl Med J, 67: 627-30, June 1964.

24. Seligman B. Bromelain: An anti-inflammatory agent. Angiology, 13: 508-510, 1962.

25. Ferrandiz J L et al. Anti-inflammatory activity and inhibition of arachidonic acid metabolism by flavonoids. Agents Action; 32: 283-287, 1991.

26. Tarayre J P et al. Advantages of a combination of proteolytic enzymes, flavonoids and ascorbic acid in comparison with nonsteroidal anti-inflammatory agents. Arzneium forsch, 27:1144-1149, 1977.

27. Yoshimoto T et al. Flavonoids and potent inhibitors of arachidonate 5 – lipoxygenase. Biochem Biophys Res Comm., 116: 612-18, 1983.

28. Weiss RF. Herbal Medicine: Beaconsfield; 1988:362

29. Grahame R et al. Devil's Claw: Pharmacological and clinical studies. Ann Rheum Dis, 1 981; 40:632.

Antioxidants and Rheumatoid Arthritis

1. Murray M, Pizzorno J. Encyclopedia of Natural Medicine (2nd edition) 1998;Prima Publishing:770-1

2. Borenstein O. Osteoarthritis clinical update. American College of Rheumatology 1999;Annual Scientific Meeting, Medscape 1999

3. McAdam P. Chicken cartilage assessed in rheumatoid arthritis. Medical Tribune, Nov1993:p8

4. Wittenborg A, et al. Effectiveness of vitamin E in comparison with diclofenac sodium in treatment of patients with chronic polyarthritis. Z Rheumatol, Aug1998;57(4):215-21

5. Edmonds SE, et al. Putative analgesic activity of repeated oral doses of vitamin E in the treatment of rheumatoid arthritis. Results of a prospective placebo controlled double blind trial. Ann Rheum Dis, Nov1997;56(11):649-55

6. Heinle AK. Selenium concentration in erythrocytes of patients with RA. Clinical and laboratory chemistry infection markers during administration of selenium. Med-Klin 1997;92(suppl 3):29-31

7. Situnayake RD. Chain breaking antioxidant status in rheumatoid arthritis: clinical and laboratory correlates. Ann Rheum Dis, Feb1991;50(2):81-6
8. Kose K, et al. Plasma selenium levels in rheumatoid arthritis. Biol Trace Elem Res, 1996;53(1-3):51-6
9. Tarp U, et al. Low selenium level in severe rheumatoid arthritis. Scand J Rheumatol, 1985;14(2):97-101.
10. Corrigan JJ Jr., et al. Effect of vitamin E on prothrombin levels in warfarin-induced vitamin K deficiency. Am J Clin Nutr, Sep1981;34(9):1701-5

Fibromyalgia

1. Intramedicine Inc. 2000-2003. www.content.intramedicine.com
2. Chang L. The association of functional gastrointestinal disorders and fibromyalgia. Eur J Surg Suppl 1998;583:32-6
3. Goldenberg DL. Fibromyalgia and chronic fatigue syndrome: are they the same? J Musculoskel Med 1990;7:19
4. Kaartinen K, Lammi K, Hypen M, et al. Vegan diet alleviates fibromyalgia symptoms. Scand J Rheumatol 2000;29:308–13
5. Gowans SE, deHueck A, Voss S, Richardson M. A randomized, controlled trial of exercise and education for individuals with fibromyalgia. Arthritis Care Res 1999;12:120–8
6. Mannerkorpi K, Nyberg B, Ahlmen M, Ekdahl C. Pool exercise combined with an education program for patients with fibromyalgia syndrome. A prospective, randomized study. J Rheumatol 2000;27:2473–81
7. Fava M, Rosenbaum JF, MacLaughlin R, et al. Neuroendocrine effects of S-adenosyl-L-methionine, a novel putative antidepressant. J Psychiatr Res 1990;24:177–84
8. Bell KM, Potkin SG, Carreon D, Plon L. S-adenosylmethionine blood levels in major depression: changes with drug treatment. Acta Neurol Scand 1994; 154(suppl):15–8
9. Puttini PS, Caruso I. Primary fibromyalgia syndrome and 5-hydroxy-L-tryptophan: a 90-day open study. J Int Med Res 1992;20:182–9
10. Moldofsky H, Warsh JJ. Plasma tryptophan and musculoskeletal pain in non-articular rheumatism ("fibrositis syndrome"). Pain 1978;5:65–71
11. Jacobsen S et al. Oral S-adenosylmethionine in priomary fibromyalgia. Double-blind clinical evaluation. Scand J Rheumatol 1991;20(4):294-302
12. Ravoni A et al. Evaluation of S-adenosylmethionine in primary fibromyalgia. A double-blind crossover study. Am J Med Nov 1987;83(5A):107-10
13. Wikner J et al. Fibromyalgia—a syndrome associated with decreased nocturnal melatonin secretion. Clin Endocrinol (Oxf). Aug 1998;49(2):179-83
14. Citera G, et al. The effect of melatonin in patients with fibromyalgia: a pilot study. Clin Rheumatol 2000;19(1):9-13
15. Russell IJ et al. Treatment of fibromyalgia syndrome with Super Malic: a randomized, double blind, placebo controlled, crossover pilot study. J Rheumatol May 1995;22(5):953-8
16. Abraham GE, Flechas JD. Management of fibromyalgia: Rationale for the use of magenesium and malic acid. J Nutr Med 1992;3:49-59
17. Eisinger J, Zakarian H, Plantamura A, et al. Studies of transketolase in chronic pain. J Adv Med 1992;5:105–13
18. Eisinger J, Bagneres D, Arroyo P, et al. Effects of magnesium, high energy phosphates, piracetam, and thiamin on erythrocyte transketolase. Magnesium Res 1994;7(1):59–61
19. Wolfe F. The clinical syndrome of fibrositis. Am J Med 1986;81(Supp 3A):7–14
20. Blunt KL, Moez HR, Rajwani MH, Guerriero RC. The effectiveness of chiropractic management of fibromyalgia patients: a pilot study. J Manipulative Physiol Ther 1997;20:389–99

21. Hains G, Hains F. Combined ischemic compression and spinal manipulation in the treatment of fibromyalgia; a preliminary estimate of dose and efficacy. J Manipulative Physiol Ther 2000;23:225–30

22. Waylonis GW. Long-term follow-up on patients with fibrositis treated with acupuncture. Ohio State Med J 1977;73:299–302

23. Deluze C, Bosia L, Zirbs A, et al. Electroacupuncture in fibromyalgia: results of a controlled trial. BMJ 1992;305(6864):1249–52

24. Berman BM, Ezzo J, Hadhazy V, Swyers JP. Is acupuncture effective in the treatment of fibromyalgia? J Fam Pract 1999;48:213–8

Premenstrual Syndrome

Mackay, H.T. and Evans, A.T. Gynecology and Obstetrics. *In Current Medical Diagnosis and Treatment* (Eds. Tierney, Jr., L.M., et al.) 33rd Annual Revision. 1994; Appleton and Large: 589-590

Murray, M. and Pizzorno, J. *Encyclopedia of Natural Medicine*. (2nd edition). Prima Publishing, 1998; 730-752 Barnhart, K.T., et al. *A Clinician's Guide to the Premenstrual Syndrome*. Med Clin North Am, 79. 1995; 1457-1472

Facchinetti, F., et al. *Oestradiol/Progesterone imbalance and the premenstrual syndrome.* Lancet, 1985; 2:1302

Munday, M.R., et al. *Correlations between progesterone, oestradiol and aldosterone levels in the premenstrual syndrome.* Clin Endocrinol. 1981; 14: 1-9

Chuong, C.J., et al. *Periovulatory beta-endorphin levels in premenstrual syndrome.* Obstet Gynecol. 1995; 83:755-760

Wynn, V., et al. *Tryptophan, depression and steroidal contraception.* J Steroid Biochem. 1975; 6: 965-970

Bermond, P. *Therapy of side effects of oral contraceptive agents with Vitamin B6.* Acta Vitaminol-Enzymol. 1982; 4: 45-54

Berman, M.K., et al. *Vitamin B6 in premenstrual syndrome.* J Am Diet Assoc. 1990; 90: 859-861

Kliejnen, J., et al. *Vitamin B6 in the treatment of premenstrual syndrome – A Review.* Br J Obstet Gynaecol 1990; 97: 847-852

Halbreich, U., et al. *Serum-prolactin in women with premenstrual syndrome.* Lancet, 1976; 2: 654-656

O-Brien, P.M., et al. *Prolactin levels in the premenstrual syndrome.* Br J Obstet Gyn. 1982; 89: 306-308

Gorbach, S.L., et al. *Diet and the excretion and enterohepatic cycling of estrogens.* Prev Med, 1987; 16: 525-531

Goldin, B.R., et al. *Estrogen patterns and plasma levels in vegetarian and omnivorous women.* New Engl J Med, 1982; 307: 1542-1547

Longcape, C., et al. *The effect of a low fat diet on oestrogen metabolism.* J Clin Endocrinal Metab., 1987; 64:1246-1250

Woods, M.N., et al. *Low-fat, high fiber diet and serum estrone sulfate in premenopausal women.* Am J Clin Nutr, 1989; 49: 1179-1183

Jones, D.Y. *Influence of dietary fat on self-reported menstrual symptoms.* Physical Behav., 1987; 40: 483-487

Aganoff, J.A., et al. *Aerobic exercise, mood states and menstrual cycle symptoms.* J Psychosom Res, 1994; 38:183-192

Choi, P.Y., et al. *Symptom changes across the menstrual cycle in competitive sportswomen, exercisers, and sedentary women.* Br J Clin Psychol, 1995; 34: 447-460

Steege, J.F., et al. *The effects of aerobic exercise on premenstrual symptoms in middle-aged women: a preliminary study.* J Psychosom Res., 1993; 37, 2: 127-133

Limon, L. *Use of alternative medicine in women's health.* Am Pharmaceutical Assoc Annual Meeting. APHA 2000: 1-5

Schildge, E. *Essay on the treatment of premenstrual and menopausal mood swings and depressive states.* Rigelh Biol Umsch, 1964; 19, 2: 18-22

Heck, A., et al. *Potential Interactions between Alternative Therapies and Warfarin.* Am J Health – Syst Pharm. 2000; 57; 13: 1221-1227

McNeil, J.R. *Interactions between herbal and conventional medicines.* Can J CME, 1999; 11,12: 97-110

Dittmar, R.W., et al. *Premenstrual syndrome, treatment with a phytopharmaceutical.* Therapiewache Gynakol,1995; 5: 60-68

Pteres-Welte, C., et al. *Menstrual abnormalities and PMS: Vitex Agnus-castus.* Therapiewache Gynakeol, 1994; 7: 49-52

Albertzazzi, P., et al. *The effect of dietary soy supplementation on hot flashes.* Obstet Gynecol., 1998; 91: 6-11

Cassidy, A., et al. *Biological effects of a diet of soy protein rich in isoflavones on the menstrual cycle of premenopausal women.* Am J Clin Nutr, 1994;60: 333-340

Patter, S.M., et al. *Soy protein and isoflavones: their effects on blood lipids and bone density inpostmenopausal women.* Am J Clin Nutr. 1998; 68 (suppl):137-139

Dalais, F.S., et al. *Dietary soy supplementation increases vaginal cytology maturation index and bone mineralcontent in postmenopausal women.* Am J Clin Nutr. 1998; 68 (suppl): 1519 (abstract)

London, R.S., et al. *Effect of a nutritional supplement on premenstrual syndrome in women with PMS: a doubleblind longitudinal study.* J Am Cell Nutr.1991; 10: 494-499

Stewart, A. *Clinical and biochemical effects of nutritional supplementation on the premenstrual syndrome.* J Reprod Med., 1987; 32: 435-441

Abraham, G.E. *Nutritional factors in the etiology of the premenstrual tension syndrome.* J Reprod Med., 1983; 28: 446-464

London, R.S., et al. *The effects of Alpha-Tocopherol on premenstrual symptomatology: A double-blind study.* II. Endocrine Correlates. J Am Col Nutr. 1984; 3: 351-356

Kaugars, G.E., et al. *Use of antioxidant supplements in the treatment of human oral leukoplakia.* Oral Surg Med Oral Pathol. 1996; 81: 5-14

Sigounas, G., et al. *DL-alpha-tocopherol induces apoptosis in erythroleukemia, prostate and breast cancer cells.* Nutr. Cancer, 1997; 28, 1: 30-35

Knecht, P. Role of Vitamin E in the prophylaxis of cancer. Ann Med., 1991; 23: 3-12London, R.S., et al.

Endocrine parameters and alpha-tocopherol therapy of patients with mammary dysplasia. Cancer Res., 1981; 41: 3811-3813

Menopause

1. Kaunitz, Andrew M., M.D. Use of Combination Hormone Replacement Therapy in Light of Recent Data From the Women's Health Initiative. Medscape Women's Health eJournal, Jul 12, 2002

2. Barclay, Laurie, M.D. Estrogen Therapy, but Not Estrogen-Progestin, Linked to Ovarian Cancer. JAMA 2002; 288:334-341, 368-369

3. British Scientists Say HRT Trial Should Continue. Reuters Health Information 2002

4. Colgan, M. Hormonal health. Apple Publishing, Canada, 1996

5. Castelli, W.P., Griffin, G.C. How to help Patients Cut Down on Saturated Fat. Postgraduate Medicine 1988; 84(3): 44-56

6. Masley, S.C. Dietary methods to Reduce LDL Levels. American Family Physician 1998; 57(6): 1299- 1306

7. Pate, R.R., et al. Physical Activity and Public Health. JAMA 1995; 273(5): 402-407

8. Kannel, W.B., et al. Effect of Weight on Cardiovascular Disease. American Journal of clinical Nutrition 1996; 63(suppl): 419S-22S

9. Patter, S M et al: Soy protein and isoflavones: their effects on blood lipids and bone density in postmenopausal women. Am J Clin Nutr 1998:68 (suppl) 137-9

10. Yoshino, G et al: Effects of gamma-oryzanol on hyperlipidemic subjects. Curr Ther Res (45), 543-552, 1989

11. Yoshino, G et al: Effects of gamma-oryzanol and probucol on hyperlipidemia. Curr Ther Res (45), 975-982, 1989

12. Murase, Y et al: Clinical studies of oral administration of gamma-oryzanol on climacteric complaints and its syndrome. Obstet Gynecol Prac (12) 147-149,1963

13. Anderson J W et al: Meta-analysis of the effects of soy protein intake on serum lipids. N Engl J Med 1995; 333:276-82

14. Messina, M: Legumes and Soybeans: overview of their nutritional profiles and health effects. Am J Clin Nutr 1999 Vol 70 (suppl); 439-50

15. Ishihara, M: Effect of gamma-oryzanol on serum lipid peroxide levels and climacteric disturbances. Asia Oceania J Obstet Gynecol (10), 317, 1984

16. Optimal Calcium Intake. JAMA 1994; 272(24)

17. Calcium supplementation and bone loss: a review of controlled clinical trials. American Journal of clinical Nutrition 1991; 54: 274S-280S

18. Osteoporosis Society of Canada. Clinical practice guidelines for the diagnosis and management of osteoporosis. CMAJ 1996

19. Supplementation with Vitamin D3 and Calcium Prevents Hip Fractures in Elderly Women. Nutrition Reviews 51(6)

20. Rates of bone loss in postmenopausal women randomly assigned to one of two dosages of vitamin D. American journal of Clinical Nutrition 1995; 61: 1140-1145

21. Effects of High-Intensity Strength Training on Multiple Risk Factors for osteoporotic Fractures. JAMA 1994; 272(24)

22. Stolze, H: An alternative to treat menopausal complaints. Gyne 3:1416,1982

23. Albertzazzi, P et al: The effect of dietary soy supplementation on hot flashes. Obstet Gynecol (91), 6- 11,1998

24. Toniolo, et al. A Prospective Study of Endogenous Estrogens and Breast Cancer in Postmenopausal Women. JNCI 1995; 87(3): 190-199

25. Lew, E.A., et al. The American Cancer Society Study; Variations in mortality by weight among 750,000 men and women. J Chronic Dis 1979; 32: 563-76

26. Tannenbaum, A. The relationship of body weight to cancer incidence Arch Pathol 1940; 30: 509

27. Dixon-Shanies, D., Shaikh, N. Growth inhibition of human breast cancer cells by herbs and phytoestrogens. Oncol Rep., 1999; 6(6): 1383-7

28. Murray, M: Remifemin: Answers to some common questions. AM J Natural Med. Vol.4 (3), April 1997

29. Many U.S. Breast Cancer Survivors Use Alternatives to HRT. J Pain Symptom Manage 2002; 23: 501-509

30. Warnecke, G: Influencing menopausal symptoms with a phytotherapeutic agent. Med Welt. 36:871- 4,1985

31. Stoll, W: Phytopharmacon influences atrophic vaginal epithelium. Double-blind study — Cimicifuga vs. estrogenic substances. Therapeuticum 1:23-31,1987

32. Gorlich,N: Treatment of ovarian disorders in general practice. Arztl Prax. 14:1742-3,1962

33. Limon, L. Use of alternative medicine in women's health. Am Pharmaceutical Assoc Annual Meeting. A Ph A, 2000. Pharmacists Conference Summaries 2000. Medscape, Inc.
34. Murkies,A L et al: Dietary flour supplementation decreases post-menopausal hot flashes: effect of soy and wheat. Maturitas (21), 189-195,1995
35. Isoflavones and Menopause. Medical Post Oct. 3, 2000
36. Cassidy, A et al: Biological effects of a diet of soy protein rich in isoflavones on the menstrual cycle of pre-menopausal women. Am J Clin Nutr (60), 333-340,1994
37. Colditz,G A: Relationship between estrogen levels, use of hormone replacement therapy and breast cancer. J Natl Cancer Inst 1998;90;11:814-823
38. John Hopkins Medical Newsletter: Health After 50,Vol 11,Issue 9 (6-7 Nov,1999)
39. Cancer and Nutrition. Simone, B. Avery Publishing Group Inc., 1992:219-23

Soy Phytoestrogens, Prevention of Breast Cancer

1. Setchell KDR, Borriello SP, Hulme P, Axelson M. Nonsteroidal estrogens of dietary origin: possible roles in hormone-dependent disease. Am J Clin Nutr 1984; 40:569-78.
2. Setchell KDR, Lawson AM, Borriello SO et al. Lignan formation in man – microbial involvement and possible roles in relation to cancer. Lancet 1981; 2: 4-8.
3. Adlercreutz H. Does fiber-rich food containing animal lignan precursors protect against both colon and breast cancer? An extension of "fiber hypothesis". Gastroenterology 1984; 86:761-6.
4. Adlercreutz H. Western diet and Western diseases: some hormonal and biochemical mechanisms and associations. Scand J Clin Lab Invest Suppl 1990; 201:3-21.
5. Setchell KDR, Adlercreutz H. Mammalian lignans and phytoestrogens: recent studies on their formation, metabolism and biological role in health and disease. In: Rowland IA, ed. The role of gut microflora in toxicity and cancer. New York: Academic Press, 1988: 315-45.
6. Lee HP, Gourley L, Duffy SW, Esteve J, Lee J, Day NE. Dietary effects on breast cancer risk in Singapore. Lancet 1991; 337:1197-200.
7. Barnes S, Grubbs C, Setchell KDR, Carlson J. Soybeans inhibit mammary tumor growth in models of breast cancer. In: Pariza MW, ed. Mutagens and carcinogens in the diet. New York: Wiley-Liss, 1990: 239-53.
8. Muir C, Waterhouse J, Mack T, Powell J, Whelan S. Cancer incidence in five continents. Vol. 5 Lyon, France: International Agency for Research on Cancer, 1987. (IARC Scientific publication no. 88).
9. Willet W. J Natl Can Inst, Vol. 88, no. 14, July 17, 1996, p.948.
10. Cancer prevention and nutritional therapies. Passwater R Keats Pub. Inc., 1983.
11. Colditz GA. Relationship between estrogen levels , use of hormone replacement therapy, and breast cancer. J Natl Can Inst, 1998; 90:11; 814-823.
12. Coward L, Barnes NC, Setchell KDR, Barnes S. The isoflavones genistein and daidzein in soy bean foods from American and Asian diets. J Agric Food Chem 1993; 41: 1961-7.
13. Adlercreutz H, Honjo A, Higashi A et al. Lignan and phytoestrogen excretion in Japanese consuming traditional diet. Scand J Clin Invest, 1988; 48:190 (abstr.).
14. Cassidy A et al. Biological effects of a diet of soy protein rich in isoflavones on the menstrual cycle of premenopausal women. Am J Clin Nutr 1994; 60:333-40.

Black Cohosh

1. Messina M. Legumes and soybeans: an overview of their nutritional profiles and health effects. Am J Clin Nutr 1999;70(suppl):439-450

2. Messina M. To recommend or not to recommend soy foods. J Am Diet Assoc. 1994;94(11):1253- 1254

3. Mills S and Bone K. Principles and Practice of Phytotherapy. Churchill Livingstone, Publisher (2000):54-6;67-8

4. Reichert RG. Phyto-Estrogens. Quarterly Review of Natural Medicine, Mar31 1994:27-33

5. Mahady GB, Fabricant D, Chadwick LR, Dietz B. Black cohosh: an alternative therapy for menopause? Nutrition in clinical care: an official publication of Tufts University 2002 Nov-Dec;5(6):283-9

6. Alternatives to Estrogen. Spectrum: The Wholistic News Magazine, Sept/Oct98;(62):19

7. Murray M and Pizzorno J. Encyclopedia of Natural Medicine (revised 2nd edition). Prima Health 1998:639-41

8. Colditz GA. Relationship between estrogen levels, use of hormone replacement therapy and breast cancer. J Natl Cancer Inst 1998;90(11):814-823

9. Kaunitz Andrew M, M.D. Use of combination hormone replacement therapy in light of recent data from the Women's Health Initiative. Medscape Women's Health eJournal, Jul12 2002.

10. Boon and Smith. Health Care Professional training program in complementary medicine:39-43

11. Bodinet C, Freudenstein J. Influence of Cimicifuga racemosa on the proliferation of estrogen receptopositive human breast cancer cells. Brest Cancer Res Treat 2002 Nov;76(1):1-10

12. McKenna, Dennis J.; Jones, Kenneth; Humphrey, Sheila; Hughes, Kerry. Black cohosh: Efficacy, Safety, and Use in Clinical and PreClinical Applications. *Alternative Therapies in Health & Medicine*; May 5, 2001; V.7, N.3: pp 93-100

13. Dixon-Shanies, D., Shaikh, N. Growth inhibition of human breast cancer cells by herbs and phytoestrogens. *Oncol Rep*, 1999 Nov-Dec; vol. 6 (6), pp. 1383-7

14. Burdette JE, Chen SN, Lu ZZ, Xu H, White BE, Fabricant DS, Liu J, Fong HH, Farnsworth NR, Constantinou AI, Van Breemen RB, Pezzuto JM, Bolton JL. Black cohosh (Cimicifuga racemosa L.) protects against menadione-induced DNA damage through scavenging of reactive oxygen species:bioassay-directed isolation and characterization of active principles. J Agric Food Chem 2002 Nov20;50(24):7022-8

15. Proc Amer Assoc Cancer Res. 44:Abst. No.2721, R910, 2003

16. Limon L. Use of alternative medicine in women's health. Am Pharmaceutical Assoc Annual Meeting. A Ph A, 2000. Pharmacists Conference Summaries 2000. Medscape, Inc.

17. Sanderoff, BT. Herbal Medicine: Use with Caution and Respect. Generations, Winter 2000/2001;24(4):p69

Ovarian Cancer

1. Huncharek M et al, Dietary fat intake and risk of epithelial ovarian cancer: A meta-analysis of 6,689 subjects from 8 observational studies. Nutrition and Cancer. 2001; 40, 2: 87-91.

2. Fleischauer A et al, Dietary antioxidants, supplements, and risk of epithelial ovarian cancer. Nutrition and Cancer. 2001; 40, 2: 92-98.

3. Carr AC and Frei B, Toward a new recommended dietary allowance for vitamin C based on antioxidant and health effects in humans. Am J Clin Nutr.1999; 69: 1086-1107.

Guarding Against Prostate Enlargement and Cancer

Berges RR, et al. Treatment of sympotomatic benign prostaic hyperplasia with beta-sitosterol: an 18 month follow-up. Br J Urol 2000 May;85(7):842-46

Boccafoschi and Annosica, S. Comparison of Serenoa repens extract with placebo by controlled clinical trial in patients with prostatic adenomatosis. Urologia 1983;50:1257-1268

Bogen KT, Keating GA. U.S. dietary exposures to heterocyclic amines. J Expo Anal Environ Epidemiol 2001 May-Jun;11(3):155-68

Braeckman J. The extract of Serenoa repens in the treatment of benign prostatic hyperplasia: A multi-center open study. Curr Ther Res 1984;55:776-785

Brawley OW, Ford LG, Thompson I, Perlman JA, Kramer BS. 5-Alpha-reductase inhibition and prostate cancer prevention. Cancer Epidemiol Biomarkers Prev 1994 Mar;3(2):177-82

Buck A. Phyto therapy for the Prostate. Br J Urol 1996;78: 325-336

Can men avoid prostate cancer? A brief review of diet and the prostate. Nutrition Health Review: The Consumer's Medical Journal 1995;72:3

Chinni SR, Li Y, Upadhyay S, Koppolu PK, Sarkar FH. Indole-3-carbinol (I3C) induced cell growth inhibition, G1 cell cycle arrest and apoptosis in prostate cancer cells. Oncogene 2001 May 24;20(23):2927-36

Clark LC, et al. Effects of selenium supplementation for cancer prevention in patients with carcinoma of the skin. A randomized-controlled trial. Nutritional Prevention of Cancer Study Group JAMA 1996;276(24):1957-1963

Coffey DS. Similarities of prostate and breast cancer: Evolution, diet and estrogens. Urology 2001 Apr;57(4

Supp I1):31-8

Di Silverio E, et al. Evidence that Serenoa repens extract displays antiestrogenic activity in prostatic tissue of benign prostatic hypertrophy. Eur Urol 21 1992; 309-314

Dreikorn K, et al Status of phyto therapeutic drugs in the treatment of benign prostatic hyperplasia [German] Urologe A. 1995;34(2):119-29

Dufour B, Choquenet C. Trial controlling the effects of Pygeum africanum extract on the functional symptoms of prostatic adenoma. Ann Urol 1984;18:193-195

Evans BAJ, et al. Inhibition of 5-alpha-reductase in genital skin fibroblasts and prostate tissue by dietary lignans and isoflavonoids. J. Endocrinology 1995; 147:295-30.

Fahim MS, et al. Zinc arginine, a 5 alph-reductase inhibitor, reduces rat ventral prostate weight and DNA without affecting testicular function. Andrologia 1993 Nov;25(6):369-375

Fitzpatrick AL, Daling JR, Furberg CD, Kronmal RA, Weissfeld JL. Hypertension, heart rate, use of antihypertensives, and ancident prostate cancer. Ann Epidemiol 2001 Nov;11(8):534-42

Gann PH, et al. Lower prostate cancer risk in men with elevated lycopene levels: results of a prospective analysis. Cancer Res 1999;59(6): 1225-1230

Giovanncci, et al. Intake of carotenoids and retinol in relation to risk of prostate cancer. J Natl Cancer Inst 1995; 87(23):1767-76

Giovannuci E. Dietary influences of 1,25(OH)2 vitamin D in relation to prostate cancer: a hypothesis. Cancer Causes Control 1998;9:567-82

Gross C, Stamey T, Hancock S, Feldman D. Treatment of early recurrent prostate cancer with 1,25- dihydroxyvitamin D3 (calcitriol). J Urol 1998; 159:2035-40

Hartmann R, et al. Inhibition of 5 alpha reductase and aromatase by PHL-00801, a combination of pygeum africanum and urtica dioica extracts. Phytomedicine, 1996;3(2):121-128

Heinonen OP, et al. Prostate cancer and supplementation with Alpha-Tocopheral and Beta-Carotene: Incidence and mortality in a controlled trial. J Natl Cancer Inst 1998;90(6):440-446

Hennenfront B, et al. American Prostate Society Quarterly1995;3:9

Kyle E, et al. Genistein-induced apoptosis of prostate cancer cells is preceded by a specific decrease in focal adhesion kinase activity. Mol Pharmacol 1997; 51:193-200

Leake A, et al. The effect of zinc on the 5 alpha-reduction of testosterone by the hyperplastic human prostate gland. J Steroid Biochem 1984 Feb; 2092:651-655

Leitzmann MF, Stampfer MJ, Wu K, Colditz GA, Willett WC, Giovannucci EL. Zinc supplement use and risk of prostate cancer. J Natl Cancer Inst 2003 Jul;95(13):1004-7

Linehan WM. Inhibition of prostate cancer metastasis: A critical challenge ahead. J Natl Cancer Inst 1995;87(5):331-332

Lipsett MB. Estrogen use and cancer risk. JAMA 1977 Mar 14;237(11);pp111:5

Lu L, et al. Effects of one-month soya consumption on circulating steroids in men: Pro. Am. Assoc. Cancer Research 1996;37:220 (abstr.)

Mattei FM, Capone M, Acconcia A. Serenoa repens extract in the medical treatment of benign prostatic hypertrophy. Urologia 1988;55:547-552

McCaleb R. Synergistic action of pygeum and nettle root extracts in prostate disease. Herbalgram 1996;40:18 Menchini-Fabris GF, et al. New perspectives of treatment of prostato-vesicular pathologies with Pygeum africanum. Arch Int Urol 1988;60:313-322

Messina M. Legumes and soybeans: an overview of their nutritional profiles and health effects. AM J Clin Nutr.1999;70(Suppl):439-50

Mitchell J, et al. Effects of phytoestrogens on growth and DNA integrity in human prostate tumor cell lines: PC-3 and LNCaP. Nutr and Cancer 2000;38(2): 223-228

Morrison HI, MacNeill IB, Miller D, Levy I, Xie L, Mao Y. The impending Canadian prostate cancer epidemic. Can J Public Health 1995 Jul-Aug;86(4)274-8

Murray M. The Healing Power of herbs (2nd edit.). Prima Publishing 1995:306-313

Naik HR, et al. An in vitro and in vivo study of anti-tumor effects of genistein on hormone refractory prostate cancer. Anticancer Res. 1994;14:2617-20

Olson KB, et al. Vitamins A and E: Further clues for prostate cancer prevention. J Natl Cancer Inst 1998;90(6):414-415

Osborn JL, Schwartz GG, Smith DC, et al. Phase II trial of oral 1,25-dihydroxyvitamin D (calcitriol) in hormone refractory prostate cancer. Urol Oncol 1995;1:195-8

Pansadoro V, Benincasa, A. Prostatic hypertrophy: Results obtained with Pygeum africanum extract. Minerva Med 1972;11:119-144

Pavon Maganto E. Zinc in prostatic physiopathology. Role of zinc in the physiology and biochemistry of the prostatic gland. Arch Esp Urol 1979 Mar; 32(2):143-52

Peterson G, et al. Genistein and biochanin A. Inhibit the growth of human prostate cancer cells but not epidermal growth factor receptor auto phosphorylation. Prostate 1993;22:335-45

Pollard M, et al. Influence of isoflavones in soy protein isolates on development of induced prostate-related cancers in L-W rats. Nutr and Cancer 1997;28(1):41-45

Pollard M, et al. Prevention and treatment of experimental prostate cancer in Lobund-Wister rats: Effects of estradiol, dihydrotestosterone and castration. Prostate 1989;15: 95-103

Prostate Cancer Research Foundation of Canada. www.prostatecancer.on.ca

Rao VA, et al. Serum and Tissue Lycopene and Biomarkers of Oxidation in Prostate Cancer Patients: A Case- Control Study. Nutrition and Cancer 1999; 33(2):159-164

Sarma AV, Schottenfeld D. Prostate cancer incidence, mortality, and survival trends in the United States: 1981- 2001. Semin Urol Oncol Feb 2002;20(1):3-9

Schweikert HU, Tunn UW, Habenicht UF, Arnold J, Senge T, Schulze H, Schröder FH, Blom JH, Ennemoser O, Horniger W, et al. Effects of estrogen deprivation on human benign prostatic hyperplasia. J Steroid Biochem Mol Biol 1993 Mar;44(4-6):573-6

Sesso HD, Paffenbarger RS Jr, Lee IM. Alcohol consumption and risk of prostate cancer: The Harvard Alumni Health Study. Int J Epidemiol 2001 Aug 30;(4):749-55

Shimizu H, et al. Cancers of the breast and prostate among Japanese and white immigrants in Los Angeles County. Br J Cancer 1991; 63:963-966

Small EJ, et al. Prospective trial of the herbal supplement PC-SPES in patients with progressive prostate cancer. J Clinical Oncology, 2000;18(21):3595-3603

Studzinski GP, Moore DC. Sunlight-can it prevent as well as cause cancer? Cancer Res 1995; 55:4014-22(review)

Sultan C, et al. Inhibition of androgen metabolism and binding by a liposterolic extract of Serenoa repens B in human foreskin fibroblasts. J Steroid Biochem 1984;20:515-519

Thompson JM, et al. Chemoprevention of prostate cancer. Semin Urol 1995;13:122-9

Willet W. Estimates of cancer deaths avoidable by dietary change. J Natl Cancer Instit 1996;86(14):p948

Wilt TJ, et al. Beta-sitosterol for the treatment of benign prostatic hyperplasia: a systematic review. Br J Urol 1999 Jun;83(a):976-83

Wilt TJ, Ishani A, Stark G, MacDonald R, Lau J, Mulrow, C. Saw Palmetto extracts for treatment of benign prostatic hyperplasia: a systemic review. JAMA 1998 Nov 11;280(18):1604-9

Lycopene

Giovannucci E et al, A Prospective Study of Tomato Products, Lycopene, and Prostate Cancer Risk. 2002. J Natl.Cancer Instit ; 94, 5 : 391-398

Vitamin D, Osteoporosis and Cancer

Brodie MJ, et al. Rifampicin and vitamin D metabolism. Clin Pharmacol Ther 1980;27(6):810-4

Chapuy MC, et al. Effect of Calcium and chole-calciferol treatment for three years on hip fractures in elderly women. Br Med J 1994;308:1081-2

Chen TC, Holick MF. Vitamin D and prostate cancer prevention and treatment. TEM 2003 Nov;14(9):423-30

Chesney RW, et al. Decreased serum 24,25-dihydroxyvitamin D_3 in children receiving glucocorticoids. Lancet 1978;2(8100):1123-5

Crowle AJ, et al. Inhibition by 1,25 dihydroxy vitamin D3, of the multiplication of virulent tubercle bacilli in cultured human macrophages. Infect Immun, 1987;55:2945-50

Dawson-Hughes B, et al. Effect of calcium and Vitamin D supplementation on bone density in men and women 65 years of age or older. N Engl J Med 1997;337:670-6

Dawson-Hughes B, et al. Rates of bone loss in postmenopausal women randomly assigned to one of two dosages of the Vitamin D. Am J Clin Nutr 1995;61:1140-5

Dawson-Hughes B. Calcium and Vitamin D requirements of elderly women. J Nutr 1996;126(Suppl4):1165S-7S

DeLuca HF. The Vitamin D story: A collaborative effort of basic science and clinical medicine. FASEB J 1988;2:224-36

Diarrhea and constipation. In: Berkow R, Fletcher AJ, Beers MH, et al, editors. The Merck Manual of Diagnosis and Therapy. 16th ed. Rahway, NJ: Merck Research Laboratories; 1992

Feldman D, et al. Vitamin D and prostate cancer. Adv Exp Med Biol 1995; 375:53-63

Fukazawa T, et al. Association of Vitamin D receptor gene polymorphism with multiple sclerosis in Japanese. J Neurol Sci 1999;166(1):47-52

Gahn PH, et al. Circulating Vitamin D metabolites in relation to subsequent development of prostate cancer. Epidemiol Biomarkers Prev 1995;5(2):121-6

Garland CF, et al. Can colon cancer incidence and death rates be reduced with Calcium and Vitamin D? Am J Clin Nutr 1991;54(Suppl 1):193S-201S

Garland CF, Garland FC, Gorham ED. Calcuim and vitamin D. Their potential roles in colon and breast cancer prevention. Ann NY Acad Sci 1999; 889:107-19

Garland FC, et al. Geographic variation in breast cancer mortality in the United States: a hypothesis involving exposure to solar radiation. Prev Med 1970;19:614-22.

Hayes C, et al. Vitamin D and multiple sclerosis. Proc Soc Exper Biol Med 1997;216:21-7

Healthnotes, 2000 Inc. Available from: URL: http://www.healthnotes.com.

Holick M. Too little vitamin D in premenopausal women: why should we care? Am J Clin Nutr. 2002; 76: 3-4.

In the news...Vitamin D and colon cancer. Harvard Women's Health Watch 2004 Feb;Vol.11(6)p7

James WP, Avenell A, Broom J, et al. A one-year trial to assess the value of Orlistat in the management of obesity. Int J Obes Relat Metab Disord 1997;21(Suppl3):24S-30S

Kállay E, Adlercreutz H, Farhan H, Lechner D, Bajna E, Gerdenitsch W, Campbell M, Cross HS. Phytoestrogens regulate vitamin D metabolism in the mouse colon: relevance for colon tumor prevention and therapy. J Nutr 1001 Nov;132(11):3490S-3493S

Knodel LC, et al. Adverse effects of hypolipidaemic drugs. Med Toxicol 1987;2(1):10-32

Lore F, et al. Vitamin D metabolites in postmenopausal osteoporosis. Horm Metab Res 1984;16:161-6

Martinez ME, et al. Calcium, Vitamin D and the occurrence of colorectal cancer among women. J Natl Cancer Instit 1996;88(19):1375-82

Mehta RG, et al. Prevention of preneoplastic mammary lesion development by a novel Vitamin D analogue, 1- alpha-hydroxyvitamin D5. J Natl Cancer Instit 1997; 89(3):212-8.

Munger KL et al. Vitamin D intake an incidence of multiple sclerosis. Neurology 2004: 62: 60-65.

Odes HS, et al. Effect of cimetidine on hepatic vitamin D metabolism in humans. Digestion 1990;46(2):61-4.

Optimal Calcium Intake: NIH consensus conference. JAMA 1994;272(24):1942-8.

Peehl DM. Vitamin D and prostate cancer risk. Eur Urol 1999;35(5-6):392-4

Rozen F, Yang XF, Huynh H, Pollak M. Antiproliferative action of Vitamin D – related compounds and insulinlike growth factor – binding protein 5 accumulation. J Natl Cancer Instit 1997;89(3):652-6

Schmidt J, Wittenhagen P, Hørder M. Molecular effects of vitamin D on cell cycle and oncogenesis. Ugeskrift for laeger 1998 Jul 20;160(30):4411-4

Shabahang M, et al. Growth inhibition of HT-29 human colon cancer cells by analogues of 1,25 dihydroxy vitamin D3. Cancer Res 1994;54:407-64

Toppet M, et al. Sequential development of vitamin D metabolites under isoniazid and rifampicin therapy. Arch Fr Pediatr 1998;45(2):145-8

Veith R. Vitamin D supplementation, 25-hydroxy Vitamin D concentrations and safety. Am J Clin Nutr 1999; 69(5):842-56

Zerwekh JE, et al. Decreased serum 24,25-Dihydroxyvitamin D concentration during long-term anticonvulsant therapy in adult epileptics. Ann Nerol 1982;12(2):184-6

Vitamin D After 45

Brodie MJ, et al. Rifampicin and vitamin D metabolism. Clin Pharmacol Ther 1980;27(6):810-4

Chapuy MC, et al. Effect of Calcium and chole-calciferol treatment for three years on hip fractures in elderly women. Br Med J 1994;308:1081-2

Chen TC, Holick MF. Vitamin D and prostate cancer prevention and treatment. TEM 2003 Nov;14(9):423-30

Chesney RW, et al. Decreased serum 24,25-dihydroxyvitamin D3 in children receiving glucocorticoids. Lancet 1978;2(8100):1123-5

Crowle AJ, et al. Inhibition by 1,25 dihydroxy vitamin D3, of the multiplication of virulent tubercle bacilli in cultured human macrophages. Infect Immun, 1987;55:2945-50

Dawson-Hughes B, et al. Effect of calcium and Vitamin D supplementation on bone density in men and women 65 years of age or older. N Engl J Med 1997;337:670-6

Dawson-Hughes B, et al. Rates of bone loss in postmenopausal women randomly assigned to one of two dosages of the Vitamin D. Am J Clin Nutr 1995;61:1140-5

Dawson-Hughes B. Calcium and Vitamin D requirements of elderly women. J Nutr 1996;126(Suppl4):1165S- 7S

DeLuca HF. The Vitamin D story: A collaborative effort of basic science and clinical medicine. FASEB J 1988;2:224-36

Diarrhea and constipation. In: Berkow R, Fletcher AJ, Beers MH, et al, editors. The Merck Manual of

Diagnosis and Therapy. 16th ed. Rahway, NJ: Merck Research Laboratories; 1992

Feldman D, et al. Vitamin D and prostate cancer. Adv Exp Med Biol 1995; 375:53-63

Fukazawa T, et al. Association of Vitamin D receptor gene polymorphism with multiple sclerosis in Japanese. J Neurol Sci 1999;166(1):47-52

Gahn PH, et al. Circulating Vitamin D metabolites in relation to subsequent development of prostate cancer. Epidemiol Biomarkers Prev 1995;5(2):121-6

Garland CF, et al. Can colon cancer incidence and death rates be reduced with Calcium and Vitamin D? Am J Clin Nutr 1991;54(Suppl 1):193S-201S

Garland CF, Garland FC, Gorham ED. Calcuim and vitamin D. Their potential roles in colon and breast cancer prevention. Ann NY Acad Sci 1999; 889:107-19

Garland FC, et al. Geographic variation in breast cancer mortality in the United States: a hypothesis involving exposure to solar radiation. Prev Med 1970;19:614-22.

Hayes C, et al. Vitamin D and multiple sclerosis. Proc Soc Exper Biol Med 1997;216:21-7

Healthnotes, 2000 Inc. Available from: URL: http://www.healthnotes.com

Holick M. Too little vitamin D in premenopausal women: why should we care? Am J Clin Nutr. 2002; 76: 3-4.

In the news…Vitamin D and colon cancer. Harvard Women's Health Watch 2004 Feb;Vol.11(6)p7

James WP, Avenell A, Broom J, et al. A one-year trial to assess the value of Orlistat in the management of obesity. Int J Obes Relat Metab Disord 1997;21(Suppl3):24S-30S

Kállay E, Adlercreutz H, Farhan H, Lechner D, Bajna E, Gerdenitsch W, Campbell M, Cross HS. Phytoestrogens regulate vitamin D metabolism in the mouse colon: relevance for colon tumor prevention and therapy. J Nutr 1001 Nov;132(11):3490S-3493S

Knodel LC, et al. Adverse effects of hypolipidaemic drugs. Med Toxicol 1987;2(1):10-32

Lore F, et al. Vitamin D metabolites in postmenopausal osteoporosis. Horm Metab Res 1984;16:161-6

Martinez ME, et al. Calcium, Vitamin D and the occurrence of colorectal cancer among women. J Natl Cancer Instit 1996;88(19):1375-82

Mehta RG, et al. Prevention of preneoplastic mammary lesion development by a novel Vitamin D analogue, 1- alpha-hydroxyvitamin D5. J Natl Cancer Instit 1997; 89(3):212-8.

Munger KL et al. Vitamin D intake an incidence of multiple sclerosis. Neurology 2004: 62: 60-65.

Odes HS, et al. Effect of cimetidine on hepatic vitamin D metabolism in humans. Digestion 1990;46(2):61-4.

Optimal Calcium Intake: NIH consensus conference. JAMA 1994;272(24):1942-8.

Peehl DM. Vitamin D and prostate cancer risk. Eur Urol 1999;35(5-6):392-4

Rozen F, Yang XF, Huynh H, Pollak M. Antiproliferative action of Vitamin D – related compounds and insulinlike growth factor – binding protein 5 accumulation. J Natl Cancer Instit 1997;89(3):652-6

Schmidt J, Wittenhagen P, Hørder M. Molecular effects of vitamin D on cell cycle and oncogenesis. Ugeskrift for laeger 1998 Jul 20;160(30):4411-4

Shabahang M, et al. Growth inhibition of HT-29 human colon cancer cells by analogues of 1,25 dihydroxy vitamin D3. Cancer Res 1994;54:407-64

Toppet M, et al. Sequential development of vitamin D metabolites under isoniazid and rifampicin therapy. Arch Fr Pediatr 1998;45(2):145-8

Veith R. Vitamin D supplementation, 25-hydroxy Vitamin D concentrations and safety. Am J Clin Nutr 1999; 69(5):842-56

Zerwekh JE, et al. Decreased serum 24,25-Dihydroxyvitamin D concentration during long-term anticonvulsant therapy in adult epileptics. Ann Nerol 1982;12(2):184-6

Calcium: Requirements, Bioavailable Forms, Physiology and Related Clinical Aspects

1. Standard Textbooks of Nutritional Science: A. Shils M, Shike M, Olson J and Ross C. Modern nutrition in health and disease. 9th ed. Lippincott Williams Wilkins 1993. B. Escott-Stump S and Mahan LK, editors. Food, nutrition and diet therapy. 10th ed. W.B. Saunders Company 2000. C. Bowman B and Russell RM, editors. Present knowledge in nutrition, 8th ed. ILSI Press 2001. D. Kreutler PA and Czajka-Narins DM, editors. Nutrition in perspective. 2nd ed. Prentice Hall Inc. 1987.

2. McKeown-Eyssen GE, et al. Dietary factors in colon cancer: international relationships. Nutr Cancer 1984; 6:160-70.

3. Levenson D, et al. A review of calcium preparations. Nutr Reviews 1994; 52:221-32.

4. Optimal calcium intake: NIH consensus panel. JAMA 1994; 272:1942-8.

5. Osteoporosis Society of Canada. Clinical practice guidelines for the diagnosis and management of osteoporosis. Can Med Assoc J 1996; 155:1113-33.

6. Nelson ME, et al. Effects of high intensity strength training on multiple risk factors for osteoporatic fractures: a randomized controlled trial. JAMA 1994; 272:1909-14.

7. Reid IR, et al. Effect of calcium supplementation on bone loss in postmenopausal women. Osteo Int.1993;1:27-31 (suppl).

8. Osteoporosis Society of Canada. Prevention and management of osteoporosis: consensus statements from the scientific advisory board of the Osteoporosis Society of Canada. CMAJ 1996Oct;155(7).

9. McCarron DA, et al. Blood pressure response to oral calcium in persons with mild to moderate hypertension: a randomized double-blind placebo-controlled crossover trial. Ann Intern Med 1985;103:825-33.

10. Meese RB, et al. The inconsistent effects of calcium supplements upon blood pressure in primary hypertension. Am J Med Sci 1987; 294:219-24.

11. Belizan JM, et al. Reduction of blood pressure with calcium supplementation in young adults. JAMA 1983; 249:1161.

12. Belizan JM, et al., Calcium supplementation to prevent hypertensive disorders of pregnancy; N Engl J Med 1991; 325:1399-405.

13. Knight KB, et al. Calcium supplementation on normotensive and hypertensive pregnant women. Am J Clin Nutr 1992; 55:891-5.

14. Heaney RP. Protein intake and bone health: the influence of belief systems on the conduct of nutritional science. Am J Clin Nutr 2000; 73(1):5-6.

15. Hotz J, et al. Behaviour of gastric secretion in acute EDTA-hypocalcemia in Man. Verh Dtsch Ges Inn Med 1971; 77:501-4.

16. Lambs L, et al. Metal ion-tetracycline interactions in biological fluids. Part 3 formation of mixed-metal ternary complexes of tetracycline, oxytetracycline, doxycycline and

minocycline with calcium and magnesium, and their involvement in the bioavailability of these antibiotics in blood plasma. Agents Actions 1984;14(5-6):743-50.

17. Kelnar CJ, et al. Hypomagnesaemic hypocalcaemia with hypokalaemia caused by treatment with high dose gentamicin. Arch Dis Child Oct 1978; 53(10):817-20.

18. Amphotericin B depletes sodium, calcium, potassium, magnesium. Physicians' Desk Reference. 53rd ed. Montvale, NJ: Medical Economics Company Inc 1999:1038.

19. Shafer RB, et al. Calcium and folic acid absorption in Patients Taking Anticonvulsant Drugs. J Clin Endocrinol Metab Dec1975; 41(06):1125-9.

20. Foxx MC, et al. The effect of anticonvulsants phenobarbital and diphenythydantoin on intestinal absorption of calcium. Acta Physiol Lat Am 1978; 29 (4-5):223-8.

21. Winnacker JL, Yeager H, Saunders JA. Rickets in children receiving anticonvulsant drugs. Biochemical and hormonal markers. Am J Dis Child 1997 Mar; 131(3):286-90

22. Kato Y, et al. Hypocalcemic action of the several types of salicylic acid analogues. Shika Kiso Igakkai Zasshi 1989Feb; 31(1):89-94.

23. Watkins DW, et al. Alterations in calcium, magnesium, iron, and zinc metabolism by dietary cholestyramine. Dig Dis Sci 1985; 30(5):477-82.

24. Frayha RA, et al. Acute colchicine poisoning presenting as symptomatic hypocalcaemia. Br J Rheumatol 1984Nov; 23(4):292-5.

25. Reid IR, et al. Evidence for decreased tubular reabsorption of calcium in glucocorticoid-treated asthmatics. Horm Res 1987; 27(4):200-4.

26. Adachi JD, Ioannidis G. Calcium and Vitamin D therapy in corticosteroid-induced bone loss: what is the evidence? Calcif Tissue Int 1999Oct; 65(4):332-6.

27. Ghishan FK, Walker F, Meneely R, et al. Intestinal calcium transport: effect of cimetidine. J Nutr 1981Dec;111(12):2157-61.

28. Edwards H, Zinberg J, King TC. Effect of cimetidine on serum calcium levels in an elderly patient. Arch Surg 1981Aug;116(8):1088-9.

29. Brodie MJ, et al. Effect of osoniazid on Vitamin D metabolism and hepatic monooxygenase activity. Clin Pharmacol Ther 1981Sept;30(3):363-7.

30. Beermann B. Thiazides and loop-diuretics therapeutic aspects. Acta Med Scand Suppl 1986;707:75-8.

31. Weberg R, et al. Mineral-metabolic side effects of low-dose antacids. Scand J Gastroenterol. 1985Aug;20(6):741-6.

32. Hanze S, et al. Studies of the effect of the diuretics furosemide, ethacrynic acid and triamterene on renal magnesium and calcium excretion. Klin Wochenschr 1967Mar;45(6):313-4.

33. Kupfer S, Kosovsky JD. Effects of cardiac glycosides on renal tubular transport of calcium, magnesium, inorganic phosphate and glucose in the dog. J Clin Investig 1965;44:1143.

34. Marchbanks CR. Drug-drug interactions with fluoroquinolones. Pharmacotherapy 1993Mar;13(2 Pt 2):23S-28S.

35. Sahai J, Healy DP, Stotka J, et al. The influence of chronic administration of calcium carbonate on the bioavailability of oral ciprofloxacin. Br J Clin Pharmacol. 1993Mar;35(3):302-4.

36. Singh N, Singh PN, Hershman JM. Effect of calcium carbonate on the absorption of levothyroxine. JAMA 2000Jun;283(21):282-5.

37. Hallberg L, Rossander-Hulthen L, Brune M, et al. Inhibition of haem-iron absorption in man by calcium. Br J Nutr 1993Mar;69(2):533-40.

38. Wood RJ, Zheng JJ. High dietary calcium intakes reduce zinc absorption and balance in humans. Am J Clin Nutr 1997Jun;65(6):1803-9

39. Reference number 39 "Peters U, Chatterjee N, McGlynn A et al. Calcium intake and colorectal adenoma in a US colorectal cancer early detection program. Am J Clin Nutr 2004; 80: 1358-65."

Calcium, Bone Density, Teenage Girls

Rozen G, Renneri G, Dodiuk-Gad R, et al. Calcium supplementation provides an extended window of opportunity for bone mass accretion after menarche. Am J Clin Nutr. 2003; 78:993-8

Vitamin K Intake Important In The Prevention Of Osteoporosis

NNFA Supplement – Mon, March 31, 2003Consumerslab.com (Vitamin K)

Clinically Relevant Aspects In The Diagnosis, Prevention and Natural Management Of Osteoporosis

Clinical practice guidelines for the diagnosis and management of osteoporosis. Canadian Medical Assoc Journal, Oct.15, 1996. (Osteoporosis Society
of Canada) Optimal Calcium Intake – NIH Consensus Conference. JAMA, 1994, 272; 24: 1942-1948
Clinical practice guidelines for the diagnosis and management of osteoporosis. Canadian Medical AssocJournal, Oct.15, 1996. (Osteoporosis Society
of Canada) Lindsay, R. The Burden of Osteoporosis: Cost. Am J Med, 98 (suppl.2A) (1995): 9-11 (suppl)
Optimal Calcium Intake – NIH Consensus Conference. JAMA, 1994, 272; 24: 1942-1948
Osteoporosis Society of Canada - Clinical practice guidelines for the diagnosis and management of osteoporosis. Canadian Medical Assoc Journal, Oct.15, 1996.

Antioxidants, Alzheimer's Disease, Dementia Risk

Grundman M. Vitamin E and Alzheimer disease: the basis for additional clinical trials. Am J Clin Nutr 2000Feb;71(2 Part 2):630S-636S
Yatim SM, et al. The antioxidant vitamin E modulates amyloid beta-peptide-induced creatine kinase activity inhibition and increased protein oxidation: implications for the free radical hypothesis of Alzheimer's disease. Neurochem Res 1999 Mar;24(3):427-35
Morris MC, et al. Vitamin E and vitamin C supplement use and risk of incident Alzheimer disease. Alzheimer Dis Assoc Disord 1998 Sep;12(3):121-6
Rivieire S, et al. Low plasma vitamin C in Alzheimer patients despite an adequate diet. Int J Geriatr Psychiatry 1998 Nov;13(11):749-54
Hake AM, Schere P. On the brink of the pandemic: epidemiology and risk factors for Alzheimer's. World Alzheimer's Congress 2000
Vatassery GT, et al. High doses of vitamin E in the treatment of disorders of the central nervous system in the aged. Am J Clin Nutri 1997: 70(5):793-801

B Vitamins and Brain Function

Abou-Saleh MT, Coppen A. The biology of folate in depression: implications for nutritional hypotheses of the psychoses. J Psychiatr Res 1986;20:91-101
Berg S. Psychological functioning in 70-and 75-year old people. Acta Psychiatr Scand 1980;Suppl 288:1-47

Bohnen N, Jolles J, Degenaar CP. Lower blood levels of vitamin B12 are related to decreased performance of healthy subjects in the Stroop Color-Word Test. Neurosci Res Commun 1992;11:53-6

Botwinick J, Storandt M. Memory, related functions and age. Springfield, IL: Charles C Thomas, 1974

Dakshinamurti K, Paulose CS, Siow YL. Neurobiology of pyridoxine. In: Reynolds RD, Leklem JE, eds. Vitamin B6: its role in health and disease. New York: Alan R Liss, Inc, 1985;99-121.

Goodwin JS, Goodwin JM, Garry PJ. Association between nutritional status and cognitive functioning in a healthy elderly population. JAMA 1983;249: 2917-21

Hertzog C, Schaie KW, Gribbin K. Cardiovasular disease and changes in intellectual functioning from middle to old age. J Gerontol 1978;33:872-83

Jacques PJ, Riggs KM. B vitamins as risk factors for age-related diseases. In: Rosenberg IH, ed. Nutritional assessment of elderly populations. Measure and function. New York: Raven Press, 1995.

Joosten E, van den Berg A, Riezler R, et al. Metabolic evidence that deficiencies of vitamin B12 (cobalamin), folate, and vitamin B6 occur commonly in elderly people. Am J Clin Nutr 1993;58:468-76

Leklem JE. Vitamin B6. A status report. J Nutr 1990;120:1503-7. 1987;83(suppl 5A):104-6

Levitt AJ, Joffe RT. Folate, vitamin B12, and life course of depressive illness. Biol Psychiatry 1989;25:867-72

Lindenbaum J, Rosenberg IH, Wilson PWF, Stabler SP, Allen RH. Prevalence of cobalamin deficiency in the Framingham elderly population. Am J Clin Nutr 1994;60:2-11

Martin DC. B12 and folate deficiency dementia. Clin Geriatr Med 1988;4:841-52

Riggs K, et al. Relations of vitamin B12, Vitamin B6, Folate, and homocysteine to cognitive performance in the Normative Aging Study. Am. J. Clin. Nutr.1996; 63:306-14

Rinn WE. Mental decline in normal aging: A review. J Geriatr Psychiatry Neurol 1988;1:144-58

Sauberlich HE. Relationship of vitamin B6, vitamin B12, and folate to neurological and neuropsychiatric disorders. In: Bendich A, Butterworth CE Jr, eds. Micronutrients in health and in disease prevention. New York: Marcel Dekker, Inc 1991:187-218.

Selhub J, Jacques PJ, Wilson PWF, Rush D, Rosenberg IH. Vitamin status and intake as primary determinants of homocysteinemia in the elderly. JAMA 1993;270:2693-8.

Shane B, Stokstad ELR, Vitamin B12 folate interrelationships. Annu Rev Nutr 1985;5:115-41

Spieth W. Slowness of task performance and cardiovascular disease. In: Welford AT, Birren JE, eds. Behavior, aging and the nervous system. Springfield, IL: Charles C Thomas, 1965:366-400

B Vitamins, Memory, Cognitive Function

1. B vitamins for staving off Alzheimer's disease. Tufts University Health & Nutrition Letter, Jan99, Vol. 16 Issue 11, p1, 2/3p.
2. Riggs K. et al. Relations of vitamin B12, Vitamin B6, Folate, and homocysteine to cognitive performance in the Normative Aging Study. Am. J. Clin.Nutr.1996; 63:306-14.
3. Martin DC. B12 and folate deficiency dementia. Clin Geriatr Med 1988;4:841-52.
4. Abou-Saleh MT, Coppen A. The biology of folate in depression: implications for nutritional hypotheses of the psychoses. J Psychiatr Res 1986; 20:91-101.
5. Sauberlich HE. Relationship of vitamin B6, vitamin B12, and folate to neurological and neuropsychiatric disorders. In: Bendich A, Butterworth CE Jr, eds. Micronutrients in health and in disease prevention. New York: Marcel Dekker, Inc, 1991:187-218.

6. Bohnen N, Jolles J, Degenaar CP. Lower blood levels of vitamin B12 are related to decreased performance of healthy subjects in the Stroop Color-Word Test. Neurosci Res Commun 1992;11:53-6.

7. Goodwin JS, Goodwin JM, Garry PJ. Association between nutritional status and cognitive functioning in a healthy elderly population. JAMA 1983;249:2917-21.

8. Joosten E, van den Berg A, Riezler R, et al. Metabolic evidence that deficiencies of vitamin B12 (cobalamin), folate, and vitamin B6 occur commonly in elderly people. Am J Clin Nutr 1993;58:468-76.

9. Lindenbaum J, Rosenberg IH, Wilson PWF, Stabler SP, Allen RH. Prevalence of cobalamin deficiency in the Framingham elderly population. Am J Clin Nutr 1994;60:2-11.

10. Leklem JE. Vitamin B6. A status report. J Nutr 1990;120:1503-7.

11. Carney MWP, Toone BK, Reynolds EH. S-Adenosylmethionine and affective disorder. Am J Med 1987;83(suppl 5A):104-6.

12. Levitt AJ, Joffe RT. Folate, vitamin B12, and life course of depressive illness. Biol Psychiatry 1989;25:867-72.

13. Shane B, Stokstad ELR, Vitamin B12 folate interrelationships. Annu Rev Nutr 1985;5:115-41.

14. Dakshinamurti K, Paulose CS, Siow YL. Neurobiology of pyridoxine. In: Reynolds RD, Leklem JE, eds. Vitamin B6: its role in health and disease. New York: Alan R Liss, Inc, 1985;99-121.

15. Selhub J, Jacques PJ, Wilson PWF, Rush D, Rosenberg IH. Vitamin status and intake as primary determinants of homocysteinemia in the elderly. JAMA 1993;270:2693-8.

16. Jacques PJ, Riggs KM. B vitamins as risk factors for age-related diseases. In: Rosenberg IH, ed. Nutritional assessment of elderly populations. Measure and function. New York: Raven Press, 1995.

17. Berg S. Psychological functioning in 70-and 75-year old people. Acta Psychiatr Scand 1980;Suppl 288:1-47.

18. Botwinick J, Storandt M. Memory, related functions and age. Springfield, IL: Charles C Thomas, 1974.

19. Hertzog C, Schaie KW, Gribbin K. Cardiovascular disease and changes in intellectual functioning from middle to old age. J Gerontol 1978;33:872-83.

20. Rinn WE. Mental decline in normal aging: A review. J Geriatr Psychiatry Neurol 1988;1:144-58. 21. Spieth W. Slowness of task performance and cardiovascular disease. In: Welford AT, Birren JE, eds. Behavior, aging and the nervous system. Springfield, IL: Charles C Thomas, 1965:366-400.

Additional Brain Nutrients
Choline

Agnoli A, et al. New strategies in the management of Parkinson's disease: A biological approach using a phospholipid precursor (CDP-Choline) Neuropsycholbiology 1982;8(6):289-96

Canty DJ, et al. Lecithin and chloine in human health and disease. Nutr Reviews 1994;52:327-339

Citicoline, Alzheimer's disease, and cognitive performance. Life Extension 2000:6(9):69,2(Alt Health Watch data base)

Encyclopedia of Nutritional Supplements. Prima Publishing 1996;Murray M:137-141

Foiravanti M, Yanagi M. Cytidinediphosphocholine (CDP-Choline) for cognitive and behavioral disturbances associated with chronic cerebral disorders in the elderly. Cochrane Syst Revi 2002;(2):000269 In: The Cochrane Library, 1,2002. Oxford: Update Software

Present Knowledge in Nutrition (5th edition). The Nutrition Foundation, Inc 1984;Choline:383-399
Secades JJ, et al. CDP-Choline: pharmacological and clinical review. Methods Find Exp Clin Pharmacol 1995;17(Suppl B):1-54
Zeisel SH, et al. Choline,an essential nutrient for humans. FASEB J 1991;5:20093-2098

Phosphatidylserine

Cenacchi T, Bertoldin T, Farina C, et al. Cognitive decline in the elderly: A double-blind, placebo-controlled multicenter study on efficacy of phosphatidylserine administration. Aging 1993;5:123-33
Crook T, Petrie W, Wells C, Massari DC. Effects of phosphatidylserine in Alzheimer's disease. Psychopharmacol Bull 1992;28:61-6
Crook TH, Tinklenberg J, Yesavage J, Petrie W, Nunzi MG, Massari DC. Effect of phosphatidylserine in age-associated memory impairment.Neurology 1991;41:644-9
Engel RR, Satzger W, Gunther W, Kathmann N, Bove D, Gerke S, et al. Double-blind cross-over study of phosphatidylserine vs. placebo in subjects with early cognitive deterioration of the Alzheimer type. Eur. Neuropsychopharmacol, 1992;2:149-55
Funfgeld EW, Baggen M, Nedwidek P, Richstein B, Mistlberger G. Double-blind study with phosphatidylserine (PS) in parkinsonian patients with senile dementia of Alzheimer's type (SKAT). Prog Clin Biol Res 1989;317:1235-46
Healthnotes Online. Healthnotes Inc, 2000
Maggioni M, Picotti GB, Bondiolotti GP, Panerai A, Cenacchi T, Nobil P, et al. Effects of phosphatidylserine therapy in geriatric patients with depressive disorders. Acta Psychiatr Scand 1990;81:265-70
Murray M. Encyclopedia of Nutritional Supplements. Rocklin, CA: Prima Publishing 1996; 356-358
Natural Products Encyclopedia. www.consumerlab.com Phosphatidylserine Nunzi MG, Milan F, Guidolin D, et al. Effects of phosphatidylserine administration on age-related structural changes in the rat hippocampus and septal complex. Pharmacopsychiat 1989;22:125-8
Valzelli L, Kozak W, Zanotti A, Toffano G. Activity of phosphatidylserine on memory retrieval and on exploration in mice. Meth Find Extl Clin Pharmacol 1987;9:657-60
Vannucchi MG, Casamenti F, Pepeu G. Decrease of acetylcholine release from cortical slices in aged rats: Investigations into its reversal by phosphatidylserine. J Neurochem 1990;55:819-25

Acetyl-L-Carnitine

Calvani M, Carta A, Caruso G, Bendetti N, Iannuccelli M. Action of acetyl-L-carnitine in neurodegeneration and Alzheimer's disease. Ann NY Acad Sci 1993;663:483-6
Cipolli C, Chiari G. Effects of L-acetylcarnitine on mental deterioration in the aged: initial results. Clin Ther 1990;132:479-510
Garzya G, Corallo D, Fiore A, Lecciso G, Tetrelli G, Zotti C. Evaluation of the effects of the L-acetylcarnitine on senile patients suffering from depression. Drugs Exp Clin Res 1990;16(2):101-6
Pettegrew JW, Klunk WE, Panchalingam K, Kanfer JN, McClure RJ. Clinical and neurochemical effects of acetyl-L-carnitine in Alzheimer's disease. Neurobiol Agin 1995;16:1-4
Sano M, Bell K, Cote L, Dooneief G, Lawton A, Legler L, et al. Double-blind parallel design pilot study of acetyl levocarnitine in patients with Alzheimer's disease. Arch Neurol 1995;49:1137-41

Savioli G, Neri M. L-acetylcarnitine treatment of mental decline in the elderly. Drugs Exp Clin Res 1994;20:169-76

Spagnoli A, Lucca U, Menasce G, Bandera L, Cizza G, Forloni G, et al. Long-term acetyl-L-carnitine treatment in Alzheimer's disease. Neurology 1991;41:172632

Tempesta E, Casella L, Pirrongelli C, Janiri L, Calvani M, Ancona L. L-acetylcarnitine in depressed elderly subjects. A cross-over study vs. placebo. Drugs Exp Clin Res 1987;8:417-23

Vecchi GP, Chiari G, Cipolli C, et al. Acetyl-L-carnitine treatment of mental impairment in the elderly: evidence from a multicenter study. Arch Gerontol Geriatr 1991;2(Suppl):159S-68S

Bacopa Monnieri (Bacopa)

Dar A, Channa S. Calcium antagonistic activity of Bacopa monniera on vascular intestinal smooth muscles of rabbit and ginea-pig. J Ethnopharmacol 1999;66(2):167-74

Dietary Supplement Information Bureau. www.content.intramedicine.com: Bacopa monnieri

Kidd PM. A review of nutrients and botanicals in the integrative management of cognitive dysfunction. Altern Med Rev 1999 Jun;4(3):144-61

Mukherjee GD et al. Clinical trial on brahmi. I. J Exp Med Sci 1966;10(1):5-11

Stough C, Lloyd J, Clarke J, Downey LA, Hutchison CW, Rodgers T, et la. The chronic effects of an extract of Bacopa monniera (Brahmi) on cognitive function in healthy human subjects. Psychopharmacology (Berl) 2001 Aug;156(4):481-4

Tripathi YB, et al. Bacopa monniera linn. As an antioxidant: Mechanism of action. Indian J Exp Biol 1996 Jun;34(6):523-6

Vohora D, Pal SN, Pillai KK. Protection from phenbytoin-induced cognitive deficit by Bacopa monniera, a reputed Indian nootropic plant. J Ethnopharmacol 2000 Aug;71(3):383-90

Huperzine A

Ashani Y, Peggins JO, Doctor BP. Mechanism of inhibition of cholinesterases by huperzine A. Biochem Biophys Res Commun, 1992:184:719-26

Bai DL, et al. Huperzine A, a potential therapeutic agent for treatment of Alzheimer's disease. Curr Med Chem, 2000 Mar;7(3):355-74

Cheng DH, Ren H, Tang XC. Huperzine A, a novel promising acetylcholinesterase inhibitor. Neuroreport 1996;8:97-101

Cheng DH, Tang XC. Comparative studies of huperzine A, E2020, and tacrine on behavior and cholinesterase activites. Pharmacol Biochem Behav 1998;60:377-86

Dworkin N. Restoring memory. Psychology Today 2000 Jul/Aug;32(4):p28

McCaleb R. Huperzia looks promising for improving memory. HerbalGram, 10/31/1995;35:p14

Pirisi, Angela. Plant wisdom: Memory moss. Yoga Journal, 08/31/1999;147:p95

Sun QQ, Xu SS, Pan JL, et al. Huperzine-A capsules enhance memory and learning performance in 34 pairs of matched adolescent students. Acta Pharmacol Sin 1999;20:601-3

Tang XC. Huperzine A (shuangyiping): A promising drug for Alzheimer's disease. Chung Kuo Yao Li Hsueh Pao, 1996 Nov;17(6):481-4

Wang Z, Ren G, Zhao Y et al. A double-blind study of huperzine A and piracetam in patients with age-associated memory impairment and dementia.In: Kanba S, Richelson E (eds.) Herbal Medicines for Nonpsychiatric Diseases. Tokyo: Seiwa Choten Publishers 1999:39-50

Xu SS, Gao, ZX, Weng Z et al. Efficacy of tablet huperzine-A on memory, cognition, and behavior in Alzheimer's disease. Chung Kuo Yao Li Hsueh Pao 1995;16:391-5

St. John's Wort

1. Boon H and Smith M, Health Care Professional Training Program in Complementary Medicine, Institute of Applied Complementary Medicine Inc., 1997.
2. Suzuki O, et.al., Inhibition of Monoamine Oxidase by Hypericin, Planta Medica 50, 1984, 272-274.
3. Holtz J, Demisch L, and Gollnick B, Investigations About Antidepressive and Mood Changing Effects of Hypericum Performatum, Planta Medica 55,1989, 643.
4. Schmidt U and Sommer H, St. John's Wort Extract in the Ambulatory Therapy of Depression. Attention and Reaction Ability are Preserved, Forschr Med 111, 1993, 339-342.
5. Johnson D, Effects of St. John's Wort Extract Jarsin. Paper Presented at the 4th International Congress on Phytotherapy, Munich, Germany, September 10-13, 1992. [Abstract SL53]; Woelk H, Multicentric Practice – Study Analyzing the Functional Capacity in Depressive Patients, Paper Presented at the 4th International Congress on Phytotherapy, Munich, Germany, September 10-13, 1992 [Abstract SL54]; Sommer H, Improvement of Phychovegetative
Complaints by Hypericum, Paper Presented at the 4th International Congress on Phytotherapy, Munich, Germany, September 10-13, 1992 [Abstract SL55]
6. Schlich D, Brauckmann F, and Schenk N, Treatment of Depressive Conditions with Hypericum, Psychol 13, 1987, 440-444
7. Harrer G and Sommer H, Treatment of Mild/Moderate Depressions with Hypericum, Phytomed 1, 1994, 3-8
8. Lavie D, Antiviral Pharmaceutical Compositions Containing Hypericin or Pseudohypericin, European
Patent Application No. 87111467.4, filed 8/8/87, European Patent Office, Publ. No. 0 256 A2. 1987,
175-177
9. Someya H, Effect of a Constituent of Hypericin Erectum on Inection and Multiplication of Epstein-Barr Virus, J Tokyo Med Coll 43, 1985, 815-826
10. Gulick R, et.al., Human Hypericism: A Photosensitivity Reaction to Hypericin (St. John's Wort), Int Conf AIDS 8, B90, 1992. [Abstract PoB 3018]
11. Murray MT, The Healing Power of Herbs (2nd edition), Prima Publishing, 1995
12. Natural Products Encyclopedia. www.consumerslab.com:St John's Wort
13. Healthnotes, Inc. 2001. www.healthnotes.com:St. John's Wort
14. Dietary Supplement Information Bureau. www.content.intramedicine.com: St. John's Wort
15. Vorbach EU, Arnoldt KH, Hubner WD. Efficacy and tolerability of St. John's Wort extract LI 160 versus imipramine in patients with severe depressive episodes versus imipramine in patients with severe depressive episodes according to ICD-10. Pharmacopsychiatry 1997;30(suppl 2):81-5
16. DeMott K. St. John's wort tied to serotonin syndrome. Clinical Psychiatry News 1998;26:p28
17. Gordon JB. SSRIs and St. John's wort: Possible toxicity? Am Fam Physician 1998;57:p950, p953
18. Lantz MS, Buchalter E, Giambanco V. St John's wort and antidepressant drug interactions in the elderly. J Geriatr Psychiatry Neurol 1999;12:7-10

19. Holzl J, Demisch L, Gollnik B. Investigations about antidepressive and mood changing effects of *Hypericum perforatum. Planta Med* 1989;55:643.

20. Chatterjee SS, Koch E, Noldner M, et al. Hyperforin with hypericum extract: Interactions with some neurotransmitter systems. *Quart Rev Nat Med* 1997;Summer:110.

21. Calapai G, Crupi A, Firenzuoli F, et al. Effects of *Hypericum perforatum* on levels of 5-hydroxytryptamine, noradrenaline and dopamine in the cortex, diencephalon and brainstem of the rat. *J Pharm Pharmacol* 1999;51:723–8.

22. Schrader E. Equivalence of St John's wort extract (Ze 117) and fluoxetine: a randomized, controlled study in mild-moderate depression. Int Clin Psychopharmacol 2999;15:61-8

23. Schrader E, Meier B, Brattstrom A. Hypericum treatment of mild-moderate depression in a placebocontrolled study: a prospective, double-blind, randomized, placebo-controlled, multicentre study. Hum Psychopharmacol 1998;13:163-9

24. Müller WE, Rolli M, Schäfer C, Hafner U. Effects of hypericum extract (LI 160) in biochemical models of antidepressant activity. *Pharmacopsychiatry* 1997;30(suppl):102–7

25. Kalb R, Trautmann-Sponsel RD, Kieser M. Efficacy and tolerability of hypericum extract WS 5572 versus placebo in mildly to moderately depressed patients. A randomized double-blind multicenter clinical trial. Pharmacopsychiatry 2001;34:96-103

26. Hansgen KD, Vesper J. Antidepressant efficacy of a high-dose hypericum extract [translated from German]. MMW Munch Med Wochenschr 1996; 138:29-33

27. Shelton RC, Keller MB, Gelenberg A, et al. Effectiveness of St. John's wort in major depression: a randomized controlled trial. JAMA 2001; 285:1978-86

28. Hypericum Depression Trial Study Group. Effect of Hypericum perforatum (St. John's wort) in major depressive disorder: a randomized controlled trial. JAMA 2002;287:1807-14

29. Schrader E. Equivalence of St John's wort extract (Ze 117) and fluoxetine: a randomized, controlled study in mild-moderate depression. Int Clin Psychopharmacol 2000;15:61-8

30. Harrer G, Schmidt U, Kuhn U, et al. Comparison of equivalence between the St. John's wort extract LoHyp-57 and fluoxetine. Arzneimittelforschung 1999;49:289-96

31. Brenner R, Azbel V, Madhusoodanan S, et al. Comparison of an extract of hypericum (L1 160) and sertraline in the treatment of depression: a double-blind, randomized pilot study. Clin Ther 2000;22:411-9

32. Philipp M, Kohnen R, Hiller KO. Hypericum extract versus imipramine or placebo in patients with moderate depression: randomized multcentre study of treatment for eight weeks. BMJ 1999;319:1534-9

33. Martinez B, Kasper S, Ruhrmann S, et al. hypericum in the treatment of seasonal affective disorders. J Geriatr Psychiatr Neurol 1994;7(suppl 1):S29-33

34. Muller WEG, et al. Effects of Hypericum Extract on the Expression of Serotonin Receptors. J Geriatric Psychiatry and Neurology. 1994;7:S63-S64

35. Rayburn WF, Gonzalez CL, Christensen HD, et al. Effect of prenatally administered hypericum (St John's wort) on growth and physical maturation of mouse offspring. Am J Obstet Gynecol 2001;184:191-5

36. Woelk H, Burkard G, Grunwald J. Benefits and risks of the hypericum extract LI 160: Drug monitoring study with 3,250 patients. J Geriatr Psychiatr neurol 1994;7(suppl 1):S34-8

37. Hubner WD, Arnoldt KH. St John's wort: a one year treatment study [in German; English abstract]. Z Phytother 2000;21:306-10

38. Schulz V, Hansel R, Tyler VE. Rational Thytotherapy: A Physicians' Guide to Herbal Medicine. 3rd ed. Berlin, Germany: Springer-Verlag 1998:p56

39. De Smet PA, Nolen WA. St. John's wort as an anti-depressant. BMJ 1996;3:241-2

40. Suzuki O, Katsumata Y, Oya M, et al. Inhibition of monoamine oxidase by hypericin. Planta Med 1984;50:272-4

41. Bladt S, Wagner H. Inhibition of MAO by fractions and constitutents of hypericum extract. J Geriatr Psychiatr Neurol 1994;7(suppl 1):S57-9

42. Thiede HM, Walper A. Inhibition of MAO and COMT by hypericum extracts and hypericin. J Geriatr Psychiatr Neurol 1994;7(suppl 1):S54-6

43. Kahn RS, et al. L-5-hydroxytryptophan in the treatment of anxiety disorders. J Affect Disord Mar1985;8(2):197-200

44. Muller WE, et al. Effects of Hypericum Extract (LI 160) in Biochemical Models of Antidepressant Activity. Pharmacopsychiatry. 1997;30(Supp 2):102-07

45. Linde K, et al. St. John's Wort for Depression--An Overview and Meta-analysis of Randomised Clinical Trials. BMJ. 1996;313m:253-58

46. Demott K. St. John's Wort Tied to Serotonin Syndrome. Clin Psychiatry News 1998;26:28.

47. Suzuki O, et al. Inhibition of Monoamine Oxidase by Hypericin. Planta Medica 1984;50:272-74.

48. Bladt S, et al. Inhibition of MAO by Fractions and Constituents of Hypericum Extract. J Geriatric Psychiatry and Neurology 1994;7:S57-S59

49. Gordon JB. SSRIs and St.John's Wort: possible toxicity? Am Fam Physician Mar1998;57(5):950,953

50. Lantz MS, Buchalter E, Giambanco V. St. John's wort and antidepressant drug interactions in the elderly. J Geriatr Psychiatry Neurol 1999;12(1):7-10.

51. Okpanyi SN, et al. Animal experiments on the psychotropic action of a hypericum extract. Arzneimittelforschung Jan1987;37(1):10-3

52. Johne A et al. Pharmacokinetic interaction of digoxin with an herbal extract from St John's wort (Hypericum perforatum) Clin Pharmacol Ther Oct1999;66(4):338-45

53. Nebel A, et al. Potential metabolic interaction between St. John's wort and Theophylline. Ann Pharmacother Apr1999;33(4):p502

54. Ruschitzka F, et al. Acute heart transplant rejection due to St. John's wort. Lancet Feb2000;355(9203):548-9

55. Rey JM, et al. Hypericum perforatum (St John;s Wort) in depression: Pest or blessing? Med J Aust Dec1998;169(11-12):583-6

56. Yue Qy, Bergquist C, Gerden B. Safety of St. John's wort (Hypericum perforatum), correspondence. Lancet 2000;355:576-7

57. Ernst E. Second thoughts about safety of St John's Wort. Lancet Dec1999;354(9195):2014-6

58. Piscitelli SC, et al. Indinavir concentrations and St. John's Wort. Lancet Feb2000;355(9203):547-8

59. Mills S, Bone K. Principles and Practice of Phytotherapy. Churchill Livingstone 2000:548-9

Coenzyme Q10 Supplementation Improvement In Early Parkinson's Disease

1. Shults, (M.D.) C.W. et al. Effects of Coenzyme Q10 in Early Parkinson Disease. *Archives of Neurology*; Vol.59, No.10: October 2002.

2. www.CNN.com. Study: Dietary supplement may slow Parkinson's.

3. Shults, Clifford W, Haas, Richard H. A possible role of coenzyme Q10 in the etiology and treatment of Parkinson's disease. *Biofactors*, 1999, Vol.9, Issue 2-4; p.267

4. Beal, M.F. Coenzyme Q10 as a possible treatment for neurodegenerative diseases. *Free Radical Research*. April 2002; 36(4): pp.455-60

5. Folkers, K. Heart failure is a dominant deficiency of Co-enzyme Q10 and challenges for future clinical research on Co Q10. *Clinical Investigator* 1993; 71 (& suppl): S51-54

6. LiHarru, G.P., Ho, L and Folkers, K. Deficiency of Co-enzyme Q10 in human heart disease. Part II. *Int J Vit Nutr Res* 42, 413, 1972

7. Folkers, K. et al. Biochemical rationale and myocardial tissue data on the effective therapy of cardiomyopathy with Co-enzyme Q10. *Proc Natl Acad Sci* 82, 901, 1985

8. Kitamua, N., et al. Myocardial tissue level of Co-enzyme Q10 in patients with cardiac failure in: Biomedical and Clinical Aspects of Co-enzyme Q10, Vol. 4 (Folkers, K. and Yamamura, Y eds.) *Elsevier Science Publ.* Amsterdam, 1984, pp. 243-252

9. Langsjoen, H., et al. Usefulness of Co-enzyme Q10 in clinical cardiology: A long-term study. *Mol Aspects Med 15* (suppl), S165-175, 1994

10. Greenberg, S. Co-enzyme Q10: a new drug for cardiovascular disease. *J Clin Pharm* 1990; 30, 7: 596-608

11. Sahelian, Ray. Supplements for Parkinson's Disease? *Better Nutrition.* October 2000; Vol.62, Issue 10: p.24

Complementary Management Of Parkinson's Disease

1. Tanner CM, et al. Parkinson disease in twins: An etiologic study. JAMA 1999;281(4):341-6

2. Shults CW, Haas RH. A possible role of coenzyme Q10 in the etiology and treatment of Parkinson's disease. Biofactors 1999;9(2-4):p267

3. Karstaedt PJ, Pincus JH. Protein redistribution diet remains effective in patients with fluctuating parkinsonism. Arch Neurol 1992;49:149–51

4. Carter JH, Nutt JG, Woodward WR, et al. Amount and distribution of dietary protein affects clinical response to levodopa in Parkinson's disease. Neurology 1989;39:552–6

5. Pincus JH, Barry KM, Dietary method for reducing fluctuations in Parkinson's disease. Yale J Biol Med 1987;60:133–7

6. Healthnotes Online 2002. healthnotes, Inc.

7. Kromhout D, Menotti A, Bloemberg B, et al. Dietary saturated and trans fatty acids and cholesterol and 25-year mortality from coronary heart disease: the Seven Countries Study. Prev Med 1995;24:308–15

8. Tell GS, Evans GW, Folsom AR, et al. Dietary fat intake and carotid artery wall thickness: the Atherosclerosis Risk in Communities (ARIC) study.Am J Epidemiol 1994;139:979–89

9. Ornish D, Brown SE, Scherwitz LW, et al. Can lifestyle changes reverse coronary heart disease? The Lifestyle Heart Trial. Lancet 1990;336:129–33

10. Burgess JR, et al. Long-chain polyunsaturated fatty acids in children with attention-deficit hyperactivity disorder. Am J Clin Nutr, Jan2000;71(1Suppl):327S-30S

11. Voigt RG, Llorente AM, Jensen CL, et al. A randomized, double-blind, placebo-controlled trial of docosahexaenoic acid supplementation in children with attention-deficit/hyperactivity disorder. J Pediatr. Aug2001;139(2):189-96

12. Laugharne J, et al. Fatty Acids and Schizophrenia. Lipids. 1996(Suppl.);31-S-163 - S-165

13. Peet M, Laugharne JD, Mellor J, Ramchand CN. Essential fatty acid deficiency in erythrocyte membranes from chronic schizophrenic patients, and the clinical effects of dietary supplementation. Prostaglandins Leukot Essent Fatty Acids. Aug1996;55(1-2):71-5

14. Stoll AL, et al. Omega 3 fatty acids in bipolar disorder; A preliminary double-blind, placebo-controlled trial. Archives of General Psychiatry. May 1999;66:407-412

15. Kahlamani L, et al. Dietary factors in relation to rheumatoid arthritis. A role for olive oil and cooked vegetables. Am J Clin Nutr 1999;70(6):1077-82

16. Rivieire S, et al. Low plasma vitamin C in Alzheimer patients despite an adequate diet. Int J Geriatr Psychiatry, Nov1998;13(11):749-54

17. Shults CW, et al. Effects of Coenzyme Q10 in early Parkinson Disease. Archives of Neurology, Oct2002;59(10):1541-1550
18. Wright JV. Interview: Alzheimer's, Parkinson's, NADH research. Jorg Birkmayer, M.D. Nutr Healing 1997;May:5–6
19. Dizdar N, Kagedal B, Lindvall B. Treatment of Parkinson's disease with NADH. Acta Neurologica Scand 1994;90:345–7
20. Fahn S. A pilot trial of high-dose alpha-tocopherol and ascorbate in early Parkinson's disease. Ann Neurol 1992;32:S128–32
21. Riekkinen P, Rinne UK, Pelliniemi TT, Sonninen V. Interaction between dopamine and phospholipids. Studies of the substantia nigra in Parkinson disease patients. Arch Neurol 1975;32:25–7
22. Funfgeld EW, Baggen M, Nedwidek P, et al. Double-blind study with phosphatidylserine (PS) in parkinsonian patients with senile dementia of Alzheimer's type (SDAT). Prog Clin Biol Res 1989;317:1235–46
23. Kinsella JE, et al. Dietary n-3 polyunsaturated patty acids and amelioration of cardiovascular disease: possible mechanisms. Am J Clin Nutr, Jul1990;52(1):1-28
24. Sato Y, Kikuyama M, Oizumi K. High prevalence of vitamin D deficiency and reduced bone mass in Parkinson's disease. Neurology 1997;49:1273–8
25. Baker AB. Treatment of paralysis agitans with vitamin B6. JAMA 1941;116:2484
26. Mars H. Metabolic interactions of pyridoxine, levodopa, and carbidopa in Parkinson's disease. Trans Am Neurol Assoc 1973;98:241–5
27. Bender DA, Earl CJ, Lees AJ. Niacin depletion in Parkinsonian patients treated with L-dopa, benserizide and carbidopa. Clin Sci 1979;56:89–93

Learning Disorders

1. Dietary Supplement Information Bureau. Jan. 30, 2002. New hope for children with learning disabilities
2. Mitchell EA, Aman MG, Turbott SH, Manku M. Clinical characteristics and serum essential fatty acid levels in hyperactive children. Clin Pediatr 1987;26:406–11
3. Stevens LJ, Zentall SS, Deck JL, et al. Essential fatty acid metabolism in boys with attention-deficit hyperactivity disorder. Am J Clin Nutr 1995; 62:761–8
4. Aman MG, Mitchell EA, Turbott SH. The effects of essential fatty acid supplementation by Efamol in hyperactive children. J Abnorm Child Psychol 1987;15:75–90
5. Birch EE, et al. A randomized controlled trial of early dietary supply of long-chain polyunsaturated fatty acids and mental development in term infants. Dev Med Child Neur. 2000;(42):174-181
6. Jorgensen MH, Hernell O, Hughes E, Michaelsen KF. Is there a relation between docosahexaenoic acid concentration in mothers' milk and visual development in term infants? J Pediatr Gastroenterol Nutr. Mar2001;32(3):293-6
7. Willatts P, Forsyth JS, DiModugno MK, et al. Effect of long-chain polyunsaturated fatty acids in infant formula on problem solving at 10 months of age. Lancet. Aug1998;352(9129):688-91
8. Uauy R, Mena P. Requirements for long-chain polyunsaturated fatty acids in the preterm infant. Curr Opin Pediatr. Apr1999;11(2):115-20

Nutritional Factors That Enhance Detoxification

1. S C Rackett et al, Diet and dermatology: the role of dietary manipulation in the prevention and treatment of cutaneous disorders. J Am Acad Dermatol;29 (3) 447-61 (1993)
2. P Lam, Defining healthy aging. Skin inc; 13 (7) 38-44 (July 2001)

3. M Murray and J Pizzorno, Encyclopedia of natural medicine (revised 2nd edition), Prima Health (pub), 1998

4. D Horrobin (ed.) Omega-6 essential fatty acids: pathophysiology and roles in clinical medicine. Wiley-Liss (pub.), New York, new York (1990)

5. Eberlein-Konig et al, Protective effect against sunburn of combine systemic ascorbic acid and d-alphatocopherol. J Am Acad Dermatology; 38 (1) 45-8 (1998)

6. M Akiyama et al, Arteriovenous haemangroma in chronic liver disease: clinical and histopathological features of four cases. Br J Dermatol; 144: 604-609 (2001)

7. Y Takagi et al, Coexistence of psoriasis and linear IgA bullous dermatosis. Br J Dermatol; 142: 513-516 (2001)

8. E Rosenberg et al, Microbiol factors in psoriasis. Arch Dermatol; 118: 1434-1444 (1982)

9. G Weber et al, The liver as a therapeutic target in dermatoses. Med Weltz; 34: 108-111 (1983)

10. S Bittiner et al, A double-blind randomized placebo-controlled trial of fish oil in psoriasis. Lancet; 1: 378- 380 (1988)

11. J Pizzorno, total wellness. Prima Publishing (pub) 1996; Chpt Decreasing toxicity: 87-162

12. M Murray and J Pizzorno, Encylcopedia of natural medicine. Prima health (pub) 1998. Chpt Detoxification: 104-125

13. G Michaelson et al, Erythrocyte glutathione peroxidase activity in acne vulgaris and the effect of selenium and vitamin E treatment. Acta Derm Venerol; 64: 9-14 (1984)

14. B Snider et al, Pyridoxine therapy for premenstrual acne flare. Arch Dermatol; 110: 103-111 (1974)

15. T Callaghan, The effect of folic acid on seborrheic dermatitis, Cutis; 3: 584-588 (1967)

16. G Andrews et al, Seborrheic dermatitis: supplemental treatment with vitamin B12, NY State J med; 1921- 1925 (1950)

17. A Nisenson, Treatment of seborrheic dermatitis with biotin and vitamin B complex, J Ped; 81: 630-631 (1972)

18. J Savolainen et al, Candida albicans and atopic dermatitis. Clin Exp Allergy; 23: 332-339 (1993)

19. H Majarmaa et al, Probiotics: a novel approach in the management of food allergy. J Allergy Clin Immunol; 99: 179-186 (1997)

20. E Isolauri et al, Probiotics: effects on immunity. Am J Clin Nutr; 73 (suppl): 444-450 (2001)

21. P Belew et al, Endotoxemia in psoriasis, Arch Dermatol; 118: 142-143 (1982)

22. R Skinner et al, Improvement of psoriasis with cholestyramine. Arch Dermatol; 118: 144 (1982)

23. F Thurman, The treatment of psoriasis with sarsparilla compound. N Engl J med; 227: 128-133 (1942)

24. J Schrezenmeir et al, Probiotics, prebiotics, and synbiotics – approaching a definition. Am J Clin Nutr; 73 (suppl): 361-364 (2001)

25. J Madara et al, Structure and function of the intestinal epithelial barrier in health and disease. Gastroenterol Pathol; 9: 306-432 (1990)

26. J Wallace, Pathogenesis of nonsteroidal anti-inflammatory drug gastropathy: recent advances. Eur J Gastro Hepatol; 5: 403-407 (1993)

27. B Crotty, Ulcerative colitis and xenbiotic metabolism. Lancet; 343: 35-38 (1994)

28. D Hollander et al, Aging-associated increase in intestinal absorption of macromolecules. Gerontology; 31: 133-137

29. D Burkitt et al, Effects of dietary fiber on stools and transit time and its role in the causation of disease. Lancet; 11: 1408-1412 (1972)

Antioxidants That Prevent Macular Degeneration

1. Jampol, L.M., et al. Age-Related Eye Disease Study Research Group (collective name-AREDS). A randomized, placebo-controlled, clinical trial of high-dose supplementation with vitamins C and E, betacarotene, and zinc for age-related macular degeneration and vision loss: AREDS report no.8. Arch Ophthalmol 2001 Oct; 119 (10): 1417-36
2. Murray, M. and Pizzorno, J. Encyclopedia of Natural Medicine (2nd edit) Prima Health 1998: 319-324
3. West, S., et al. Are antioxidants or supplements protective of age-related macular degeneration? Arch Ophthalmol. 1994. 112: 222-227
4. Eye Disease Case-Control Study Group. Antioxidant status and neovascular age-related macular degeneration. Arch Ophthalmol. 1993, 111: 104-109
5. Patient Risk Factors; Antioxidants and Maculopathy. Nurses" Drug Alert 23, 1999; 6: 45
6. Olson, R. J. Supplemental antioxidant vitamins and minerals in patients with macular degeneration. J Am Coll Nutr, 1991; 10: 550/Abstract 52
7. Newsome, D.A., et al. oral zinc in macular degeneration. Arch Ophthalmol. 1988; 106: 192-198
8. Halliwell, B., and Gutteridge, J. Free Radicals in Biology and Medicine (2nd edit.), Oxford University Press, 1991; 218-266
9. Stur, M., et al. Oral zinc and the second eye in age-related macular degeneration. Invest Ophthalmol. 1996, 37: 1225-1235
10. Hammond, Jr., B.R. et al. Density of the human crystalline lens is related to the macular pigment carotenoids, lutein and zeaxanthin. Optom Vis Sci., 1997; 74; 7: 499-504
11. Landrum, J.T., et al. The macular pigment: A possible role in protection from age-related macular degeneration. Adv Pharmacol, 1997; 38: 537-556
12. Landrum, J.T. et al. Macular pigment stereomers in individual eyes. Invest Ophthalmol Vis Sci. 1995; 38: 1795-1801
13. Hammond, B.R., et al. Dietary modification of human macular pigment density. Invest Ophthalmol Vis Sci, 1997; 38: 1795-1801
14. Seddon, J.M., et al. Dietary Carotenoids, Vitamin A, C, and E and advanced age-related macular degeneration. JAMA 1994; 272: 1413-1420
15. Dagnelie, G., et al. Lutein improves visual function in some patients with retinal degeneration: a pilot study via the Internet. Optometry 2000, 71; 3: 147-164Seddon, J.M., et al. Dietary Carotenoids, Vitamin A, C, and E and advanced age-related macular degeneration. JAMA 1994; 272: 1413-1420
16. Seddon, J.M., et al. Dietary Carotenoids, Vitamin A, C, and E and advanced age-related macular degeneration. JAMA 1994; 272: 1413-1420
17. Mares-Perlmen, J.A., et al. Serum antioxidants and age-related macular degeneration in a populationbased case control study. Arch Ophthalmol, 1988; 113: 1518-1523
18. Young, R.W., Solar radiation and age-related macular degeneration. Surv Ophthalmol 1988; 32: 252-59
19. Katz, M.L., Parker, K.R., Handelman, G.J., et al. Effects of antioxidant nutrient deficiency on the retina and retinal pigment epithelium of albino rats a light and electron microscopic study. Exp Eye Res 1982; 34: 339-59
20. Scharrer, A., et al. Anthocyanosides in the treatment of retinopathies. Klin Monatsbl Augenheilked. 1981; 178: 386-389
21. Caselli, L., et al. Clinical electro-retinographic study on the activity of anthocyanosides. Arch Med Int. 1985; 37: 29-35
22. Lebuisson, D.A., et al. Treatment of senile macular degeneration with ginkgo biloba extract: A preliminary double-blind versus placebo study. Presse Med. 1986; 15: 1556-1558

23. Corbe, C., et al. Light vision and Chorioretinal circulation: Study of the effect of procyanidolic oligomers. J Fr Ophthalmol, 1988; 11: 453-460
24. Wegmann, R., et al. Effects of anthocyanosides on photoreceptors: Cytoenzymatic aspects. Ann Histochim 1969, 14: 237-256
25. Murray, M. The Healing Power of Herbs (2nd edit). Prima Publishing, 1995: 50-59
26. DeFeudis, F.V., (ed.). Ginkgo biloba extract (Egb-761): Pharmacological Activities and Clinical Applications. Elsevier, Paris; 1991
27. Soyeux, A., et al. Endotelon: Diabetic retinopathy and hemorrheaology (preliminary study) Bull Soc Ophthalmol Fr., 1987; 87: 1441-1444
28. Proto, F., et al. Electrophysical study of Vitis Vinifera procyanoside oligomers effects on retinal function in myopic subjects. Ann OH Clin Ocul. 1988; 11: 453-460
29. Murray, M., and Pizzorno, J. Encyclopedia of Natural Medicine, 2nd edition. (Prima Publishing) 1998: 319-24
30. Varma, S., Scientific basis for medical therapy of cataracts by antioxidants. Am J Clin Nutr. 1991, 53; 1:335-345 (suppl)
31. Robertson, J., et al. A possible role for Vitamin C and E in cataract prevention. Am J Clin Nutr. 1991, 53; 1:346-351 (suppl)
32. Bouton, S., et al. Vitamin C and the aging eye. Arch Int Med, 1939; 63: 930-945
33. Atkinson, D., Malnutrition as an etiological factor in senile cataract. EENT Monthly, 1952, 31: 79-83
34. Ringwold, A., et al. Senile cataract and ascorbic acid loading. Acta Opthalmol. 1985; 63: 277-280
35. Jacques, P.F., et al. Epidemiologic evidence of a role for the antioxidant vitamins and carotenoids in cataract prevention. Am J Clin Nutr 1991, 53; 1:352-355 (suppl)
36. Robertson, J., et al. A possible role for vitamin C and E in cataract prevention. Am J Clin Nutr 1991, 53; 1:346-351 (suppl)
37. Lyle, B.J., et al. Antioxidant intake and risk of incident age-related nuclear cataracts in the Beaver Dam study. Am J Epidemiol. 1999, 149: 801-809
38. Rouhiainen, P., et al. Association between low plasma Vitamin E concentration and progression of early cortical lens opacities. Am J Epidemiol. 1996, 144: 496-500
39. Teikari, J.M., et al. Long-term supplementation with alpha-tocopherol and beta-carotene and age-related cataract. Acta Ophthalmol Scan, 1997; 75:634-640
40. Lyle, B.J., et al. Antioxidant intake and risk of incident age-related nuclear cataracts in the Beaver Dam study. Am J Epidemiol. 1999, 149: 801-809
41. Jacques, P.F., et al. Epidemiologic evidence of a role for the antioxidant vitamins and carotenoids in cataracts prevention. Am J Clin Nutr 1991, 53;1: 352-355 (suppl)
42. Chasen-Taber, L, et al. A prospective study of carotenoid and vitamin A intakes and risk of cataract extraction in U.S. women. Am J Clin Nutr 1999, 70; 4: 509-516
43. Brown, L., et al. A prospective study of carotenoid intake and risk of cataract extraction in U.S. men. Am J Clin Nutr. 1999, 70; 4: 517-524
44. Reiter, R.J., et al. Oxygen radical detoxification process during aging: The functional importance of melatonin. Aging Clinical Exp Res, 1995; 7: 340-351
45. Chaundry, P.S., et al. Inhibition of human lens aldose reductase by flavonoids, sulindac and indomethacin. Biochem Pharmacol 1983, 32; 1995-1998

Grape Seed Extract

1. Schwitters B, Masquelier J. OPC in Practice: Biflavanols and their Applications. Rome, Italy: Alfa,Omega; 1993.
2. Murray M. The Healing Power of Herbs. 2nd edition. Rocklin, CA: Prima Publishing; 1995. p. 184-91.

3. Henriet JP. Veno-lymphatic insufficiency. Phlebologie 1993;46:313-25.
4. Lagrue G, Oliver-Martin F, Grillot A. A study of the effects of procyanidolic oligomers on capillary resistance in hypertension and in certain nephropathies. Sem Hosp Paris 1981;57:1399-401.
5. Gomez Trillo JT. Varicose veins of the lower extremities:symptomatic treatment with a new vasculotrophic agent. Prensa Med Mex, 1973;38:293-6.
6. Soyeux A, et al. Endotelon: Diabetic retinopathy and hemorrheology (preliminary study). Bull Soc Ophthalmol Fr 1987;87:14441-4
7. Proto F, et al. Electrophysical study of vitis vinefera procyanoside oligomers effects on retinal function in myopic subjects. Ann OH Clin Ocul 1988;114:85-93.
8. Corbe C, Boissin JP, Siou A. Light vision and chorioretinal circulation: study of the effect of procyanidolic oligomers (Endotelon). J Fr Ophthalmol 1988;11:453-60.
9. Boissin JP, Corbe C, Siou A. Chorioretinal circulation and dazzling: use of procyanidol oligomers. Bull Soc Ophthalmol Fr 1988;88:173-4,177-9.
10. Masquelier J, Dumon MC, Dumas J. Stabilization of collagen by procyanidolic oligomers. Acta Therap 1981;7:101-5.
11. Tixier JM, Godeau G, Robert AM, Hornebeck W. Evidence by in vivo and in vitro studies that binding to pycnogenols to elastin affects its rate of degradation by elastases. Biochem Pharmocol 1984;33(24):3933-9.
12. Maffei F, Facino R, Carinin M, et al. Free radicals scavenging action and anti-enzyme activities of procyanidines from Vitis vinefera. Arzniem Forsch 1994;44:592-601.
13. Murray M. Encyclopedia of Nutritional Supplements. Rocklin, CA: Prima Publishing; 1996. p. 320-31.

Lipoic Acid

1. Murray M. Encyclopedia of Nutritional Supplements. Rocklin, CA: Prima Publishing; 1996. p. 343-6.
2. Kagan VE, Shvedova A, Serbinova E, Khan S, Swanson C, Powell R, et al. Dihydrolipoic acid-A universal antioxidant both in the membrane and in the aqueous phase. Reduction of peroxyl, ascorbyl and chromanoxyl radicals. Biochem Pharmacol 1992;44:1637-49.
3. Barbiroli B, Medori R, Tritschler HJ, Klopstock T, Seibel P, Reichmann H, et al. Lipoic (thioctic) acid increases brain energy availability and skeletal muscle performance as shown by in vivo 31P-MRS in a patient with mitochondrial cytopathy. J Neurol. 1995;242:472-7.
4. Packer L. Antioxidant properties of lipoic acid and its therapeutic effects in prevention of diabetes complications and cataracts. Annals NY Acad Sci 1994;738:257-64.
5. Kahler W, Kuklinski B, Ruhlmann C, Plotz C. Diabetes mellitus: a free radical-associated disease. Results of adjuvant antioxidant supplementation. Z Gesamte Inn Med 1993;48(5):223-32.
6. Nagamatsu M, Nickander KK, Schmelzer JD. Lipoic acid improves nerve blood flow, reduces oxidative stress, and improves distal nerve conduction in experimental diabetic neuropathy. Diabetic Care 1995;18:1160-7.
7. Jacob S, Henriksen EJ, Schiemann AL, Simon I, Clancy DE, Tritschler HJ, et al. Enhancement of glucose disposal in patients with type 2 diabetes by alpha-lipoic acid. Arzneim Forsch 1995;45(8):872-4.
8. Kawabata T, Packer L. Alpha-lipoate can protect against glycation of serum albumin, but not low density lipoprotein. Biochem Biophys Res Comm 1994;203,99-104.
9. Suzuki YJ, Tsuchiya M, Packer L. Lipoate prevents glucose-induced protein modifications. Free Rad Res Comms 1992;17:211-7.

10. Fuchs J, Schofer H, Milbradt R, et al. Studies on lipoate effect on blood redox state in human immunodeficiency virus infected patients. Arzneim Forsch 1993;43:1359-1362.
11. Baur A, Harrer T, Peukert M. Alpha-lipoic acid is an effective inhibitor of human immuno-deficiency virus (HIV-1) replication Klin Wochenschr 1991; 69:722-4.
12. Suzuki YJ, Aggarwal BB, Packer L. Alpha-lipoic acid is a potent inhibitor of NF-kB activation in human T cells. Biochem Biophys Res Comm 1992; 189:1709-15.

Bilberry

1. Kuhnau J, The flavonoids, A Class of Semi-essential Food Components: Their Role in Human Nutrition, World Rev Nutr Diet 1976;24:117-91.
2. Gabor M, Pharmacologic Effects of Flavonoids on Blood Vessels, Angiologica 1972;9:355-74.
3. Havsteen B, Flavonoids, A Class of Natural Products of High Pharmacological Potency, Biochem Pharmacol 1983;32:1141-8.
4. Monboisse JC, et. al. Non-enzymatic Degradation of Acid Soluble Calf Skin Collagen by Superoxide Ion: Protective Effect of Flavonoids, Biochem Pharmacol 1983;32:53-8.
5. Monboisse JC, Braquet P, Borel JP. Oxygen-free Radicals as Mediators of Collagen Breakage. Agents Actions 1984;15:49-50.
6. Rao CN, Rai VH, And Steinman B, Influence of Bioflavonoids on the Collagen Metabolism in Rats with Adjuvant Induced Arthritis. Ital J Biochem 1981;30:54-62.
7. Ronziere MC, et. al., Influence of Some Flavonoids on Reticulation of Collagen Fibrils in Vitro. Biochem Pharmacol 1981;30:771-6.
8. Middleton E, The Flavonoids, Trends Pharm Sci 1984;5:335-8.
9. Amella M, et. al., Inhibition of Mass Cell Histamine Release by Flavonoids and Bioflavonoids. Planta Medica 1985;51:16-20.
Jonadet M, et. al., Anthocyanosides Extracted from Vitis Vinifera, Vaccinium Myrtillus and Pinus Maritimus, I. Elastese-inhibiting Activities in Vitro, II. Compared Angioprotective Activities in Vivo, J Pharm Belg 1983;38:41-6.
10. Detre A, et. al., Studies on Vascular Permeability in Hypertension: Action of Anthocyanosides. Clin Physiol Biochem 1986;4:143-9.
11. Sujet Normal Therapie 1964;19:171-85.
12. Terrasse J and Moinade S, Premiers Resultats Obtenus Avec un Nouveau Facteur Vitaminique P "les Anthocyanosides" Extraits du Vaccinium Myrtillus, Presse Med 1964;72:397-400.
13. Sala D, Rolando M, Rossi PL and Pissarello L, Effects of Anthocyanosides on Visual Performances at Low Illumination. Minerva Oftalmol 21, 283-285, 1979. Gloria E and Peria A, Effect of Anthocyanosides on the Absolute Visual Threshold, Ann Ottalmol Clin Ocul 1966;92:595-607.
14. Junemann G, On the Effect of Anthocyanosides on Hemeralopia Following Quinine Poisoning. Klin Monatsbl Augenheilkd 1967;151:891-6.
15. Caselli L, Clinical and Electroretinographic Study on Activity of Anthocyanosides. Arch Med Int 1985;37:29-35.
16. Wegman R, Maeda K, Troche P, and Bastide P. Effects of Anthocyanosides on Photoreceptors, Cytoenzymatic Aspects. Ann Histochim 1969; 14:237-56.
17. Bravetti G, Preventive Medical Treatment of Senile Cataract with Vitamin E and Anthocyanosides: Clinical Evaluation. Ann Ottalmol Clin Ocul 1989;115:109.
18. Scharrer A and Ober M, Anthocyanosides in the Treatment of Retinopathies. Klin Monatsbl Augenheilkd 1981;178:386-9.

19. Mian E, et.al., Anthocyanosides and the Walls of Microvessels, Further Aspects of the Mechanism in the Action of their Protective Effect in Syndromes due to Abnormal Capillary Fragility. Minerva Med 1977;68:3565-81.

20. Ghiringhelli G, Gregoratti F, and Marastoni F, Capillarotropic Activity of the Anthocyanosides in High Doses in Phlebopathis Stasis. Min Cardioangiol 1978;26:255-76.

21. Murray MT, The Healing Power of Herbs (2nd edition), Prima Publishing, 1995.

22. Dietary Supplement Information Bureau. www.content.intramedicine.com: Bilberry

23. Jayle GE, et al. Study concerning the action of athocyanoside extracts of Vaccinium myrtillus on nightvision. Ann Occul Paris. 1965; 198 (6): 556-62.

24. Moranzonni P, et al. Vaccinium myrtillus. Fitoterapia. 1996; vol LXVII (1): 3-29

Horsechestnut Seed

1. Mills S, Bone K. Principles and Practice of phytotherapy. Churchill Livingstone 2000;Horsechestnutseed:448-55

2. Schulz V et al. Rational Phytotherapy. Berlin:Springer-Verlag;1998:129-38

3. Chandler RF. Horse chestnut. Canadian Pharm J 1993;Jul/Aug:297-300

4. Dinsdale, M. Horse Chestnut. Better Nutriiton, Feb2000;62(2):32

5. Guillaume M, Padioleau F. Venotonic effect, vascular protection, anti-inflammatory and free radical scavenging properties of horse chestnut extract. Arzneim-Forsch Drug Res 1994;44:25-35

6. Sirtori, CR. Aescin: pharmacology, pharmacokinetics and therapeutic profile. Pharmacol Res 2001 Sep;44(3):183-93

7. Herbal Help for Tired Swollen Legs. Environmental Nutrition, Jun2001;24(6):p7

8. Brunner F, Hoffmann C, Schuller-Petrovic S. Responsivemenss of human varicose saphenous veins to vasoactive agents. Br J Clin Pharmacol 2001 Mar;51(3):219-24

9. Bone, Kerry. Phytotherapy Review & Commentary: Horse-chestnut—A safe and effective vein treatment. Townsend Letter for Doctors & Patients, May2000;202:p152

10. Pittler, MH, Ernst E. Horse chestnut seed extract for chronic venous insufficiency. Cochrane Database Syst Rev 2002;(1):pp.CD003230

11. Pittler MH, Ernst E. Horse-chestnut seed extract for chronic venous insufficiency. A criteria-based systematic review. Arch Dermatol 1998 Nov; 134(11):1356-60

12. Morien, K. Horse Chestnut Effective in Chronic Venous Insufficiency. HerbalGram, Winter 99;45:p22

13. Koch R. Comparative study of Venostasin and Pycnogenol in chronic venous insufficiency. Phytotherapy Res 2002 Mar;12(Suppl 1):S1-5

14. Rothkopf M, et al. New findings on the efficacy and mode of action of the horse chestnut saponins escin. Arzneim-Forsch/Drug Res 1976;26 (2):225-35

15. **Guillaume M et al. Veinotonic effect, vascular protection, anti-inflammatory and free radical scavenging properties of horse chestnut extract. Arzneim-Forsch/Drug Res 1994;44(1):25-35

16. Tyler, VE. Herbs of Choice: The Terapeutic Use of Phytomedicinals. Binghampton, NY; Pharmaceutical Products Press, 1994:112-3

17. Blumental M, Busse WR, Goldberg A et al. (eds.) The Complete Commission E Monographs: Therapeutic Guide to Herbal Medicines. Boston, MA: Integrative Medicine Communications, 1988:148-9

18. Hellberg K, Ruschewski W, de Vivie R. Medikamentoes bedingtes post-operatives Nierenversagen nach herzchirugischen. Eingriffen. Thoraxchirurgie 1975;23:396-9

19. Wilhelm K, Feldmeier C. Postoperative und posttraumatische Oedemprophylaxe und-therapie. Laborchemische Untersuchungen ueber die Nierenvertraeglichkeit von beta-Aescin. Med Klin 1975;70:2079-83

20. Newall CA, et al. Herbal Medicines: A Guide for Health Care Professionals. London: The Pharmaceutical Press 1996:166-7

21. Heck AM et al. Potential interactions between alternative therapies and warfarin. Am J health Syst Pharm, Jul2000;57(13):1221-7

22. Heck AM, DeWitt BA, Lukes AL. Am J Helath Syst Pharm 2000 Jul 1;57(13):p1221-7;Quiz p1228-30

23. Akopov SE et al. Mechanisms of platelet-induced angioplastic reactions: Potentiation of calcium sensitivity. Can J Physiol Pharmacol. Jul 1997;75(7):849-52

24. Dworschak E et al. Medical activities of aesculus hippocastaneum (Horse-chestnut) Saponins. Adv Exp Med Biol 1996;404:471-4

Green Tea

Benzie IF, Szeto YT, Strain JJ, Tomlinson B. Consumption of green tea causes rapid increase in plasma antioxidant power in humans. Nutr Cancer 1999;34:83–7

Blot WJ, Chow WH, and McLaughlin, JK: Tea and cancer: a review of the epidemiological evidence. Eur J Cancer Prev 1996;5:425-438

Bushman JL. Green Tea and Cancer in Humans: A Review of the Literature.. Nutrition and Cancer 1998;31(3):151-159

Chung FL, Morse MA, Eklind KI, Xu Y. Inhibition of the tobacco-specific nitrosamine-induced lung tumorigenesis by compounds derived from cruciferous vegetables and green tea. Ann NY Acad Sci 1993;686:186-202

Fujiki H, Suganuma M, Okabe S, Komori A, Sueoka E, et al. Japanese green tea as a cancer preventive in humans. Nutr Rev 1996;54:S67-S70

Gensler HL, Timmermann BN, Valcic S, Wachter GA, Dorr R, et al. Prevention of photocarcinogenesis by topical administration of pure epigallocatechin gallate isolated from green tea. Nutr Cancer 1996;26:325-335

Graham HN. Green tea composition, consumption, and polyphenol chemistry. Prev Med 1992;21:334–50

International Agency for Research on Cancer. Coffee, Tea, Matè, Methylxanthines, and Methylgloxyal. 1990 Lyon , France: Int Agency Res Cancer 1991:207-271. (IARC Monogr 51)

Khan SG, Katiyar SK, Agarwal R, Mukhtar H. Enhancement of antioxidant and phase II enzymes by oral feeding of green tea polyphenols in drinking water to SKH-1 hairless mice: possible role in cancer chemoprevention. Cancer Res 1992;52:4050-4052

Komori A, Yatsunami J, Okabe S, Abe S, Hara K, et al. Anticarcinogenic activity of green tea polyphenols. Jpn J Clin Oncol 1993;23:186-190

Kono S, Shinchi K, Ikeda N, et al. Green tea consumption and serum lipid profiles: A cross-sectional study in Northern Kyushu, Japan. Prev Med 1992;21:526–31

La Vecchia C, Negri E, D'Avanzo B, Franceschi S: Food temperature gastric cancer. Int J Cancer 46, 432-434

Mukhtar H, Katiyar SK, Agarwal R. Green tea and skin – anticarcinogenic effects. J Invest Dermatol 1994;102:3-7

Sagesaka-Mitane Y, Milwa M, Okada S. Platelet aggregation inhibitors in hot water extract of green tea. Chem Pharm Bull 1990;38:790–3

Sasazuki S, Komdama H, Yoshimasu K, et al. Relation between green tea consumption and severity of coronary atherosclerosis among Japanese men and women. Ann Epidemiol 2000;10:401–8

Serafini M, Ghiselli A, Ferro-Luzzi A. In vivo antioxidant effect of green tea in man. Eur J Clin Nutr 1996;50:28–32

Stensvold I, Tverdal A, Solvoll K, et al. Tea consumption. Relationship to cholesterol, blood pressure, and coronary and total mortality. Prev Med 1992;21:546–53

Stoner G, Mukhtar H. Polyphenols as cancer chemopreventive agents. J Cell Biochem 1995; 22:169-180

Tsubono Y, Tsugane S. Green tea intake in relation to serum lipid levels in middle-aged Japanese men and women. Ann Epidemiol 1997;7:280–4

Valcic S, Timmermann BN, Alberts DS, Wachter GA, Krutzsch M, et al. Inhibitory effect of six green tea catechins and caffeine on the growth of four selected human tumor cell lines. Anticancer Drugs 1996;7:461-468

Yamaguchi Y, Hayashi M, Yamazoe H, et al. Preventive effects of green tea extract on lipid abnormalities in serum, liver and aorta of mice fed an atherogenic diet. Nip Yak Zas 1991;97:329–37

Yu G, Hsieh C, Wang L, Yu S, Liu X, et al. Green tea consumption and risk of stomach cancer: a populationbased case-control study in Shanghai, China. Cancer Causes Control 1995;6:532-538

Detoxification and Immune Function After 40
Reishi MushroomExtract

American Herbal Products Association. Use of Marker Compounds in Manufacturing and Labeling Botanically Derived Dietary Supplements. Silver Spring, MD: American Herbal Products Association; 2001 el-Mekkawy S, et al. Anti-HIV-1 and Anti-HIV-1-protease Substances from Ganoderma lucidum. Phytochemistry. 1998 Nov;49(6):1651-57

Eo SK, et al. Antiherpetic Activities of Various Protein Bound Polysaccharides Isolated from Ganoderma lucidum. J Ethnopharmacol. 1999 Dec;68(1-3):175-81

Hijikata Y, et al. Effect of Ganoderma lucidum on Postherpetic Neuralgia. Am J Chin Med. 1998;26(3-4):375-81 Hikino H, et al. Mechanisms of Hypoglycemic Activity of Ganoderan B: A Glycan of Ganoderma lucidum Fruit Bodies. Planta Med. 1999 Oct;55(5):423-28

Horner WE, et al. Basidiomycete Allergens: Comparison of Three Ganoderma Species. Allergy. 1993 Feb;48(2):110-16

Jong SC, et al. Medicinal Benefits of the Mushroom Ganoderma. Adv Appl Microbiol. 1992;37:101-34

Kanmatsuse K, et al. Studies on Ganoderma lucidum. I. Efficacy Against Hypertension and Side Effects. Yakugaku Zasshi. 1985 Oct;105(10):942-47

Lee SY. Cardiovascular Effects of Mycelium Extract of Ganoderma lucidum: Inhibition of Sympathetic Outflow as a Mechanism of Its Hypotensive Action. Chem Pharm Bull.(Tokyo). 1990 May; 38(5):1359-64

Lin JM, et al. Radical Scavenger and Antihepatotoxic Activity of Ganoderma formosanum, Ganoderma lucidum and Ganoderma neo-japonicum. J Ethnopharmacol. 1995 Jun;47(1):33-41

McGuffin M ed, et al. Botanical Safety Handbook. Boca Raton: CRC Press; 1997:55.

Sone Y, et al. Structures and Antitumor Activities of the Polysaccharides Isolated from Fruiting Body and the Growing Culture of Mycelium of Ganoderma lucidum. Agr Biol Chem. 1985;49:2641-53

Su C. Potentiation of ganodermic acid S on prostaglandin E(1)-induced cyclic AMP elevation in human platelets. Thromb Res. 2000 Jul;99(2):135-45

Teow SS. Effective Dosage of Ganoderma Nutriceuticals in the Treatment of Various Ailments. in: 1996 Taipei International Ganoderma Research Conference. Abstracts: Taipei International Convention Center. Taipei, Taiwan. 1996 Aug Wang SY. The Anti-tumor Effect of Ganoderma lucidum is Mediated by Cytokines Released From Activated Macrophages and T Lymphocytes. Int J Cancer. May1997;70(6):699-705

Yun TK. Trial of a New Medium-term Model Using Benzo(a)pyrene Induced Lung Tumor in Newborn Mice. Anticancer Res. May1995;15(3):839-45

Astragalus

American Herbal Products Association. Use of Marker Compounds in Manufacturing and Labeling Botanically Derived Dietary Supplements. Silver Spring, MD: American Herbal Products Association; 2001

Chen LX, Liao JX, Guo WQ. Effects of Astragalus membranaceus on Left Ventricular Function and Oxygen Free Radical in Acute Myocardial Infarction Patients and Mechanism of Its Cardiotonic Action. Chung Kuo Chung Hsi I Chieh Ho Tsa Chih. 1995 Mar;15(3):141-3

Geng CS, et al. Advances in Immuno-pharmacological Studies on Astragalus membranaceus. Chung Hsi I Chieh Ho Tsa Chih. 1986;6(1):62-64

Geng CS, et al. Advances in Immuno-pharmacological Studies on Astragalus membranaceus. Chin J Integ Trad West Med. 1986;6:62

Griga IV. Effect of a Summary Preparation of Astragalus cicer on the Blood Pressure of Rats with Renal Hypertension and on the Oxygen Consumption by the Tissues. Farm Zh. 1977;6:64-66

Lei ZY, Qin H, Liao JZ. Action of Astragalus membranaceus on Left Ventricular Function of Angina Pectoris. Chung Kuo Chung Hsi I Chieh Ho Tsa Chih. Apr1994;14(4):199-202,195

Leung A, et al. Encyclopedia of Common Natural Ingredients Used in Foods, Drugs, and Cosmetics. New York: Wiley-Interscience Publication; 1996:50-53.

PDR for Herbal Medicines, 2nd edition. Montvale, NJ: Medical Economics Company; 2000:56

Shi HM, et al. Intervention of Lidocaine and Astragalus membranaceus on Ventricular Late Potentials. Zhongguo Zhong Xi Yi Jie He Za Zhi. 1994 Oct;14(10):598-600

Zhang YD, et al. Effects of Astragalus (ASI, SK) on Experimental Liver Injury. Yao Hsueh Hsueh Pao. 1992;27(6):401-06

Milk Thistle

American Herbal Products Association. Use of Marker Compounds in Manufacturing and Labeling Botanically Derived Dietary Supplements. Silver Spring, MD: American Herbal Products Association; 2001

Carrescia O, et al. Silymarin in the Prevention of Hepatic Damage by Psychopharmacologic Drugs. Experimental Premises and Clinical Evaluations. Clin Ter. 1980;95(2):157-64.

Dehpour AR, et al. Liquorice Components Protect Liver Damage Induced by Actaminophen. Poster Presentation, 48th Annual Meeting of the International Congress of the Society of Medicinal Plant Research, P2A/23. 2000 Sep PDR for Herbal Medicines, 2nd edition. Montvale, NJ: Medical Economics Company; 2000:518.

Schopen RD, et al. Therapy of Hepatoses. Therapeutic Use of Silymarin. Med Welt. 1969;21:691-98

Shear NH, Malkiewicz IM, Klein D, et al. Acetaminophen-induced Toxicity to Human Epidermoid Cell Line A431 and Hepatoblastoma Cell Line Hep G2, In Vitro, is Diminished by Silymarin. Skin Pharmacol. 1995;8(6):279-91

Sonnenbichler J, Scalera F, Sonnenbichler I, et al. Stimulatory Effects of Silibinin and Silicristin from the Milk Thistle Silybum marianum on Kidney Cells.J Pharmacol Exp Ther. Sep1999;290(3):1375-83.

Valenzuela A, et al. Selectivity of Silymarin on the Increase of the Glutathione Content in Different Tissues of the Rat. Planta Medica. 1989;55:1550-52.

Valenzuela A, et al. Silymarin Protection Against Hepatic Lipid Peroxidation Induced by Acute Ethanol Intoxication in the Rat. Biochem Pharm. 1985;34:2209-12

Varga M, et al. Ethanol Elimination in Man Under Influence of Hepatoprotective Silibinin. Blutalkohol. Nov1991;28(6):405-08.

Vogel G, et al. Protection by Silibinin Against Amanita Phalloides Intoxication in Beagles. Toxicol Appl Pharm. 1984;73:355-62

Indole-3-Carbinol

Barcelo S, Gardiner JM, Gescher A. Chipman JK. CYP2E1-mediated mechanism of anti-genotoxicity of the broccoli constituent sulforaphane.Carcinogenesis 1996;17:277-82

Beecher CW. Cancer preventive properties of varieties of Brassica oleracea: a review. Am J Clin Nutr 1994 May;59(5suppl):1166S-70S

Bell MC, Crowley-Nowick P, Bradlow HL, et al. Placebo-controlled trial of indole-3-carbinol in the treatment of CIN. Gynecol Oncol 2000:78;123-9

Bradfield CA, Bjeldanes LF. Effect of dietary indole-3 carbinol on intestinal and hepatic monooxygenase, gluatathione-S-Transferase and epoxide hydrolase activities in rat. Food Chem Toxicol 1984;22:977-82

Bradlow HL, Michnovicz JJ, Halper M., et al. Long-term responses of women to indole-3-carbinol or a high fiber diet. Cancer Epidemiol Biomarkers Prev 1994;3:591-5

Bradlow HL, Sepkovic DW, Telang NT, Osborne MP. Indole-3-carbinol. A novel approach to breast cancer prevention. Ann NY Acad Sci 1999;889:204-13

Bradlow HL, Sepkovic DW, Telang NT, Osborne MP. Indole-3-carbinol. A novel approach to breast cancer prevention. Ann NY Acad Sci 1995;768:180-200

Bradlow HL, Sepkovic DW, Telang NT, Osborne MP. Multifunctional aspects of the action of indole-3-carbinol as an antitumor agent. Ann NY Acad Sci 1999;889:204-13

Broadbent TA, Broadbent HS. The chemistry and pharmacology of indole-3-carbinol (indole-3-methanol) and 3-(methoxymethyl) Indole. [Part I]. Curr Med Chem 1998;5:337-52

Broadbent TA, Broadbent HS. The chemistry and pharmacology of indole-3-carbinol (indole-3-methanol) and 3-(methoxymethyl) Indole. [Part II]. Curr Med Chem 1998;5:469-91

Broadbent TA, Broadbent HS. The chemistry and pharmacology of indole-3-carbinol (indole-3-methanol) and 3-(methoxymethyl) Indole. [Part I]. Curr Med Chem 1998;5:337-52

Broadbent TA, Broadbent HS. The chemistry and pharmacology of indole-3-carbinol (indole-3-methanol) and 3-(methoxymethyl) Indole. [Part II]. Curr Med Chem 1998;5:469-91

Dhinmi SR, Li Y, Upadhyay S, Koppolu PK, Sarkar FH. Indole-3-carbinol (I3C) – induced cell growth inhibition,G1 cell cycle arrest and apoptosis in prostate cancer cells. Oncogene 24May2001;20(23):2927-36

Hecht SS. Chemoprevention of cancer by isothiocyanates, modifiers of carcinogen metabolism. J Nutr 1999;129:7688-94S

Hendrich S. Bjeldanes, LF. Effects of dietary cabbage, Brussels sprouts, Ilicium verum, Schizandra chinensis and alfa alfa on the benzopyrene metabolic enzyme system in mouse liver. Food Chem Toxicol, 1983;21:479-86

Jin L, Qi M, Chen DZ, et al. Indole-3-carbinol prevents cervical cancer in human papilloma virus type 16 (HPV16) transgenic mice. Cancer Res, 1999;59:3991-7

Loub WD, et al. Aryl hydrocarbon hydroxylase induction in rat tissues by naturally occurring indoles of cruciferous plants. JNCI, 1975;54:985-8

Maheo L, Morel F, Langouet S, et al. Inhibition of cytochromes P-450 and induction of glutathione Stransferases by sulforaphane in primary human and rat hepatocytes. Cancer Res, 1997;57:3649-52

McDanell R, et al. Differential induction of mixed-function oxidase (MFO) activity in rat liver and intestine by diets containing processed cabbage. Food chem. Toxicol, 1987;25:363-8

Meng Q, Qi M, Chen D.X. et al. Suppression of breast cancer invasion and migration by indole-3-carbinol: associated with up-regulation of BRCA1 and E-cadherin/catenin complexes. J Mol Med, 2000;78:155-65

Michnovicz JJ, Bradlow, H.L. (1990) Induction of estradiol metabolism by dietary indole-3-carbinol in humans. JNCI, 1990;82:947-9

Michnovicz JJ. Increased estrogen 2-hydroxylation in obese women using oral indole-3-carbinol. Int J Obes Relat Metab Disord, 1998;22:227-9

Osborne MP, et al. Increase in the extent of estradiol 16 alpha-hydroxylation in human breast tissue: A potential biomarker of breast cancer risk. JNCI, 1993;85:1917-20

Plumb GW, Lambert N, Chambers SJ, et al. Are whole extracts and purified glucosinolates from cruciferous vegetables antioxidants? Free Radic Res, 1996;25:75-86

Rosen CA, Woodson GE, Thompson JW, et al. Preliminary results of the use of indole-3-carbinol for recurrent respiratory papillomatosis. Otolaryngol Head Neck Surg, 1998;118:810-5

Sabinsa Corporation. Indole-3-Carbinol Product Manual (www.sabinsa.com)

Stoewsand GS, et al. Protective effects of dietary Brussels sprouts against mammary carcinogenesis in Sprague-Dawley rats. Cancer Lett, 1988;39:199-207

Stoewsand GS. Bioactive organosulfur phytochemicals in Brassica oleracea vegetables – a review. Food Chem Toxicol, 1995;33:537-43

Talaley P, Zhang Y. Chemoprotection against cancer by isothiocyanates and glucosinolates. Biochem Soc Trans, 1996;24:806-10

Tiwari RK., et al. Selective responsiveness of human breast cancer cells to indole-3-carbinol, a chemopreventive agent. JNCI, 1994;86(2):126-31

Verhoeven DT, Goldbohm RA, van Poppel G, et al. A review of mechanisms underlying anticarcinogenicity by brassica vegetables. Chem Biol Interact 1997;103:79-129 [review]

Verhoeven DT, Goldbohm RA, van Poppel, G., et al. Epidemiological studies on brassica vegetables and cancer risk. Cancer Epidemiol Biomarkers Prev, 1996;5:733-48 [review]

Yuan F, Chen DZ, Liu K, et al. Anti-estrogenic activities of indole-3-carbinol in cervical cells. Implication for prevention of cervical cancer. Anticancer Res, 1999;19(3A):1673-80

Zeligs M. The Cruciferous Choice. Townsend Letter for Doctors & Patients. Aug/Sept 2001; (217/218):p47-48

Vitamins and Minerals

American Academy of Pediatrics Committee on Infectious Diseases. Vitamin A treatment of measles. Pediatrics 1993,91:1014–5

Anderson R. The immunostimulatory, anti-inflammatory an anti-allergic properties of ascorbate. Adv Nutr Res1984;6:19–45 [review]

Banic S. Immunostimulation by vitamin C. Int J Vitam Nutr Res Suppl 1982;23:49–52 [review]

Bendich A. Antioxidant vitamins and immune responses. In: Chandra RK, ed. Nutrition and immunology. New York: Alan R Liss Inc, 1988:125-48

Bendich A. Beta-carotene and the immune response. Proc Nutr Soc 1991;50:263–74

Berger MM, Spertini F, Shenkin A, et al. Trace element supplementation modulates pulmonary infection rates after major burns: a double-blind, placebo-controlled trial. Am J Clin Nutr 1998;68:365–71

Bresee JS, Fischer M, Dowell SF, et al. Vitamin A therapy for children with respiratory syncytial virus infection: a multicenter trial in the United States. Pediatr Infect Dis J 1996;15:777–82

Chandra RK. Effect of vitamin and trace-element supplementation on immune responses and infection in elderly subjects. Lancet 1992;340:1124–7

Chavance M, Herbeth B, Lemoine A, et al. Does multivitamin supplementation prevent infections in healthy elderly subjects? A controlled trial. Int J Vitam Nutr Res 1993;63:11–6

Chew BP. Role of carotenoids in the immune response. J Dairy Sci 1993;76:2804–11

Coodley GO, Coodley MK, Lusk R, et al. Beta-carotene in HIV infection: an extended evaluation. AIDS 1996;10:967–73

de la Fuente M, Ferrandez MD, Burgos MS, et al. Immune function in aged women is improved by ingestion of vitamins C and E. Can J Physiol Pharmacol 1998;76:373–80

De Waart FG, Portengen L, Doekes G, et al. Effect of 3 months vitamin E supplementation on indices of the cellular and humoral immune response in elderly subjects. Br J Nutr 1997;78:761–74

Delafuente JC, Prendergast JM, Modigh A. Immunologic modulation by vitamin C in the elderly. Int J Immunopharmacol 1986;8:205–11

Eicher-Pruiett SD, Morrill JL, Blecha F, Higgins JJ, Anderson NV, Reddy PG. Neutrophil and lymphocyte response to supplementation with vitamins C and E in young calves. J Dairy Sci 1992;75:1635-42

Esterbauer H, Dieber-Rotheneder M, Striegl G, Waeg G. Role of vitamin E in preventing the oxidation of lowdensity lipoprotein. Am J Clin Nutr 1991;53(suppl):314S-21S

Fawzi WW, Mbise R, Spiegelman D, et al. Vitamin A supplements and diarrheal and respiratory tract infections among children in Dar es Salaam, Tanzania. J Pediatr 2000;137:660–7

Fawzi WW, Mbise RL, Fataki MR, et al. Vitamin A supplementation and severity of pneumonia in children admitted to the hospital in Dar es Salaam, Tanzania. Am J Clin Nutr 1998;68:187–92

Frei B, England L, Ames BN. Ascorbate is an outstanding antioxidant in human blood plasma. Proc Natl Acad Sci U S A 1989;86:6377-81

Fryburg DA, Mark RJ, Griffith BP, et al. The effect of supplemental beta-carotene on immunologic indices in patients with AIDS: a pilot study. Yale J Biol Med 1995;68:19–23.

Fuller CJ, Faulkner H, Bendich A, et al. Effect of beta-carotene supplementation on photosuppression of delayed-type hypersensitivity in normal young men. Am J Clin Nutr 1992;56:684–90

Gerber WF, Lefkowitz SS, Hung CY. Effect of ascorbic acid, sodium salicylate, and caffeine on the serum interferon level in response to viral infection. Pharmacology 1975;13:228

Girodon F, Lombard M, Galan P, et al. Effect of micronutrient supplementation on infection in institutionalized elderly subjects: a controlled trial. Ann Nutr Metab 1997;41:98–107

Glasziou PP, Mackerras DEM. Vitamin A supplementation in infectious diseases: a meta-analysis. BMJ 1993;306:366–70

Golstein JL, Ho YK, Basu SK, Brown MS. Binding site on macrophages that mediated uptake and degradation of acetylated low density lipoprotein, producing massive cholesterol deposition. Proc Natl Acad Sci U S A 1979;76:333-7

Hemilä H. Vitamin C and common cold incidence: a review of studies with subjects under heavy physical stress. Int J Sports Med 1996;17:379–83

Hemilä H. Vitamin C and the common cold. Br J Nutr 1992;67:3–16

Hughes DA, Wright AJ, Finglas PM, et al. The effect of beta-carotene supplementation on the immune function of blood monocytes from healthy male nonsmokers. J Lab Clin Med 1997;129:309–17

Jeng Kee-Ching G. et all. Supplementation with vitamins C and E enhances cytokine production by peripheral blood mononuclear cells in healthy adults. 1996;64:97=60-5

Jialal I, Grundy SM. Preservation of the endogenous antioxidants in low-density lipoprotein by ascorbate but not Probucol during oxidative modifications. J Clin Invest 1991;87:597-601

Jialal I, Vega GI, Grundy SM. Physiologic levels of ascorbate inhibit the oxidative modification of low-density lipoprotein. Atherosclerosis 1990;83:185-91

Kazi N, Radvany R, Oldham T, et al. Immunomodulatory effect of beta-carotene on T lymphocyte subsets in patients with resected colonic polyps and cancer. Nutr Cancer 1997;28:140–5

Kennes B, Dumont I, Brohee D, et al. Effect of vitamin C supplements on cell-mediated immunity in old people. Gerontology 1983;29:305–10

Kjolhede CL, Chew FJ, Gadomski AM, et al. Clinical trial of vitamin A as adjuvant treatment for lower respiratory tract infections. J Pediatr 1995;126:
807–12Knodell RG, Tate MA, Akl BF, et al. Vitamin C prophylaxis for posttransfusion hepatitis: Lack of effect in a controlled trial. Am J Clin Nutr 1981;34(1):20–3

Knudsen PJ, Dinarello CA, Storm TB. Progtaglandins posttranscriptionally inhibit monocyte expression of interleukin 1 activity by increasing intracellular cyclic adenosine monophosphate. J Immunol 1986;31:89-94

Kowdley KV, Meydani SN, Cornwall S, Grand RJ, Mason JB. Reversal of depressed T-lymphocyte function with repletion of vitamin E deficiency. Gastroenterolgy 1992;102:2139-42

Marchant CE, Law NS, van der Veen C, Hardwick SJ, Carpenter KLH, Mitchison MJ. Oxidized low-density lipoprotein is cytotoxic to human monocyte-macrophages: protection with lipophilic antioxidants. FEBS Lett 1995;358:175-8

Marcus SL, Petrylak DP, Dutcher JP, et al. Hypovitaminosis C in patients treated with high-dose interleukin 2 and lymphokine-activated killer cells. Am J Clin Nutr 1991;54(suppl):1292S-7S

Meydani SN, Barklund MP, Liu S, et al. Vitamin E supplementation enhances cell-mediated immunity in healthy elderly subjects. Am J Clin Nutr 1990;52:557–63

Meydani SN, Barklund MP, Liu S, Meydani M, et al. Vitamin E supplementation enhances cell-mediated immunity in healthy elderly subjects. Am J Clin Nutr 1990;52:557-63

Meydani SN, Hayek M, Coleman L. Influence of vitamins E and B6 on immune response. Ann N Y Acad Sci 1992;669:125-30

Meydani SN, Meydani M, Blumberg JB, et al. Vitamin E supplementation and in vivo immune response in healthy elderly subjects: a randomized controlled trial. JAMA 1997;277:1380–6

Meydani SN, Meydani M, Verdon CP, Shapiro AC, Blumberg JB, Hayes KC. Vitamin E supplementation suppresses prostaglandin E2 synthesis and enhanced the immune response of aged mice. Mech Ageing Dev 1986;34:191-201

Mohsenin V, Dubois AB, Douglas JS. Effect of ascorbic acid on response to methacholine challenge in asthmatic subjects. Am Rev Respir Dis 1983;127:143-7

Murata A. Virucidal activity of vitamin C for prevention and treatment of viral diseases. In Proceedings of the First Intersectional Congress of IAMS, vol 3. Science Council Japan, 1975, 432

Murata T, Tamai H, Morinobu T, et al. Effect of long-term administration of beta-carotene on lymphocyte subsets in humans. Am J Clin Nutr 1994;60:597–602

Murphy S, West KP Jr, Greenough WB 3d, et al. Impact of vitamin A supplementation on the incidence of infection in elderly nursing-home residents: a randomized controlled trial. Age Ageing 1992;21:435–9

Penn ND, Purkins L, Kelleher J, et al. The effect of dietary supplementation with vitamins A, C and E on cellmediated immune function in elderly long-stay patients: a randomized controlled trial. Age Ageing 1991;20:169–74

Pike J, Chandra RK. Effect of vitamin and trace element supplementation on immune indices in healthy elderly. Int J Vitam Nutr Res 1995;65:117–21

Pinnock CB, Douglas RM, Badcock NR. Vitamin A status in children who are prone to respiratory tract infections. Aust Paediatr J 1986;22:95–9

Quinlan KP, Hayani KC. Vitamin A and respiratory syncytial virus infection. Serum levels and supplementation trial. Arch Pediatr Adolesc Med 1996;150:25–30

Ross AC. Vitamin A supplementation as therapy--are the benefits disease specific? Am J Clin Nutr 1998;68:8–9[review]

Santos MS, Leka LS, Ribaya-Mercado JD, et al. Short- and long-term beta-carotene supplementation do not influence T cell-mediated immunity in healthy elderly persons. Am J Clin Nutr 1997;66:917–24

Santos MS, Meydani SN, Leka L, et al. Natural killer cell activity in elderly men is enhanced by beta-carotene supplementation. Am J Clin Nutr 1996;64:772–7

Semba RD. Vitamin A, immunity, and infection. Clin Infect Dis 1994;19:489–99 [review].

Steinberg D, Parthasarathy S, Carew TE, Khoo JC, Wiztum JL. Beyond cholesterol: modifications of modified low-density lipoprotein that increase its atherogenicity. N Engl J Med 1989;320:915-24

Stephensen CB, Franchi LM, Hernandez H, et al. Adverse effects of high-dose vitamin A supplements in children hospitalized with pneumonia. Pediatrics 1998;101(5):E3 [abstract]

Tengerdy RP, Mathias MM, Nockels CF. Effect of vitamin E on immunity and disease resistance. In: Prasad A, ed. Vitamins, nutrition and cancer. Basel, Switzerland: Karger, 1986:123-33

Topika J, Binkova B, Sram RJ, Erin AN. The influence of alpha-tocopherol and pyritinol on oxidative DNA damage and lipid peroxidation of human lymphocytes. Mutat Res 1989;225:131-6

Weimann BJ, Weiser H. Effects of antioxidant vitamins E, C and B-carotene on immune functions in MRL/lpr mice and rats. Ann N Y Acad Sci 1992;669:390-2

Ziemlanski S, Wartanowicz M, Klos A, Raczka A, Klos M. The effect of ascorbic acid and alpha-tocopherol supplementation on serum proteins and immunoglobulin concentration in elderly. Nutr Re Int 1986;2:1-5

Milk Thistle (*Silybum Marianum*)

1. Foster S. Milk Thistle. Silybum marianum. Houston, TX: American Botanical Council;1997:p7

2. Awang D. Milk thistle. Can Pharm J 1993;422:403-4

3. Wagner H. Antihepatotoxic flavonoids. Plant Flavonoids in Biology and Medicine: Biochemical, Pharmacological, and Sturcture-Activity Relationships (Cody V, Middleton E, Harbourne jV, eds.) Alan R. Liss, New York 1986:p545-58

4. Adzet T. Polyphenolic compounds with biological and pharmacological activity. Herbs Spices Med Plants 1986;1:167-84

5. Hikino H, Kiso Y, Wagner H, Fiebig. Antihepatotoxic actions of flavanolignans from silybum marianum fruits. Planta Medica 1984;50:248-50

6. Wagner H. Plant constituents with antihepatotoxic activity. Natural Products as Medicinal Agents (Beal JL and Reinhard E, eds.) Hippokrates-Verlag, Stuttgart, Germany 1981

7. Vogel G et al. Protection against Amanita phalloides intoxication in beagles. Toxicol appl Pharm 1984;73:355-62

8. Vogel G et al. Studies on pharmacodynamics, site and mechanism of action of silymarin, the antihepatotoxic principle from Silybum marianum (L.)Gaert. Arzneimittel-Forsch 1975;25:179-85

9. Valenzuela A et al. Silymarin protection against hepatic lipid peroxidation induced by acute ethanol intoxication in the rat. Biochem Pharm 1985;34:2209-12

10. Hikino H, Kiso Y. Natural products for liver diseases. Economic and Medicinal Plant Research 1988;2:39-72

11. Valenzuela A, Aspillaga M, Vial S, Guerra R. Selectivity of silymarin on the increase of the glutathione content in different tissues of the rat. Planta Medica 1989;55:420-2

12. Campos R, Garrido A, Guerra R, Valenzuela A. Silybin dihemisuccinate protects against gluta thione depletion and lipid peroxisation induced by acetaminophen in rat liver. Planta Medica 1989;55:417-9

13. Fiebrich F, Koch H. Silymarin, an inhibitor of prostaglandin synthetase. Experientia 1979;35:148-50

14. Fiebrich F, Koch H. Silymarin, an inhibitor of prostaglandin synthetase. Experientia 1979;35:150-2

15. Sonnenbichler J et al. Stimulatory effect of silibinin on the DNA synthesis in partially hepatectomized rat livers: Non-response in hepatoma and othr malignant cell lines. Biochem Pharm 1986;35:538-41

16. Sonnenbichler J, Zetl I. Biochemical effects of the flavonolignan silibinin on RNA, protein and DNA synthesis in rat livers. Plant Flavonoids in Biology and Medicine: Biochemical, Pharmacological, and Structure–Activity Relationships (Cody V, Middleton E, and Harbourne JB, eds.) Alan R. Liss, New York 1986:319-31

17. Magliulo P, Carosi G, Minoli L, Gorini S. Studies on the regenerative capacity of the liver in rats subjected to partial hepatectomy and treated with silymarin. Arzneimittelforschung 1973;23:161-7

18. Desplaces A et al. The effects of silymarin on experimental phalloidin poisoning. Arzneimittel-Forsch 1975;25:89-96

19. Muzes G, Deak G, Land I et al. Effect of the bioflavonoid silymarin on the in vitro activity and expression of superoxide dismutase (SOD) enzyme. Acta Physiologica Hungarica 1991;78(1):3-9

20. Schopen RD, Lange OK: Therapy of hepatoses, Therapeutic use of silymarin. Med Welt 1970;21:691-8

21. Ferenci P et al. Randomized controlled trial of silymarin treatment in patients with cirrhyosis of the liver. J Hepatol 1989;9:105-13

22. Deak G et al. Immunomodulator effect of silymarin therapy in chronic alcoholic liver diseases. Orv Hetil 1990;131:p1291-2 p1295-6

23. Buzzelli G, Moscarella S, Giusti A et al. A pilot study on the liver protective effect of silybinphosphatidylcholine complex (IdB1016) in chronic active hepatitis. International Journal of Clinical Pharmacology Tehrapy and Toxicology 1993;31(9):456060

24. Lirussi F, Okolicsanyi L. Cytoprotection in the nineties: Experience with ursodeoxycholic acid and silymarin in chronic liver disease. Acta Physiologica Hungarica 1992;80(1-4):363-7

25. Berenguer J et al. Double-blind trial of silymarin versus placebo in the tratment of chronic hepatitis. Muench Med Wochenschr 1971;119:240-60

26. Weiss RF. Herbal Medicine. Gothenburg, Sweden: Ab Areanum 1988:362

27. Hruby C. Silibinin in the treatment of deathcap fungus poisoning. Forum 1984;6:23-6

28. Faulstich II, Jahn W, Wieland T. Silybin inhibition of amatoxin uptake in the perfused rat liver. Arzneimittelforshung 1980;30(1):452-4

29. Tuchweber B, Sieck R, Trost w. Prevention of silybin of phalloidin-induced acute hepatotoxicity. Toxicology and Applied Pharmacology 1979;51:265-75

30. Salami HA, Sarna S. Effect of silymarin on chemical, functional and morphological alterations of the liver. Scandinavian Journal of Gastroenterology 1982;17:517-21

31. Palasciano G, Portincasa P, Palmieri V et al. The effect of silymarin on plasma levels of malondialdehyde in patients receiving long-term treatment with psychotropic drugs. Current Therapeutic Research 1994;55(5)537-45

32. Nassauto G et al. Effect of silibinin on biliary lipid composition. Experimental and clinical study. J Hepatal 1991;12:290-95

33. Kock HP et al. Silymarin: Potent inhibitor of cyclic AMP phosphodiesterase. Meth Find Exp Clin Pharm 1985;7:409-13

34. Weber G et al. The liver, a therapeutic target in dermatoses. Med Welt 1983;34:108-11

35. Blumenthal M, Brusse WR, Goldber A et al. The Complete German Commission E Monographs. Austin, TX: American Botanical Council 1998:p685

36. Health care professional training program in complementary medicine. Boon H and Smith M. Institute of Applied Complementary Medicine Inc. 1997:241-5

37. Wagner H et al. The chemistry of silymarin (silybin), the active principle of the fruits of silybum marianum (L.). Gaertn Arzneim-Forsch Drug Res 1968;18:688-96

38. Brown DJ. Herbal Prescriptions for Better Health. Rocklin, CA:Prima Publishing 1996:151-8

39. Murray MT. The Healing Power of herbs. Rocklin, CA:Prima Publishing 1992:p246

40. Brown D. Silymarin educational monograph. Townsend Newsletter for Doctors 1994;136:1282-5

41. Tyler VE. Herbs of Choice. The Therapeutic Use of Phytomedicinals. Binghamton, NY: Pharmaceutical Products Press 1994:p209

42. The Botanical Pharmacy. Quarry Health Books2000. Boon H and Smith M:250-4

43. Beckmann-Knopp S, Rietbrock S, Weyhenmeyer R et al. Inhibitory effects of silibinin on cytochrome P-450 enzymes in human liver microsomes. Pharmacol Toxicol Jun2000;86(6):2506

44. Venkataramanan R, Ramachandran V, Komoroski BJ et al. Milk Thistle, a herbal supplement, drecreases the activity of CYP3A4 and uridine disphosphoglucuronosyl transferase in human hepatocyte cultures. Drug Metab Dispos Nov2000;28(11):1270-3

45. Zhao J et al. Tissue distribution of silibinin, the major active constituent of silymarin, in mice and its association with enhancement of phase II enzymes: Implications in cancer chemoprevention. Carcinogenesis Nov1999;20(11):2101-8

46. Healthnotes Online. Healthnotes Inc, 2000. www.healthnotes.com: Milk Thistle

47. Natural Products Encyclopedia. www.consumerslab.com: Milk Thistle

48. Dietary Supplement Information Bureau. www.content.intramedicine.com: Thistle

49. Salmi HA, Sarna S. Effect of silymarin on chemical, functional and morphological alterations of the liver. A double-blind controlled study. Scand J Gastroenterol 1982;17:517-21

50. Feher J, Desk G, Muzes G et al. Liver protective action of silymarin therapy in chronic alcoholic liver diseases [in Hungarian]. Orv hetil 1989;130:2723-7

51. Fintelmann V, Albert A. Proof of the therapeutic efficacy of LegalonW for toxic liver illnesses in a double-blind trial [translated from German]. Therapiewoche 1980;30:5589-94

52. Trinchet JC, Coste T, Levy VG et al. Treatment of alcoholic hepatitis with silymarin. A double-blind comparative study in 116 patients [translated from French]. Gastroenterol Clin Biol 1989;13:120-4

53. Bunout D, Hirsch SB, Petermann MT et al. Controlled study of the effect of silymarin on alcoholic liver disease [translated from Spainch]. Rev Med Chil 1992;120:1370-5

54. Allain H, Schuck S, lebreton S et al. Aminotransferase levels and silymarin in de novo tacrine-treated patients with Alzheimer's disease. Dement Geriatr Cogn Disord 1999;10:181-5

55. Giannola C, Buogo F, Forestiere G et al. A two-center study on the effects of silymarin in pregnant women and adult patients with so-called minor hepatic insufficiency [in Italian]. Clin Ther 1985;114:129-35

56. Albrecht M, Frerick H, Kuhn U et al. Therapy of toxic liver pathologies with Legalon [in German]. Z Klin Med 1992;47:87-92

57. Adverse Drug Reactions Advisory Committee. An adverse reaction to the herbal medication in milk thistle (Silybum marianum). Med J Aust 1999;170:218-9

Cruciferous Vegetables and Their Indole-3-Carbinol Content Help Reduce Cancer Risk

1. Hecht, S.S. Chemoprevention of cancer by isothiocyanates, modifiers of carcinogen metabolism. *J Nutr* 1999; 129: 7688-74S

2. Verhoeven, D.T., Goldbohm, R.A., van Poppel, G., et al. A review of mechanisms underlying anticarcinogenicity by brassica vegetables. *Chem Biol Interact* 1997; 103: 79-129 [review]

3. Verhoeven, D.T., Goldbohm, R.A., van Poppel, G., et al. Epidemiological studies on brassica vegetables and cancer risk. *Cancer Epidemiol Biomarkers Prev* 1996; 5: 733-48 [review]

4. Talaley, P., Zhang, Y. Chemoprotection against cancer by isothiocyanates and glucosinolates. *Biochem Soc Trans* 1996; 24: 806-10

5. Maheo, L., Morel, F., Langouet, S., et al. Inhibition of cytochromes P-450 and induction of glutathione S-transferases by sulforaphane in primary human and rat hepatocytes. *Cancer Res* 1997; 57: 3649- 52

6. Barcelo, S., Gardiner, J.M., Gescher, A. Chipman, J.K. CYP2E1-mediated mechanism of antigenotoxicity of the broccoli constituent sulforaphane. *Carcinogenesis* 1996; 17: 277-82

7. Plumb, G.W., Lambert N., Chambers, S.J., et al. Are whole extracts and purified glucosinolates from cruciferous vegetables antioxidants? *Free Radic Res* 1996; 25: 75-86

8. Dhinmi, S.R., Li, Y., Upadhyay, S., Koppolu, P.K., Sarkar, F.H. Indole-3-carbinol (I3C) – induced cell growth inhibition, G1 cell cycle arrest and apoptosis in prostate cancer cells. *Oncogene* 2001, May 24; 20 (23): 2927-36

9. Stoewsand, G.S. Bioactive organosulfur phytochemicals in Brassica oleracea vegetables – a review. *Food Chem Toxicol* 1995; 33: 537-43

10. Broadbent, T.A., Broadbent, H.S. The chemistry and pharmacology of indole-3-carbinol (indole-3- methanol) and 3-(methoxymethyl) Indole. [Part I]. *Curr Med Chem* 1998; 5: 337-52

11. Broadbent, T.A., Broadbent, H.S. The chemistry and pharmacology of indole-3-carbinol (indole-3- methanol) and 3-(methoxymethyl) Indole. [Part II].*Curr Med Chem* 1998; 5: 469-91

14. Beecher, C.W. Cancer preventive properties of varieties of Brassica oleracea: a review. *Am J Clin Nutr.* 1994 May; 59 (5 suppl): 1166S-1170S

15. Loub, W.D., et al. (1975) Aryl hydrocarbon hydroxylase induction in rat tissues by naturally occurring indoles of cruciferous plants. *JNCI*, 54: 985-988

16. McDanell, R., et al. (1987) Differential induction of mixed-function oxidase (MFO) activity in rat liver and intestine by diets containing processed cabbage. Food chem. *Toxicol* 25: 363-368

17. Hendrich, S. and Bjeldanes, LF. (1983) Effects of dietary cabbage, Brussels sprouts, Ilicium verum, Schizandra chinensis and alfa alfa on the benzopyrene metabolic enzyme system in mouse liver. *Food Chem Toxicol* 21: 479-486

18. Osborne, M.P., et al. (1993) Increase in the extent of estradiol 16 alpha-hydroxylation in human breast tissue: A potential biomarker of breast cancer risk. *JNCI* 85: 1917-20

19. Michnovicz, J.J. Increased estrogen 2-hydroxylation in obese women using oral indole-3-carbinol. *Int J Obes Relat Metab Disord* 1998; 22: 227-9
20. Bradlow, H.L., Michnovicz, J.J., Halper, M. et al. Long-term responses of women to indole-3-carbinol or a high fiber diet. *Cancer Epidemiol Biomarkers Prev* 1994; 3: 591-5
21. Tiwari, R.K. et al. (1994) Selective responsiveness of human breast cancer cells to indole-3-carbinol, a chemopreventive agent. *JNCI*, 86(2): 126-31
22. Stoewsand, G.S., et al. (1988) Protective effects of dietary Brussels sprouts against mammary carcinogenesis in Sprague-Dawley rats. *Cancer Lett* 39:199-207
23. Michnovicz, J.J. and Bradlow, H.L. (1990) Induction of estradiol metabolism by dietary indole-3- carbinol in humans. *JNCI*, 82: 947-949
24. Bradfield, C.A. and Bjeldanes, L.F. (1984) Effect of dietary indole-3 carbinol on intestinal and hepatic monooxygenase, gluatathione-S-Transferase and epoxide hydrolase activities in rat. *Food Chem Toxicol* 22: 977-982
25. Bradlow, H.L., Sepkovic, D.W., Telang, N.T., Osborne, MP. Indole-3-carbinol. A novel approach to breast cancer prevention. *Ann NY Acad Sci* 1999;889: 204-13
26. Bradlow, H.L., Sepkovic, D.W., Telang, N.T., Osborne, M.P. Indole-3-carbinol. A novel approach to breast cancer prevention. *Ann NY Acad Sci* 1995;768: 180-200
27. Bradlow, H.L., Sepkovic, D.W., Telang, N.T., Osborne, M.P. Multifunctional aspects of the action of indole-3-carbinol as an antitumor agent. *Ann NY Acad Sci* 1999; 889: 204-13
28. Meng, Q., Qi M, Chen, D.X., et al. Suppression of breast cancer invasion and migration by indole-3- carbinol: associated with up-regulation of BRCA1 and E-cadherin/catenin complexes. *J Mol Med* 2000; 78: 155-65
29. Bell, M.C., Crowley-Nowick, P., Bradlow, H.L, et al. Placebo-controlled trial of indole-3-carbinol in the treatment of CIN. *Gynecol Oncol* 2000: 78;123-9
30. Yuan, F., Chen, D.Z., Liu, K., et al. Anti-estrogenic activities of indole-3-carbinol in cervical cells. Implication for prevention of cervical cancer. *Anticancer Res* 1999; 19(3A): 1673-80
31. Jin, L, Qi, M., Chen, D.Z., et al. Indole-3-carbinol prevents cervical cancer in human papilloma virus type 16 (HPV16) transgenic mice. *Cancer Res* 1999; 59: 3991-7
32. Rosen, C.A., Woodson, G.E., Thompson, J.W., et al. Preliminary results of the use of indole-3- carbinol for recurrent respiratory papillomatosis. *Otolaryngol Head Neck Surg* 1998; 118:810-15
33. Zeligs, M. The Cruciferous Choice. *Townsend Letter for Doctors & Patients*. Aug/Sept 2001, issue 217/218. p. 47-48
34. Sabinsa Corporation. *Indole-3-Carbinol Product Manual* (www.sbinsa.com)

Reishi Mushroom Extract And Immune Support

1. Jong, S.C., et al. Medicinal Benefits of the Mushroom Ganoderma. Adv Appl Microbiol. 1992; 37: 101-34
2. Herbs To The Rescue. Nutrition News, 11/30/92; V.XVI N.11; p.4
3. Jones, Kenneth, Reishi (Ganoderma): Longevity Herb of the Orient; Part 2. Townsend Letters for Doctors & Patients; 11/20/92; N.112; p.1008-1012
4. Leung, A.y., Foster, S. Encyclpedia of Common natural Ingredients Used in Foods, Drugs, and Cosmetics, 2nd ed. New York: John Wiley & Sons, 1996, 255-60
5. Hobbs, C. Medicinal Mushrooms. Santa Cruz, C.A., Botanica Press, 1995, 96-107
6. Ikekawa, T., et al. 1968. Antitumor Action of Some Basidiomycetes, Especially Phellinus linteus. Japan J Can Res 59: 155157.
7. Morishige, Fukumi (lecture), 1988. In Becoming Healthy with Reishi, III. Kampo I-Yaku Shimbun, Toyo-Igaku Sha Co., Ltd., Tokyo; 12-20. Trans.
8. Tsukagoshi, S., et al. 1984. Krestin (PSK). Cancer Treat Rev 11 (2): 131-135.

9. Teikoku Chemical Industry Co., Ltd. 1982. Mushroom Glycoproteins as neoplasm Inhibitors. Japanese Patent No. 82 75,926, May 12, 1982; in Chem Abstr 97:4431 1j.

10. Lingzhi. In Chang, H-M. and p. P-H. But, editors. 1986. Pharmacology and Applications of Chinese Materia Medica. Vol I. Singapore: World Scientific;642-653

11. Nakashima, S., et al. 1979. Effect of Polysaccharrides from Ganoderma applanatum on immune Responses I. Enhancing Effect on the Induction of Delayed Hypersensitivity in Mice. Microbiol Immunol 23 (6): 501-513

12. Li Shih-chen. 1933. Pen T-sao Kang Mu. Shang Wu Printer, Shanghai. Trans.

13. Liu, B, and Y-S Bau. 1980. Fungi Pharmacopoeia (Sinica). The Kinoko Company, Oakland, California; 168-169

14. Lin, J.M., et al. Radical Scavanger and Antihepatotoxic Activity of Ganoderma formosanum, Ganoderma lucidum and Ganoderma neo-japonicum. J Ethnopharmacol. Jun 1995; 47 (1): 33-41

15. Wang, S.Y, Hsu, M.L., Hsu, H.C., Tzeng, C.H., Lee, S.S., Shiao, M.S., Ho, C.K. The anti-tumor effect of Ganoderma lucidum is mediated by cytokines released from activated macrophages and T lymphocytes. Int J Cancer 1997 Mar 17; 70 (6): 699-705

16. Lee, J.M., Kwon, H., Jeong, h., Lee, J.W., Lee, S.Y., Baek, S.J., Surh, Y.J. Inhibition of lipid peroxidation and oxidative DNA damage by Ganoderma lucidum [In Process Citation]. Phytother Res 2001 May; 15 (3): 245-9

17. Wang, S.Y. The Anti-tumor Effect of Ganoderma lucidum is mediated by Cytokines Released From Activated macrophages and T Lymphocytes. Int J Cancer. May 1997; 70 (6): 699-705

18. Sone, Y., et al. Structures and Antitumor Activities of the Polysaccharides isolated from Fruiting Body and the Growing Culture of Mycelium of Ganoderma lucidum., Agr Biol Bhem. 1985; 49: 2641-53.

19. Tizard, I.R. 1984. Immunology: An Introduction. Saunders, Philadelphia; 94 and 323.

20. Hayward, A.R. 1988, Immune Deficiency Disease. In Allergic Diseases from Infancy to Adulthood. Bierman, C. Warren and David s. Pearlman, editors. W.B. Saunders, 2nd edition, 1988; 34.

21. Tasaka, T., et al. 1988. Anti-allergic constitutents in the culture medium of Ganoderma lucidum (I). Inhibitory effect of oleic acid on histamine release. Agents and Actions 23 (3/4): 153-156

22. Tasaka, T., et al. 1988. Anti-allergic constitutents in the culture medium of Ganoderma lucidum (II). The Inhibitory effect of cyclooctasulpher on histamine release. Agents and Actions 23 (3/4): 157-160

23. Lee, S.Y. Eo, S.K., et al. Antiherpetic Activities of Various protein Bound Polysaccarides isolated from Ganoderma lucidum. J Ethnopharmacol. Dec 1999; 68 (1-3): 175-81

24. Hijikata, y., et al. Effect of Ganoderma lucidum on Postherpetic Neuralgia, Am J Chin Med. 1998; 26 (3-4): 375-81

25. el-Mekkawy, S., et al. Anti-HIV-1 and Anti-HIV-1-protease Substances from Ganoderma lucidum. Phytochemistry. Nov 1998; 49 (6): 1651-57

26. Willard, T., and K. Jones. 1990. Reishi Mushroom. Sylvan Press, Issaquah, Washington, 1990.

27. Cohen, m. 1988. Paths to wholeness in HIV Infection: A Comprehensive approach. In AIDS, Immunity and Chinese Medicine. Proceedings of the Ninth Annual symposium of the Oriental healing Arts Institute, oct. 23, 1988, Long Beach, Califonia. B.C. Enger and E.R. Long, editors. O.H.A.I., Long Beach, California, 1989; 92-102

28. Pers. Comm.., Dharmananda, Ph.D., Institute of Traditional medicine, Portland, Oregon, **March,** 1992

29. Chen, W.C., Hau, D.M., Lee, s.S. Effects of Ganoderma lucidum and krestin on cellular immunoceompetnece in gamma-ray-irradiated mice. Am J Chin med 1995; 23 (1): 71-80

30. Kammatsuse, K., Kajiware, N., Hayashi, K. Studies on Ganaderma lucidum: I. Efficacy against hypertension and side effect. Yakugaku Zasshi 1985; 105: 531-3

31. Jin, H., Zhang, G., Cao, X., et al. Treatment of hypertension by ling zhi combined with hyptensor and its effects on arterial, arteriolar and capillary pressure and microcirculation. In: Nimmi H., Xiu R.J., Sawada, T., Zheng, C. (eds). Microcirculatory Approach to Asian Traditional Medicine. New york:Eslevier Science, 1996, 131-8

32. lee, S.y. Cardiovascular Effects of Mycelium Extract of Ganoderma lucidum; inhibition of sympathetic Outflow as a Mechanism of its hypotensive Action. Chem Pharm Bull. (Tokyo). May 1990; 38 95): 1359-64

33. Su, C. Potentiation of ganodermic acid S on prostaglandin E (1)-induced cyclic AMP elevation in human platelets. Thromb Res. Jul 2000; 99 (2): 135-45

34. Jong, S.C., et al. Medicinal Benefits of the Mushroom Ganodermal. Adv Appl Microbiol. 1992; 37:101-34

35. Sahley, Billie, J. Reishi Mushroom, Healing Herb of the Future. MMRC Health Educator Reports;01/31/97; p.1-2

36. Tamura, T., et al. Fermentation product as food for patients with liver failure. In Chem Abstr108(13):110853m.

37. Hirotani, M., et al. 1986. Ganoderic Acids T., S. and R., New Triterpenoids from the Cultured Myceliaof Ganoderma lucidum. Chem Pharm Bull 134 95): 2282-2285

38. Gong, Z. and Z.-B. Lin. 1981. The Pharmacological Study of Lingzhi (Ganoderma lucidum) and the Research of Therapeutical Principle of "Fuzheng Guben" in Traditional Chinese Medicine. Pei-Ching I Hseuh Yuan Hseuh Paoi 13: 6-10. Trans.

39. Lin, J.-M., Lin c.-C., et al. Radical scavenger and antihepatotoxic activity of Ganoderma formosanum, Ganoderma lucidum and Gonoderma neo-japonicum. J Ethnopharm 47: 33-41, 1995

40. Hobbs, C. Medicinal Mushrooms. Santa Cruz, CA: Botanica Press, 1995, 96-107

41. McGuffin, M., ed. Et al. Botanical Safety Handbook. Boca Raton: CRC Press: 1997: 55

42. Horner, W.E., et al. Basidiomycete Allergens: Comparison of Three Ganoderma Species. Allergy. Feb 1993; 48 (2): 110-16

43. Lee, S.Y. Cardiovascular Effects of Mycelium Extract of Ganoderma lucidum: Inhibition of Sympathetic Outflow as a Mechanism of its Hypotensive Action. Chem Pharm Bull. (Tokyo). May 1990; 38 (50: 1359-64

44. Kanmatsuse, k., et al. Studies on Ganoderma lucidum. I. Efficacy Against Hypertension and Side Effects. Yakugaku Zasshi. Oct 1985; 105 (10): 942-47

45. Hikino, H., et. Al. Mechanisms of Hypoglycemic Activity of Ganoderan B: A Glycan of Ganoderma lucidum Fruit Bodies. Planta Med. Oct 1999; 55 (5):423-28

46. Tao, J. et al. Experimental and Clinical Studies on Inhibitory Effect of Ganoderma lucidum On Platelet Aggregation. J Tongji Med Univ. 1990; 10 (4): 240-43

Astragalus (Astragalus Membranaceus Moench)

1. Foster, S., Chongxl, Y. Herbal Emissaries. Bringing Chinese Herbs to the West. Rochester, VT; Healing Arts Press, 1992: 356

2. Zhao, K.S., Manoinin, C., Doria, G. Enhancement of the immune response in mice by Astragalus membranaceous extracts. Immunopharmacology. 1990: 20(3): 225-233

3. Sun, Y, et al. Preliminary observations on the effects of the Chinese medicinal herbs Astragalus membranaceous and Ligustrum lucid on lymphocyte blastogenic responses. Journal of Biological Response Modifiers. 1983; 2: 227-237

4. Geng, C.S., et al. Advances in Immuno-pharmacological Studies on Astragalus membranaceous. Chung, Hsi, i Chieh Ho Tsa Chih. 1986; 6 (1): 62-64

5. Chen, LX, Liao, JX., Guo, WQ. Effects of Astragalus membranaceous on left Ventribular Function and Oxygen Free Radical in Acute Myocardial Infarction Patients and Mechanism of its Cardiotonic Action. Chung Kuo, Chung Hsi, I Chieh Ho Tsa Chih. Mar 1995; 15 (3): 141-3

6. Sun, Y, Change, YH, Uy, Gq, et al. Effect of Fu-zheng therapy in the management of malignant diseases. Chinese Med Journal, 1981; 61: 97-101

7. Leung, AY, Foster, S. Encyclopedia of Common Natural Ingredients Used in Food, Drugs, and Cosmetics. 2nd ed. Toronto/New York: John Wiley and Sons Inc; 1996: 649

8. Chevallier, A. The Encyclopedia of Medicnal Plants. London: Readers Digest; 1996: 336

9. Zhao, K W, Kong, HY. Effect of Astragalan on secretion of tumour necrosis factor in human peripheral blood monomuclear cells. Chung-Kuo Chung Hsi i Chieh, Ho Tsa Chih. 1993

10. Luo, HM, Dai, RH, Li Y. Nuclear cardiology study on effective ingredients of Astragalus membranaceous in treating heart failure. Chung-Kuo Chung His i Chieh, Ho Tsa Chih. 1995; 15 (12): 709-9

11. Hirotani, M, Zhou, Y, Rui, H, Furuya, T. Cycloartane triterpene glycosides from the hairy root cultures of Astragalus membranaceous. Phytochemistry. 1994; 37 (5): 1403-7

12. Weng, XS. Treatment of leucopenia with pure astragalus preparation – an analysis of 115 leucopenic cases 9Chinese). Chung-Kuo Chung Hsi i Chieh, Ho Tsa Chih. 1995; 15 (8): 462-4

13. Chu, DT, et al. Immunotherapy with Chinese medicinal herbs. II. Reversal of cyclophosphamideinduced immune suppression by administration of fractionated Astragalus membranaceus in vivo. Journal of Clinical Laboratory Immunology. 1988; 25: 125-129

14. Chen, YC. Experimental studies on the effects of danggui buxue decoction on IL-2 production of blood-deficient mice (Chinese). Chung-Kuo Chung Hsi i Chieh. 1994; 19 (12): 739-41, 763

15. Liang, H, Zhang, Y, Geng, B. The effect of astragalus polysaccharides (APS) on cell medicated immunity (GMI) in burned mice. Chung-Hua Cheng Hsing Shao Shang Wai Ko Tsa Chih.

16. Hou, YD, Ma, GL, Wu, SH, Li, HT. Effect of radix Astrageli seu Hedysari on the interferon system. Chinese Medical Journal. 1981; 94: 35-40

17. Jin, R, Wan, LL, Mitsuishi, T. Effects of shi-ka-ron and Chinese herbs in mice treated with anti-tumor agent mito mycin C (Chinese). Chung-Kuo Chung Hsi i Chieh, Ho Tsa Chih. 1995; 15 (2) 101-3

18. Sugiura, H, Nishida, H, Indaba, R, Iwata, H. Effects of exercise in the growing stage in mice and of Astragalus membranaceous on immune functions (Japanese). Nippon Eiseigaku Zasshi – Japanese Journal of hygiene, 1993; 47 (6): 1021-31

19. Yang, YZ, Jin, PY, Guo Q, et al. Effect of Astragalus membranaceous on natural killer cell activity and induction of a- and g- interferon in patients with coxsackie B viral myocarditis. Chinese Medical Journal 1990; 103 (4): 304-307

20. Yang, YZ, Guo, Q, Jin, PY, et al. Effect of Astragalus membranaceous injection on Coxsackie B-2 virus infected rat beating heart cell culture. Chinese Medical Journal. 1987; 100-595

21. Hou, YD. Study on the biological active ingredients of Astragalus membranaceous. Chung His i Chieh Ho Tsa Chih. 1984; 4:420

22. Zhang, Xq, et al. Studies of Astragalus membranaceous on antiinfluenza virus activity, interferon induction and immunostimulation in mice. Chinese Journal of Microbiology and Immunology. 1984; 4:92

23. Research Group of Common Cold and Bronchitis. Investigation into Astragalus membranaceous. II. A research on some of its mechanism of reinforcing the Qi (vital energy.) Journal of Traditional Chinese Medicine. 1980; 3:67

24. Shi, HM, Dai, RH, Fan, WH. Intervention of lidocaine and Astragalus membranaceous on ventricular late potentials (Chinese). Chung-Kuo Chung Hsi i Chieh, Ho Tsa Chih. 1994; 14 (10): 598-600

25. Li, SQ, Yuan, RX, Gao, H. Clinical observation of the treatment of ischemic heart disease with Astragalus membranaceous (Chinese). Chung-Kuo Chung Hsi i Chieh, Ho Tsa Chih. 1995; 15 (2): 77-80

26. Lei, ZY, Qin, H, Liao, JZ. Action of Astragalus membranaceous on left ventricular function of antina pectoris (Chinese). Chung-Kuo Chung Hsi I Chieh, Ho Tsa Chih. 1994; 14 (4): 199-202

27. Cha, RJ, Zeng, DW, Chang, QS. Non-surgical treatment of small cell lung cancer with chemo-radioimmunotherapy and traditional Chinese medicine (Chinese). Chung-Hua Nei Ko Tsa Chih – Chinese Journal of Internal medicine. 1994; 33 (7): 462-6

28. Lau, BH, Ruckle, HC, Botolazzo, T, Lui, PD. Chinese medicinal herbs inhibit growth of murine renal cell carcinoma. Cancer Biotherapy. 1994; 9 (2):153-61

29. Chu, DT, Lin, JR, Wong, W. The in vitro potentiation of LAK cell cytotoxidicty in cancer and AIDS patients induced by F3 – a fractionated extract of Astragalus membranaceous (Chinese). Chung-Hun Chung Liu Tsa Chih – Chinese Journal of Oncology. 1994; 16 (3): 167-71

30. Hong, C, Ku, J, et al. Astragalus membranaceous stimulates human sperm motility in vitro. American journal of Chinese Medicine. 1992; 20: 289-94

31. Murray, MT. The Healing Power of Herbs. Rocklin, CA: Prima Publishing; 1992: 246

32. Zhao, KS, et al. Enhancement of the Immune Response in Mice by Astragalus membranaceous Extracts. Immunopharmacology. 1990; 20 (3): 225-33

33. Chu, DT, et al. Immune Resoration of Local Xenogeneic Graft-versus-host Reaction in Cancer Patients in In-vitro and Reversal of Cyclophosphamide-induced Immune suppression in the Rat in Vivo by Fractionated Astragalus membranaceous. Chung Hsi i Chieh Ho Tsa Chih. Jun 1989; 9: 351- 54.

Prebiotics (FOS and other Oligosaccharides)

1. Tomomatsu H. Health effects of oligosaccharides. Prog Food Nutr Sci 1983;7:29-37.

2. Molis C, Flourie B, Ourne F, Gailing MF, Lartique S, Guibert A, et al. Digestion, excretion, and energy value of fructooligosaccharides in healthy humans. Am J Clin Nutr 1996;64:324-8.

3. Alles MS, Hautvast JG, Nagengast FM, Hartemink R, Van Laere KM. Fate of fructo-oligosaccharides in the human intestine. Br J Nutr 1996;76:211-21.

4. Duggan C, Gannon J, Walker WA. Protective nutrients and functional foods for the gastrointestinal tract. Am J Clin Nutr 2002:75(5):789-808.

5. Gibson GR, Beatty EH, Wang X, Cummings JH. Selective stimulation of bifidobacteria in the human colon by oligofructose and mutin. Gastroenterology 1995;106:975-82.

6. Bouhnik Y, Fluorié B, Dagay-Abensour L, Pochart P, Gramet G, Durand M, et al. Administration of transgalacto-oligosaccharides increases faecal Bifidobacteria and modifies colonic fermentation metabolism in healthy humans. J Nutr 1997; 127: 444-8.

7. Bouhmik Y, et al. Short-chain fructo-oligosaccharide administration dose-dependently increases fecal bifodobacteria in healthy humans. J Nutr 1999;129:113-6.

8. Roberfroid M. Dietary fibre, inulin and oligosaccharides. Crit Rev Good Sci Nutr 1993;33:103-48 [review].

9. Tomomatsu H. Health effects of oligosaccharides. Food Technology 1994;48(10):61-5.

10. Gibson GR, Beatty ER, Wang X, Cummings JH. Selective stimulation of bifidobacteria in the human colon by oligofructose and inulin. Gastroenterology 1995;108:975-82.

11. Jackson KG, Taylor GRJ, Clohessy AM, Wlliams CM. The effect of the daily intake of inulin on fasting lipid, insulin and glucose concentrations in middle-aged men and women. Br J Nutr 1999;82:23-30.

12. Yamashita, K, Kawai, K, and Itakura, M. Effects of fructo-oligosoccharides on blood glucose and serum lipids in diabetic subjects. Nutr Res 1984;4:961-6.

13. Roberfroid M. Prebiotics: preferential substrates for specific germs. Am J Clin Nutr.2001;73(Suppl 2):406S-9S.

14. Isolauri E, Sutas Y, Kankaanpaa P, Arvilommi H, Salminen S. Probiotics; effects on immunity. Am J Clin Nutr 2001:73(Suppl 2):444S-50S.

15. Wollowski I, Rechkemmer G, Pool-Zobel BL. Protective role of probiotics and prebiotics in colon cancer. Am J Clin Nutr 2001;73(Suppl 2):451S-5S.

16. Roberfroid M. Dietary fibre, inulin and oligofructose. A review comparing their physiological effects. Crit Rev Food Sci Nutr 1993;33:103-48.

17. Healthnotes online. 2000 Healthnotes, Inc. (www.healthnotes.com):FOS

Boosting Your Immune System with Vitamin C and Vitamin E Supplementation

1. Tengerdy RP, Mathias MM, Nockels CF. Effect of vitamin E on immunity and disease resistance. In: Prasad A, ed. Vitamins, nutrition and cancer. Basel, Switzerland: Karger, 1986:123-33.

2. Bendich A. Antioxidant vitamins and immune responses. In: Chandra RK, ed. Nutrition and immunology. New York: Alan R Liss Inc, 1988:125-48.

3. Kowdley KV, Meydani SN, Cornwall S, Grand RJ, Mason JB. Reversal of depressed T-lymphocyte function with repletion of vitamin E deficiency. Gastroenterolgy 1992;102:2139-42.

4. Meydani SN, Hayek M, Coleman L. Influence of vitamins E and B6 on immune response. Ann N Y Acad Sci 1992;669:125-30.

5. Meydani SN, Barklund MP, Liu S, Meydani M, et al. Vitamin E supplementation enhances cellmediated immunity in healthy elderly subjects. Am J Clin Nutr 1990;52:557-63.

6. Mohsenin V, Dubois AB, Douglas JS. Effect of ascorbic acid on response to methacholine challenge in asthmatic subjects. Am Rev Respir Dis 1983;127:143-7.

7. Marcus SL, Petrylak DP, Dutcher JP, et al. Hypovitaminosis C in patients treated with high-dose interleukin 2 and lymphokine-activated killer cells. Am J Clin Nutr 1991;54(suppl):1292S-7S.

8. Ziemlanski S, Wartanowicz M, Klos A, Raczka A, Klos M. The effect of ascorbic acid and alphatocopherol supplementation on serum proteins and immunoglobulin concentration in elderly. Nutr Re Int 1986;2:1-5.

9. Eicher-Pruiett SD, Morrill JL, Blecha F, Higgins JJ, Anderson NV, Reddy PG. Neutrophil and lymphocyte response to supplementation with vitamins C and E in young calves. J Dairy Sci1992;75:1635-42.

10. Weimann BJ, Weiser H. Effects of antioxidant vitamins E, C and B-carotene on immune functions in MRL/lpr mice and rats. Ann N Y Acad Sci 1992;669:390-2.

11. Meydani SN, Meydani M, Verdon CP, Shapiro AC, Blumberg JB, Hayes KC. Vitamin E supplementation suppresses prostaglandin E2 synthesis and enhanced the immune response of aged mice. Mech Ageing Dev 1986;34:191-201.

12. Topika J, Binkova B, Sram RJ, Erin AN. The influence of alpha-tocopherol and pyritinol on oxidative DNA damage and lipid peroxidation of human lymphocytes. Mutat Res 1989;225:131-6.

13. Knudsen PJ, Dinarello CA, Storm TB. Progtaglandins posttranscriptionally inhibit monocyte expression of interleukin 1 activity by increasing intracellular cyclic adenosine monophosphate. J Immunol 1986;31:89-94.

14. Golstein JL, Ho YK, Basu SK, Brown MS. Binding site on macrophages that mediated uptake and degradation of acetylated low density lipoprotein, producing massive cholesterol deposition. Proc Natl Acad Sci U S A 1979;76:333-7.

15. Steinberg D, Parthasarathy S, Carew TE, Khoo JC, Wiztum JL. Beyond cholesterol: modifications of modified low-density lipoprotein that increase its atherogenicity. N Engl J Med 1989;320:915-24.

16. Marchant CE, Law NS, van der Veen C, Hardwick SJ, Carpenter KLH, Mitchison MJ. Oxidized lowdensity lipoprotein is cytotoxic to human monocyte macrophages: protection with lipophilic antioxidants. FEBS Lett 1995;358:175-8.

17. Esterbauer H, Dieber-Rotheneder M, Striegl G, Waeg G. Role of vitamin E in preventing the oxidation of low-density lipoprotein. Am J Clin Nutr 1991;53(suppl):314S-21S.

18. Frei B, England L, Ames BN. Ascorbate is an outstanding antioxidant in human blood plasma. Proc Natl Acad Sci U S A 1989;86:6377-81.

19. Jialal I, Vega GI, Grundy SM. Physiologic levels of ascorbate inhibit the oxidative modification of lowdensity lipoprotein. Atherosclerosis 1990;83:185-91.

20. Jialal I, Grundy SM. Preservation of the endogenous antioxidants in low-density lipoprotein by ascorbate but not Probucol during oxidative modifications. J Clin Invest 1991;87:597-601.

21. Jeng Kee-Ching G. et all. Supplementation with vitamins C and E enhances cytokine production by peripheral blood mononuclear cells in healthy adults. 1996;64:97=60-5.Tomomatsu H. Health effects of oligosaccharides. Prog Food Nutr Sci 1983;7:29-37.

22. Molis C, Flourie B, Ourne F, Gailing MF, Lartique S, Guibert A, et al. Digestion, excretion, and energy value of fructooligosaccharides in healthy humans. Am J Clin Nutr 1996;64:324-8.

Vitamin E and Beta-Carotene Can Boost the Immune System in Older Persons

1. Meydani SN, et al. Antioxidants and immune response in aged persons: Overview of present evidence. 1995. Am J Clin Nutr; 62; (suppl): 1462-76.

2. National Research Council. Recommended dietary allowances. 10th. Ed. Washington, DC: National Academy Press, 1989.

3. Garry PJ, Goodwin JS, Hunt WC, Hooper EM, Leonard AG. Nutritional status in a healthy elderly population: dietary and supplemental intakes. Am J Clin Nutr 1982;36:319-31.

4. Ryan AS, Craig L, Finn SC. Nutrient intakes and dietary patterns of older Americans: a national study. J Gerontol 1992;47:M145-50.

5. Panemangalore M, Lee CJ. Evaluation of the indices of retinol and alpha-tocopherol status in freeliving elderly. J Gerontol 1992;1992:B98-104.

6. Vatssery GT, Johnson GJ, Krezowski AM. Changes I vitamin E concentrations in human plasma and platelets with age. J Am Coll Nutr 1983;4:369-75.

7. Wilson TS, Datta SB, Murrell JS, Andrews CT. Relationship of vitamin C to mortality in a geriatric hospital: a study of the effect of vitamin C administration. Age Aging 1973;2:163-71.

8. Wilson TS, Weeks MM, Mukheyee J, Murrell S, Andrews CT. A study of vitamin C levels in the aged and subsequent mortality, J Gerontol 1982;14:17-24.

9. Linderman RD, Clark ML, Colemore JP. Influence of age and sex on plasma and red cell zinc concentration. J Gerontol 1971;26:358-63.

10. Meydani SN, Hayek M. Vitamin E and the immune response. In: Chandra RK, ed. Nutrition and immunology. St John's, Canada: ARTS Biomedical Publishers and Distributors, 1992:105-28.

11. Chavance M, Brubacher G, Herbeth B, et al. Immunological and nutritional status among the elderly. In: de Weck AL, ed. Lymphoid cell functions in aging. Interlaken: Eurage, 1984;231-7.

12. Chavance M, Brubacher G Herbert B, et al. Immunological nutritional status among the elderly. In: Chandra RK, ed. Nutritional immunity and illness in the elderly. New York: Pergamon Press,1985:137-42.

13. Bostick RM, Potter JD, McKenzie DR, et al. Reduced risk of colon cancer with high intake of vitamin E: the Iowa Women's Health Study. Cancer Res 1993;53:4230-7.

14. Longnecker MP, Martin-Morena JM, Knet P, et al. Serum alpha-tocopherol concentration in relation to subsequent colorectal cancer: pooled data from five cohorts. J Natl Cancer Inst 1992;84:430-5

15. Prasad JS. Effect of vitamin E supplementation on leuckocyte function. Am J Clin Nutr 1980;33:606-8.

16. Zheng W, Blot J, Diamond EL, et al. Serum micronutrients and the subsequent risk of oral and pharyngeal cancer. Cancer Res 1993;53:795-8

Ginseng

1. Boon H, Smith M. The Botanical Pharmacy. Quarry Health Books 2000:180-99

2. Murray M. The healing Power of Herbs. Prima Publishing 1995:265-79, 314-20

3. Chang H, But P. Pharmacology and Applications of Chinese Materia Medica. World Scientific, Philadelphia PA 1986:p773

4. Teegarden R. Chinese Tonic Herbs. Japan Publishing Inc NY 1985:p197

5. Bensky D, Gamble A. Chinese Herbal Medicine Materia Medica. Eastland Press, Seattle WA 1986:p556

6. Fulder SJ. Ginseng and the hypothalmic-pituitary control of stress. American Journal of Chinese Medicine 1981;0:112-8

7. Hiai S, Yokoyama H Oura H. Features of ginseng saponins-induced corticosterone secretion. Endocrinologia Japonica 1979;26:737-40

8. Hiai S, Yokoyama H, Oura H, Kawashima Y. Evaluation of corticosterone secretion-inducing effects of ginsenosides and their prosapogenins and sopogenins. Chemical and Pharmaceutical Bulletin 1983;31:168-74

9. Fulder S. The drug the builds Russians. New Science 1980;21:576-9

10. Avakian EV et al. Effect of panax ginseng on energy substrates during exercise. Fed Proc 1980;39:287

11. Avakian EV et al. Effect of panax ginseng extract on erergy metabolism during exercise in rats. Planta Medica 1984;50:p151

12. McNaughton L et al. A comparison of Chinese and Russian ginseng as ergogenic aids to improve various factets of physical fitness. Int Clin Nutr Rev 1989;9:32-7

13. See DM, Broumand N, Sahl L, Tilles JG. In vitro effects of Echinacea and ginseng on natural killer and antibody-dependent cell cytotoxicity in healthy subjects and chronic fatigue syndrome or acquired immunodeficiency syndrome patients. Immunopharmacology 1997;35(3):229-35

14. Liu J, Wang S, Liu H et al. Stimulatory effect of saponins from Panax ginseng on immune function of lymphocytes in the elderly. Mechanisms of Ageing and Development 1995;83(1):43-53

15. Bohn B, Nebe CT, Birr C. Flow-cytometric studies with Eleutherococcus senticosus extract as an immunomodulatory agent. Arzneimittelforschung 1987;37(10):1193-6

16. Jie YH, Cammisuli S, Baggiolini M. Immunomodulatory effects of Panax ginseng C.A. Meyer in the mouse. Agents and Actions 1984;15:386-91

17. Yun TK, Yun YS, Han IW. Anti-carcinogenic effect of long-term oral administration of newborn mice exposed to various chemical carcinogens.Cancer Detection and Prevention 1983;6:515-25

18. Yeung HW, Cheung K, Leung KN et al. Immunopharmacology of Chinese medicine. I. Ginsenginduced immuno suppression in virus infected mice. American Journal of Chinese Medicine 1982;10:44-54

19. Kang M, Yoshimatsu H, Oohara A et al. Ginsenoside Rg1 modulates ingestive behavior and thermal response induced by interleukin-1 beta in rats. Physiology and Behaviour 1995;57(2):393-6

20. Scaglione F, Cattaneo G, Alessandria M, Cogo R. Efficacy and safety of the standardized Ginseng extract G115 for potentiating vaccination against the influencza syndrome and protection against the common cold. [Published erratum appears in Drugs Exp Clin Res 1996;22(6):p338].
Drugs Under Experimental and Clinical Research 1996;22(2):65-72

21. Healthnotes Online. Healthnotes Inc. 2000; www.healthnotes.com: Ginseng

22. Punnonen R, Lukola A. Oestrogen-like effects of ginseng. British Mecial Journal 1980;281:p1110

23. Palmer BV, Montgomer ACV, Monteiro JC. Ginseng and mastalgia. [Letter] British Medical Journal 1978;1:p1284

24. Salvati G, Genovesi G, Marcellini L et al. Effects of Panax Ginseng: C.A. Meyer, Saponins on male fertility. Panminerva Med 1996;38(4):249-54

25. Chen, X, Lee TJ. Ginsenosides-induced nitric oxide-mediated relaxation of the rabbit corpus cavernosum. British Journal of Pharmacology 1995;115(1):15-8

26. Sotaniemi EA, Haapakoski E, Rautio A. Ginseng therapy in non-insulin-dependent diabetic patients. Diabetes Care 1995;18(10):1373-5

27. Vukson V et al. American ginseng reduces postprandial glycemia in nondiabetic subjects and subjects with type 2 diabetes mellitus. Arch Int Med 2000;160:1009-1013

28. Farnsworth NR, Kinghorn AD, Soejarto D, Waller DP. Siberian ginseng (Eleuthrococcus sentricosus): Current status as an adaptogen. In: Wagner H, hikino H, Farnsworth NR, eds. Economic and Meidicinal Plant Research. Academic Press Orlando FL: 1985:155-215

29. Ben-Hur et al. Effect of Panax ginseng and Eleutherococcus S. on survival of cultural mammalian cells after ionizing radiation. Am J Chin Med 1981;9:48-56

30. Kupin VI et al. Stimulation of the immunological reacitivty of cancer patients by eleutherococcus extract. Vopr Onkol 1986;32:21-6 [in Russia]

31. Salvati G et al. Effects of Panax ginseng C.A. Meryer saponins on male fertility. Panminerva Med 1996;38:249-54

32. Colgan M. Optimum Sports Nutrition. Advanced Research Press 1993:p310

33. Brown DJ. Herbal Prescriptions for Better health. Prima Publishing Rocklin CA 1996;129-38

34. Miller LG. Herbal Medicinals: Selected clinical considerations focusing on known or potential drugherb interactions. Arch Intern Med 1998;158(20):2200-11

35. McNeil JR. Interactions between hebal and conventional medicines. Can J Cont Med Edu 1999;11(12):97-110

36. Heck A et al. Potential interactions between alternative therapies and warfarin. Am J Health Syst Pharm 2000;57(13):1221-7
37. McRae S. Elevated serum digoxin levels in a patient taking digoxin and Siberian ginseng. Can Med Assoc J 1996;155:293-295
38. Yun TK et al. Preventive effect of ginseng intake against various human cancers: A case-control study on 1987 pairs. Cancer Epidem Biomarkers Prev 1995;4:401-8
39. Liberti LE, der Marderosian A. Evaluation of commercial ginseng products. Journal of Pharmaceutical Sciences. 1978;67:1487-9
40. Cui JF, Garle M, Bjorkhem I, Eneroth P. Determination of aglycones of ginsenosides in ginseng preparations sold in Sweden and in urine samples from Sweidsh athletes consuming ginseng. Scandinavian Journal of Clinical and Laboratory Investigation. 1996;56(2):151-60
41. Cui J, Garle M, Eneroth P, Bjorkhem I. What do commercial ginseng preparations contain? [Letter] Lancet 1994;344(8915):p134
42. Walker AF. What is in ginseng? [Letter:comment] Lancet 1994;344(8922):p619
43. Watt J, Bottomley MB, Read MTF. Olympic athletics medical experience, Seoul – personal views. British Journal of Sports Medicine 1989;23(2):76-9

N-Acetylcysteine

1. Murray M, Pizzoino J. Encyclopedia of Natural Medicine. 2nd edition. Rocklin, CA: Prima Publishing; 1998. p. 104-25;199-210.
2. Staal FJ, Ela SW, Roederer M, Anderson MT, Herzenberg LA, Herzenberg LA. Glutathiore deficiency and human immunodeficiency virus infection. Lancet 1992;339:909-12.
3. Favier A, Sappey C, Leclerc P, Faure P, Micoud M. Antioxidant status and lipid peroxidation in patients infected with HIV. Chem Biol Interact 1994;91:165-80.
4. Marmor M, Alcabes P, Titus S, Frenkel K, Krasinski K, Penn A, et al. Low serum thiol levels predict shorter times-to-death among HIV-infected injecting drug users. AIDS 1997;11:1389-93.
5. Roberts RL, Aroda VR, Ank BJ. N-acetylcysteine enhances antibody-dependent cellular cytotoxicity in neutrophils and mononuclear cells from healthy adults and human immunodeficiency virus-infected patients. J Infect Dis 1995;172(6):1492-502.
6. Breitkreutz R, Pittack N, Thomas Nebe C, Schuster D, Brust J, Beichert M, et al. Improvement of immune functions in HIV infection by sulfur supplementation: two randomized trials. J Mol Med 2000;78(1):55-62.
7. Roederer M, Staal FJ, Raju PA, Ela SW, Herzenberg LA. Cytokine-stimulated human immunodeficiency virus replication is inhibited by N-acetyl-L-cysteine. Proc Natl Acad Sci 1990;87:4884-8.
8. Robinson MK, Hong RW, Wilmore DW. Glutathione deficiency and HIV infection. Lancet 1992;339:1603–4.
9. De Rossa SC, Zaretsky MD, Dubs JG, et al. N-acetylcysteine replenishes glutathione in HIV infection. Eur J Clin Invest 2000;30,10:915-29.
10. The Merck Manual. 16th edition. San Diego, CA: Merck Research Laboratories; 1992. p. 906-9.
11. Ballatori N, Lieberman MW, Wang W. N-acetylcysteine as an antidote in methylmercury poisoning. Environ Health Perspect 1998;106(5):267-71.
12. Flora SJ. Arsenic-induced oxidative stress and its reversibility following combined administration of N-acetylcysteine and meso 2,3-dimercaptosuccinic acid in rats. Clin Exp Pharmacol Physiol 1999;26(11):865-9.

13. Kleinveld HA, Demacker PNM, Stalenhoef AFH. Failure of N-acetylcysteine to reduce low-density lipoprotein oxidizability in healthy subjects. Eur J Clin Pharmacol 1992;43:639-42.

14. Healthnotes 2000. Healthnotes Inc. (www.healthnotes.com): Drug Interactions Summary for NAcetylcysteine.

15. Brumas V, Hacht B, Filella M, Berthon G. Can N-acetylcysteine affect zinc metabolism when used as a paracetamol antidote? Agents Action 1992;36:278-8.

16. Herzenberg LA, De Rosa SC, Dubs JG, Roederer M, Anderson MT, Ela SW, et al. Glutathione deficiency is associated with impaired survival in HIV disease. Proc Natl Acad Sci 1997;94:1967-72.

Chromium

1. Standard Textbooks of Nutritional Science:- Shils M, Shike M, Olson J, Ross C. Modern Nutrition in Health and Disease. 9th ed. Baltimore, MD:
Lippincott Williams & Wilkins; 1993.- Escott-Stump S, Mahan LK, editors. Food, Nutrition and Diet Therapy. 10th ed. Philadelphia, PA:
W.B. Saunders Company; 2000.- Bowman B, Russell RM, editors. Present Knowledge in Nutrition, 8th ed. Washington, DC:.ILSIPress; 2001.- Kreutler
PA, Czajka-Narins DM, editors. Nutrition in Perspective. 2nd ed. Upper Saddle River, NJ: Prentice Hall Inc.; 1987.

2. Fisher J. The Chromium Program. New York, NY: Harper and Row; 1990.

3. Murray M. Encyclopedia of Nutritional Supplements. Rocklin, CA: Prima Publishing; 1996. p. 194-8.

4. Mertz W. Chromium in human nutrition: a review. J Nutr 1993;123:626-33.

5. Abraham AS, Brooks BA, Eylath U. The effects of Chromium supplementation on serum glucose and lipids in patients with and without non-insulin dependent diabetes. Metabolism 1992;41:768-71.

6. Mossop RT. Effects of Chromium (III) on fasting blood glucose, cholesterol, and cholesterol HDL levels in diabetics. Centr Afr J Med 1983;29:80-2.

7. Rabinowitz MB, Gonick HC, Levin SR, et al. Effect of Chromium and yeast supplements on carbohydrate metabolism in diabetic men. Diabetes Care 1983;6:319-27.

8. Anderson RA. Chromium, glucose tolerance, and diabetes. Biological Trace Element Research 1992;32:19-24.

9. Lee NA, Reasner CA. Beneficial effect of Chromium supplementation on serum triglyceride levels in NIDDM. Diabetes Care 1994;17:1449-52.

10. Offenbach E, Pistunyer F. Beneficial effect of Chromium-rich yeast on glucose tolerance and blood lipids in elderly patients. Diabetes 1980;29:919-25.

11. Press RI, Geller J, Evans GW. The effect of Chromium picolinate on serum cholesterol and apolipoprotein fractions in human subjects. Western J Med 1993;152:41-5.

12. Wang MM, Fox EA, Stoecker BJ, Menendez CE, Chan SB. Serum cholesterol of adults supplemented with brewer's yeast or Chromium Chloride. Nutr Res 1989;9:989-98.

13. Roeback JR, Hla KM, Chambless LE, Fletcher RH. Effects of Chromium supplementation on serum high-density lipoprotein cholesterol levels in men taking beta-blockers. Annals Int Med 1991;115:917- 24.

14. Lefavi RG, Wilson GD, Keith RE, Anderson RA, Blessing DL, Hames CG, et al. Lipid-lowering effect of a dietary Chromium (III) Nicotinic Acid complex in male athletes. Nutr Res 1993;13:239-49.

15. Lavie CJ, O'Keefe JH, Blonde L, et al. High-density lipoprotein cholesterol: recommendations for routine testing and treatment. Postgrad Med 1990;87(7):36-44,47,51

16. McCarthy MG. Hypothesis: Sensitization of insulin-dependent hypothalamic glucoreceptors may account for the fat-reducing effects of Chromium Picolinate. J Optimal Nutr 1993;21:36-53.

17. Evans GW, Pouchnik DJ. Composition and biological activity of chromium-pyridine carbosylate complexes. J Inorgranic Biochemistry 1993;49:177-87.

18. Katts GR, Ficher JA, Blum K. The effects of Chromium Picolinate supplementation on body composition in different age groups. *Age* 1991;14(4):138 (Abstract #40).

19. Anderson RA, Cheng N, Bryden NA, Polansky MM, Cheng N, Chi J et al. Elevated intakes of supplemental Chromium improves glucose and insulin variables in individuals with type 2 diabetes. Diabetes 1997; 11:1786-91.

20. Revina A, et al. Reversal of corticosteroid-induced diabetes mellitus with supplemental Chromium. Diab Med 1999; 16(2):164-7.

21. Anderson RA. Chromium, as an essential nutrient for humans. Regul Toxicol Pharmacol 1997;26(Suppl Pt 2): 35S-41S.

22. Schrauzer GN, Shrestha KP, Flores MP. Somatopsychological effects of Chromium supplementation. J Nutr Med 1992;3:43-8.

23. Cerulli J, Grabe DW, Gauthier I, Malone M, McGoldrick MD. Chromium Picolinate toxicity. Ann Pharmacother 1998;32:438-41.

24. Healthnotes 1998-2002. Available from: URL: http://www.healthnotes.com.

25. Studies presented at the Annual Scientific Sessions of the American Diabetes Association, San Francisco, CA, 1996.

26. Kozlovsky AS, Moser PB, Reiser S, Anderson RA. Effects of diets high in simple sugars on urinary chromium losses. Metabolism 1986;35(6):515-8.

27. Anderson RA, Bryden NA, Polansky MM. Urinary Chromium excretion and insulinogenic properties of carbohydrates. Am J Clin Nutr 1990;51(5):864-8.

Magnesium

1. Standard Textbooks of Nutritional Science:- Shils M, Shike M, Olson J, Ross C. Modern Nutrition in Health and Disease. 9th ed. Baltimore, MD: Lippincott Williams & Wilkins; 1993.- Escott-Stump S, Mahan LK, editors. Food, Nutrition and Diet Therapy. 10th ed. Philadelphia, PA: W.B. Saunders Company; 2000.- Bowman B, Russell RM, editors. Present Knowledge in Nutrition, 8th ed. Washington, DC:.ILSI Press; 2001.- Kreutler PA, Czajka-Narins DM, editors. Nutrition in Perspective. 2nd ed. Upper SaddleRiver, NJ: Prentice Hall Inc.; 1987.

2. Murray M. Encyclopedia of Nutritional Supplements. Rocklin, CA: Prima Publishing; 1996.

3. Witterman JCM, et al. Reduction of blood pressure with oral magnesium supplementation in women with mild to moderate hypertension. Am J Clin Nutr 1994; 60:129-35.

4. Motoyama T, Sano H, Fukuzaki H. Oral Magnesium supplementation in patients with essential hypertension. Hypertension 1989;13:227-32.

5. McLean RM. Magnesium and its therapeutic uses: a review. Am J Med 1994;96:63-76.

6. Altura BM. Basic biochemistry and physiology of Magnesium: a brief review. Magnes Trace Elem 1991;10:167-71.

7. Purvis JR, Movahed A. Magnesium disorders and cardiovascular disease. Clin Cardiol 1992;15:556-68.

8. Altura BM. Ischemic heart disease and Magnesium. Magnesium 1988;7:57-67.

9. Perticone F, Borelli D, Ceravolo R, Mattioli PL. Antiarrhythmic short-term protective Magnesium treatment in ischemic dilated cardiomyopathy. J Am Coll Nutr 1990;9:492-9.

10. Galland LD, Baker SM, McLellan RK. Magnesium deficiency in the pathogenesis of mitral valve prolapse. Magnesium 1986;5:165-74.

11. Fernandes JS, et al. Therapeutic effect of a Magnesium salt in patients suffering from mitral valvular prolapse and latent tetany. Magnesium 1985:4:283-9.

12. White JR, Campbell RK. Magnesium and diabetes: a review. Ann Pharmacother 1993;27:775-80.

13. Djurhuus MS, Skott P, Hother NO, Klitgaard NA, Beck NH. Insulin increases renal Magnesium excretion: a possible cause of Magnesium depletion in hyperinsulinaemic states. Diabetic Med 1995;12:664-9.

14. Consensus Statement, Magnesium supplementation in the treatment of diabetes. Diabetes Care 1996;19(Suppl. 1):S93-5.

15. Paolisso G, Sgambato S, Gambardella A, Pizza G, Tesauro P, Varricchio M, et al. Daily Magnesium supplements improve glucose handling in elderly subject. Am J Clin Nutr 1992;55:1161-7.

16. Clauw DJ, et al. Magnesium deficiency in the eosinophilia-myalgia syndrome. Arth Rheum 1994;9:1331-4.

17. Hicks JT. Treatment of fatigue in general practice: a double-blind study. Clin Med J 1964:85-90.

18. Friedlander HS. Fatigue as a presenting symptom: management in general practice. Curr Ther Res 1962;4:441-9.

19. Facchinetti F, Borella P, Sances G, et al. Oral Magnesium successfully relieves premenstrual mood changes. Obstet Gynecol 1991;78:177-81.

20. Goei GS, Abraham GE. Effect of nutritional supplement, Optivite, on symptoms of premenstrual tension. J Repro Med 1983;28;527-31.

21. Tucker K, et al. Magnesium intake is associated with bone mineral density in elderly women. J Bone Mineral Res 1995;(Suppl):10S-46S.

22. Abraham, GE, Grewal, H. A total dietary program emphasizing Magnesium instead of Calcium effect on the mineral density of calcaneous bone in postmenopausal women on hormonal therapy. J Reprod Med 1990;5:503-7.

23. Stendig-Lindberg G, Tepper R, Leichter I. Trabecular bone density in a two-year controlled trial of peroral Magnesium in osteoporosis. Magnes Res 1993;2:155-63.

24. Rude RK, Adams JS, Ryzen E, Endres DB, Niimi H. Low serum concentration of 1,25-dihydroxyvitamin D in human Magnesium deficiency. J Clin Endo Metabol 1985;61:933-40.

25. Conradt A, Weidinger H, and Algayer H. ON: The role of Magnesium in fetal hypertrophy, pregnancy-induced hypertension, and preeclampsia. Mag Bull 1984;6:68-76.

26. Kiss V, et al. Effect of maternal Magnesium supply on spontaneous abortion and premature birth and on intrauterine fetal development: experimental epidemiological study. Mag Bull 1981; 3:73-9.

27. Spatling L, Spatling G. Magnesium supplementation in pregnancy. A double-blind study. Br J Obstet Gynaecol 1988;95:120-5.

28. Rudnicki M, Frolich A, Rasmussen WF, McNair P. The effect of Magnesium on maternal blood pressure in pregnancy-induced hypertension. A randomized double-blind placebo-controlled trial. Acta Obstet Gynecol Scand 1991;70:445-50.

29. Martin RW, Morrison JC. Oral Magnesium for tocolysis. Contemp Ob/Gyn 1987;30:111-8.

30. Johansson G, Backman U, Danielson BG, Fellstrom B, Ljunghall S, Wikstrom B. Biochemical and clinical effects of the prophylactic treatment of renal Calcium stones with Magnesium Hydroxide. J Urol 1980;124:770-4.

31. Wunderlich W. Aspects of the influence of Magnesium ions on the formation of calcium oxalate. Urol Res 1981;9:157-60.

32. Hallson P, Rose G, Sulaiman SM. Magnesium reduces Calcium oxalate crystal formation in human whole urine. Clin Sci 1982;62:17-9.

33. Johansson G, Backman U, Danielson B, et al. Magnesium metabolism in renal stone formers. Effects of therapy with magnesium hydroxide. Scand J Urol Nephrol 1980; 53:125-30.

34. Prien E, Gershoff S. Magnesium oxide-pyridoxine therapy for recurrent calcium oxalate calculi. J Urol 1974:509-12.

35. Gershoff S, Prien E. Effect of daily MgO and Vitamin B6 administration to patients with recurring Calcium Oxalate stones. Am J Clin Nutr 1967;20:33-7.

36. Reavley N. The New Encyclopedia of Vitamins, Minerals, Supplements and Herbs. New York, NY: M. Evans and Company Inc.; 1998.

37. Healthnotes 1998-2002. Available from: URL: http://www.healthnotes.com

38. Seelig MS. Auto-immune complications of D-penicillamine - a possible result of Zinc and Magnesium depletion and of Pyridoxine inactivation. J Am Coll Nutr 1982;1(2):207-14.

39. Berton G, et al. Metal ion-tetracycline interactions in biological fluids. 2. potentiometric study of Magnesium complexes with tetracycline, oxytetracycline, doxycycline, and minocycline, and discussion of their possible influence on the bioavailability of these antibiotics in blood plasma. J Inorg Biochem 1983;19(1):1-18.

40. Kes P, Reiner Z. Symptomatic hypomagnesemia associated with gentamicin therapy. Magnes Trace Elem 1990;9(1):54-60.

41. Jacobson ED, Faloon WW. Malabsorptive effects of neomycin in commonly used doses. A Am Med Assoc 1961;175:187-90.

42. Barton CH, Pahl M, Vaziri ND, Cesario T. Renal Magnesium wasting associated with amphotericin B therapy. Am J Med 1984;77(3):471-4.

43. Watkins DW, Khalafi R, Cassidy MM, Vahouny GV. Alterations in Calcium, Magnesium, Iron, and Zinc metabolism by dietary cholestyramine. Dig Dis Sci 1985;30(5):477-82.

44. Rolla G, Bucca C, Bugiani M, Oliva A, Branciforte L. Hypomagnesemia in chronic obstructive lung disease: effect of therapy. Magnes Trace Elem 1990;9(3):132-6.

45. Blum M, Kitai E, Ariel Y, et al. Oral contraceptive lowers serum Magnesium. Harefuah. 1991;121(10):363-4.

46. Seelig MS. Increased need for Magnesium with the use of combined estrogen and Calcium for osteoporosis treatment. Magnes Res 1990;3(3):197-215.

47. Gearhart MO, Sorg TB. Foscarnet-induced severe hypomagnesemia and other electrolyte disorders. Ann Pharmacother 1993;27(3):285-9.

48. Kupfer S, Kosovsky JD. Effects of cardian glycosides on renal tubular transport of Calcium, Magnesium, inorganic phosphate and glucose in the dog. J Clin Invest 1965;44:1132-43.

49. Ghamdi SM, Cameron EC, Sutton RA. Magnesium deficiency: pathophysiologic and clinical overview. Am J Kidney Dis 1994;24(5):737-52.

50. Norman DA, et al. Jejunal and ileal adaptation to iterations in dietary Calcium: changes in Calcium and Magnesium absorption and pathogenetic role of parathyroid hormone and 1,25-dihydroxyvitamin D. J Clin Invest 1981;67(6):1599-603.

51. Spencer H, et al. Magnesium-phosphorus interactions in man. Trace substances in environmental health-XIII. Hemphill DD editor. Columbia: Univ.Missouri; 1979.

Selenium

1. Standard Textbooks of Nutritional Science:- Shils M, Shike M, Olson J, Ross C. Modern Nutrition in Health and Disease. 9th ed. Baltimore, MD:
Lippincott Williams & Wilkins; 1993.- Escott-Stump S, Mahan LK, editors. Food, Nutrition and Diet Therapy. 10th ed. Philadelphia, PA:W.B. Saunders

Company; 2000.- Bowman B, Russell RM, editors. Present Knowledge in Nutrition, 8th ed. Washington, DC:.ILSI Press; 2001.- Kreutler PA, Czajka-Narins DM, editors. Nutrition in Perspective. 2nd ed. Upper Saddle River, NJ:Prentice Hall Inc.; 1987.

2. Schrauzer GN, White DA, Schneider CJ. Cancer mortality correlation studies III. Statistical associations with dietary Selenium intakes. Bioinorganic Chem 1977;7:23-56.

3. Shamberger RJ, Willis CE. Selenium distribution and human cancer mortality. Clin Lab 1971;2:211-21.

4. Russo MW, et al. Plasma Selenium levels and the risk of colorectal adenomas. Nutr and Cancer 1997; 28(2):125-9.

5. Simone C. Cancer and Nutrition. Garden City Park, NY: Avery Publishing Group Inc.; 1992.

6. Murray M. Encyclopedia of nutritional supplements. Rocklin, CA: Prima Publishing; 1996. p. 222-8.

7. Burk RF. Selenium. In: Nutrition Foundation. Nutrition reviews: present knowledge in nutrition. 5th ed. Washington DC: Nutrition Foundation Inc,; 1984. p. 519-27.

8. Hocman G. Chemoprevention of cancer: selenium. Int 5 Biochem 1998;20:123-32.

9. Blot WJ, Li JY, Taylor PR, Guo W, Dawsey S, Wang GQ, et al. Nutrition intervention trials in Linxian China: supplementation with specific vitamin/mineral combinations, cancer incidence, and disease-specific mortality in the general population. J Natl Cancer Inst 1993;85:1483-92.

10. Blot WJ, Li JY, Taylor PR, Li B. Lung cancer and vitamin supplementation. N Engl J Med 1994;331(9):614.

11. Clark LC, Combs GF, Turnbull BW, Slate EH, Chalker DK, Chow J, et al. Effects of selenium supplementation for cancer prevention in patients with carcinoma of the skin. A randomized controlled trial. Nutritional Prevention of Cancer Study Group. JAMA 1996;276(24):1957-63.

12. Yoshizawa K, Willett WC, Morris SJ, Stampfer MJ, Spiegelman D, Rimm EB, et al. Study of prediagnostic selenium levels in toenails and the risk of advanced prostate cancer. J Natl Cancer Inst 1998;90:1219-24.

13. Kiremidjian-Schumacher, L, Stotzky G. Selenium and immune responses. Environmental Res 1987;42:277-303.

14. Kiremidjian-Schumacher L, Roy M, Wishe HI, Cohen MW, Stotzky G. Supplementation with selenium and human immune cell functions; II, effect on cytotoxic lymphocytes and natural killer cells. Biol Trace Elem Res 1994;41:115-27.

15. Roy M, Kiremidjian-Schumacher L, Wishe HI, Cohen MW, Stotzky G. Supplementation with selenium and human immune cell functions. I. Effect on lymphocyte proliferation and interleukin-2 receptor expression. Biol Trace Elem Res 1994;41:103-14.

16. Delmas-Beauvieux MC, Peuchant E, Couchouron A, Constans J, Sergeant C, Simonoff M, et al. The enzymatic antioxidant system in blood and glutathione status in HIV-infected patients: effects of supplementation with selenium or beta-carotene. Am J Clin Nutr 1996;64:101-7.

17. Marmor M, Alcabes P, Titus S, Frenkel K, Krasinski K, Penn A, et al. Low serum thiol levels predict shorter times to death among HIV-infected injecting drug users. AIDS 1997;11:1389-93.

18. Hendler S. The doctors' vitamin and mineral encyclopedia. Simon and Schuster 1990:1983-92.

19. Tarp U, Overvad K, Thorling EB, Graudal H, Hansen JC. Selenium treatment in rheumatoid arthritis. Scand J. Rheumatol 1985:14:364-8.

20. Munthe E, Aaseth J. Treatment of rheumatoid arthritis with selenium and Vitamin E. Scan J Rheumatol 1984;53(Suppl):103S.

21. Tarp U, Overvad K, Hansen JC, Thorling EB. Low selenium levels in severe rheumatoid arthritis. Scand J Rheumatol 1985;14:97-101.

22. Hinks L, et al. Trace element status in eczema and psoriasis. Clin Exp Derm 1987;12:93-7

23. Heinle K, Adam A, Gradl M, Wiseman M, Adam O. Selenium concentration in erythrocytes of patients with rheumatoid arthritis. Clinical and laboratory chemistry infection markers during administration of selenium. Med Klin 1997;92(3):29-31.

24. Karakucuk S, Ertugrul Migra G, Faruk Ekinciler O. Selenium concentrations in serum, lens and aqueous humor of patients with senile cataracts. Acta Ophthalmol Scand 1995;73(4):329-32.

25. Reavley N. The new encyclopedia of vitamins, minerals, supplements and herbs. M Evans and Company Inc. 1998:294-303.

26. Contempre B, Dumont JE, Ngo B, Thilly CH, Diplock AT, Vanderpas J. Effects of selenium supplementation in hypothyroid subjects of an iodine and selenium deficient area: the possible danger of indiscriminate supplementation of iodine deficient subjects with selenium. J Clin Endocrinal Metabol 1991;73:213-5.

27. Peretz A, Neve J, Vertongen F, Famaey JP, Molle L. Selenium status in relation to clinical variables and corticosteroid treatment in rheumatoid arthritis.
J Rheumatol Dec 1987;14(6):1104-7.

28. Heese HD, Lawrence MA, Dempster WS, Pocock F. Reference concentrations of serum selenium and manganese in health nulliparas. S Afr Med J 1988;73(3):163-5.

29. Healthnotes 1998-2002. Available from: URL: http://www.healthnotes.com.

Zinc

1. Standard Textbooks of Nutritional Science:- Shils M, Shike M, Olson J, Ross C. Modern Nutrition in Health and Disease. 9ᵗʰ ed. Baltimore, MD: Lippincott Williams & Wilkins; 1993. - Scott-Stump S, Mahan LK, editors. Food, Nutrition and Diet Therapy. 10th ed. Philadelphia, PA: W.B. Saunders Company; 2000.
-Bowman B, Russell RM, editors. Present Knowledge in Nutrition, 8th ed. Washington, DC:.ILSI Press; 2001. - Kreutler PA, Czajka-Narins DM, editors.
Nutrition in Perspective. 2nd ed. Upper Saddle River, NJ: Prentice Hall Inc.; 1987.

2. Murray M. Encyclopedia of nutritional supplements. Rocklin, CA: Prima Publishing; 1996. p. 181-9.

3. Fahim MS, Fahim Z, Der R, Harman J. Zinc treatment for the reduction of hyperplasia of the prostate. Fed Proc 1976;35:361.

4. Leake A, Chrisholm GD, Busuttil A, Habib FK. Subcellular distribution of zinc in the benign and malignant human prostate: evidence for a direct zinc androgen interaction. Acta endocrinol 1984;105:281-8.

5. Leake A, Chisholm GD, Habib FK. The effect of zinc on the 5-alpha-reduction of testosterone by the hyperplastic human prostate gland. J Steroid Biochem 1984;20:651-5.

6. Wallae AM, Grant JK. Effect of zinc on androgen metabolism in the human hyperplastic prostate. Biochem Soc Trans 1975;3:540-2.

7. Judd AM, MacLeod RM, Login IS. Zinc acutely selectively and reversibly inhibits pituitary prolactin secretion. Brain Res 1984;294:190-2.

8. Login IS, Thorner MO, MacLeod RM. Zinc may have a physiological role in regulating pituitary prolactin secretion. Neuroendocrinology 1983;37:317-20.

9. Farnsworth WF, et al. Interaction of prolactin and testosterone in the human prostate. Urol Res 1981;9:79-88.

10. Pories WJ, Henzel JH, Rob CG, Strain WH. Acceleration of wound healing in man with zinc sulphate given by mouth. Lancet 1969;1:1069.

11. Greaves MW, Ive FA. Double-blind trial of zinc sulphate in the treatment of chronic venous leg ulceration. Br J Derm 1972;87:632.

12. Frommes DJ. The healing of gastric ulcers by zinc sulphate. Med J Aust 1975;2:793.

13. Young B, Ott L, Kasarskis E, Rapp R, Moles K, Dempsey R, et al. Zinc supplementation is associated with improved neurologic recovery rate and visceral protein levels of patients with severe closed head injury. J Neurotrauma 1996;1:25-34.

14. Hendler S. The doctors' vitamin and mineral encyclopedia. New York, NY: Simon and Schuster; 1990. p. 205-6.

15. Lieberman S, Bruning N. The real vitamin and mineral book. Garden City Park, NY: Avery Publishing Group; 1997. p. 148-54.

16. Tikkiwal M, Ajmera RL, Mathur NK. Effect of zinc administration on seminal zinc and fertility of oligospermic males. Ind J Phys Pharmacol 1987;31:30-4.

17. Takihara H, Cosentino MJ, Cockett AT. Zinc sulfate therapy for infertile males with or without varicocelectomy. Urology 1987;29:638-41.

18. Netter A, Hartoma R, Nahoul K. Effect of zinc administration on plasma testosterone, dihydrotestosterone and sperm count. Arch Androl 1981;7:69-73.

19. Newsome DA, Swartz M, Leone NC, Elston NC, Miller E. Oral zinc in macular degeneration. Arch ophthalmol 1988;106:192-8.

20. Stur M, Tihl M, Reitner A, Meisinger V. Oral zinc and the second eye in agerelated macular degeneration. Invest ophthalmol Vis Sci 1996;37:1225-35.

21. Boukaiba N, Flament C, Acher S, Chappuis P, Piau A, Fusselier M, et al. A physiological amount of zinc supplementation: effects on nutritional, lipid And thymic status in an elderly population. Am J Clin Nutr 1993;57:566-72.

22. Devine A, Rosen C, Mohan S, Baylink D, Prince R. Effects of zinc and other nutritional factors on insulin-like growth factor-1 and insulin-like growth Factor binding proteins in postmenopausal women. Am J Clin Nutr 1998;68(1):200-6.

23. Mossad SB, Macknin ML, Medendorp SV, Mason P. Zinc gluconate lozenges for treating the common cold. Ann Int Med 1996;125:81-8.

24. Garland ML, Hagmeyer KO. The role of zinc lozenges in treatment of the common cold. Ann Pharmacother 1998;32:93-6.

25. Reavley N. The new encyclopedia of vitamins, minerals, supplements, and herbs. New York, NY: M. Evans and Company Inc.; 1998. p. 324.

26. Sturniolo GC, Montino MC, Rossetto L, Martin A, D'Inca R, D'Odorico A, et al. Inhibition of gastric acid secretion reduces zinc absorption in man. J Am Coll Nutr 1991;10(4):372-5.

27. Mapp RK, McCarthy TJ. The effect of zinc sulphate and of bicitropeptide on tetracycline absorption. S Afr Med J 1976;50(45):1829-30.

28. Penttila O, Hurme H, Neuvonen PJ. Effect of zinc sulphate on the absorption of tetracycline and doxycycline in man. Eur J Clin Pharmacol 1975;9(2-3):131-4.

29. Golik A, Zaidenstein R, Dishi V, Blatt A, Cohen N, Cotter G, et al. Effects of captopril and enalapril on zinc metabolism in hypertensive patients. J Am Coll Nutr 1998;17(1):75-8.

30. Powanda MC. Clofibrate-induced alterations in zinc, iron and copper metabolism. Biochem Pharmacol 1978;27(1):125-27.

31. Fontaine J, Neve J, Peretz A, et al. Effects of acute and chronic prednisolone treatment on serum zinc levels in rats with adjuvant arthritis. Agents Actions 1991;33(3-4):247-53.

32. Fell GS, et al. Urinary zinc levels as an indicator of muscle catabolism. Lancet 1973Feb;1(7798):280-2

33. Solecki TJ, Aviv A, Bogden JD. Effect of a chelating drug on balance and tissue distribution of four essential metals. Toxicology 1984;31:207-16.

34. Wester PO. Urinary zinc excretion during treatment with different diuretics. Acta Med Scand 1980;208(3):209-12.

35. Dorea JG, Ferraz E, Queiroz EF. Effects of anovulatory steroids on serum levels of zinc and copper. Arch Latinoam Nutr 1982;32(1):101-10.
36. Lu JX, Combs GF Jr. Penicillamine: pharmacokinetics and differential effects on zinc and copper status in chicks. J Nutr 1992;122(2):355-62.
37. Mountokalakis T, Dourakis S, Karatzas N, Maravelias C, Koutselinis A. Zinc deficiency in mild hypertensive patients treated with diuretics. J Hypertens Suppl 1984;2(3):S571-2.
38. Hurd RW, Van Rinsvelt HA, Wilder BJ, Karas B, Maenhaut W, De Reu L. Selenium, zinc, and copper changes with valproic acid: possible relation to Drug side effects. Neurology 1984;34(10):1393-5.
39. Baum MK, Javier JJ, Mantero-Atienza E, Beach RS, Fletcher MA, Sauberlich HE, et al. Zidovudine-associated adverse reactions in a longitudinal study Of asymptomatic HIV-1-infected homosexual males. J Acquir Immune Defic Syndr 1991;4(12):1218-26.
40. Cossack ZT, van den Hamer CJ. Kinetics of copper absorption in zinc-overload states and following the withdrawal of zinc supplement: the role of endogenous zinc status. J Pediatr Gastroenterol Nutr 1987;6(2):296-301.
41. Hoogenradd TU, Van den Hamer CJ. 3 years of continuous oral zinc therapy in 4 patients with Wilson's Disease. Acta Neurol Scand 1983;67(6):356-64.
42. Solomons NW, Jacob RA. Studies on the bioavailability of zinc in humans: effects of heme and nonheme iron on the absorption of zinc. Am J Clin Nut 1981;34(4):475-82.
43. Rossander-Hulten L, Brune M, Sandstrom B, Lonnerdal B, Hallberg L. Competitive inhibition of iron absorption by manganese and zinc in humans. Am J Clin Nutr 1991;54(1):152-6.

Drug-Nutrient Interactions

Drug-Nutrient Interactions In General

McNeill JR. Interactions between herbal and conventional medicines. Can J CME 1999,11;12:97-110

Boullata J, Pharm D, Nace M. Safety issues with herbal medicine. Pharmacotherapy 2000, 20; 3: 257-269

Bleeding Disorders

McNeill JR. Interactions between herbal and conventional medicines. Can J CME 1999, 11;12:97-110

Heck A, et al. Potential interactions between alternative therapies and warfarin. Am J Health-Syst Pharm 2000,57;13:1221-7

Canadian Guidelines for Cardiac Rehabilitation and cardiovascular Disease Prevention, 11th ed. Canadian Association of Cardiac Rehabilitation 1999

Boon H, Smith M. Health Care Professional Training Program in Complementary Medicine. Institute of Applied Complementary Medicine Inc. 1997

Kinsella, JE, et al. Dietary n-3 polyunsaturated fatty acids and amelioration fo cardiovascular disease: possible mechanisms. Am J Clin Nutr 1990,;52:1-28

Mills S, Bone K. 30 Principles and Practice of Phytotherapy. Churchill Livingstone: 199-200 (Garlic)

Miller LG. Herbal Medicinals: Selected clinical considerations focusing on known or potential drug-herb interactions. Arch Intern Med 1998;158;20:2200-11

McNeill JR. Interactions between herbal and conventional medicines. Can J CME 1999, 11;12:97-110

Reavley N. New Encyclopedia of vitamins, Minerals, Supplements and Herbs. M. Evans and Company, Inc. NY 1998, Bookman Press (Australia)

Heart Function Disorders

McNeill JR. Interactions between herbal and conventional medicines. Can J CME 1999, 11;12:97-110

McRae S. Elevated serum digoxin levels in a patient taking digoxin and Siberian ginseng. Can Med Assoc J 1996,155:293-5

Heck A, et al. Potential interactions between alternative therapies and warfarin. Am J Health-Syst Pharm 2000,57;13:1221-7

Cupp MJ. Herbal Remedies: adverse effects on drug interactions. Am Fam Physician 1999,59;5:1239-45

Other Special Considerations

Miller LG. Herbal Medicinals: Selected clinical considerations focusing on known or potential drug-herb interactions. Arch Intern Med 1998;158;20: 2200-11Rand V, Hughes E. Botanicals: the wildcard in your patinet's list of medications. The 50th annual meeting of the Am Acad Family Phys Sci Assembly Sept16-20 1998

Patti ME, et al. Activation of the hexosamine pathway of glucosamine in vivo induces insulin resistance of early postreceptor insulin signaling events in skeletal muscle. Diabetes 1999;48;8:1562-71

Escher M, Desmeules J, Giostra E, et al. Hepatitis associated with kava, a herbal remedy for anxiety. BMJ 2001;322:139.

Kraft M, Spahn TW, Menzel J, et al. Fulminant liver failure after administration of the herbal antidepressant kava-kava. Dtsch Med Wochenschr 2001;126:970--2.

Saß M, Schnabel S, Kröger J, Liebe S, Schareck WD. Acute liver failure from kava-kava---a rare indication for liver transplantation. Z Gastroenterol 2001;39:491.

Campo JV, McNabb J, Perel JM, Mazariegos GV, Hasegawa SL, Reyes J. Kava-induced fulminant hepatic failure. J Am Acad Child Adolesc Psychiatry 2002;41:631--2.

Humbertston C, Akhtar J, Krenzelok E. Acute hepatitis induced by kava kava, an herbal product derived from *Piper methysticum*. J Clin Toxicol 2001;39:549.

Russmann S, Lauterburg BH, Helbling A. Kava hepatotoxicity. Ann Intern Med 2001;135:68--9.

Food and Drug Administration. Letter to health-care professionals: FDA issues consumer advisory that kava products may be associated with severe liver injury. Rockville, Maryland: U.S. Department of Health and Human Services, Food and Drug Administration, 2002. Available at http://www.cfsan.fda.gov/~dms/addskava.html.

Strahl S, Ehret V, Dahm HH, Maier KP. Necrotizing hepatitis after taking herbal remedies. Dtsch Med Wochenschr 1998;123:1410--4.

Walker AM. The relation between voluntary notification and material risk in dietary supplement safety. Food and Drug Administration docket 00N-1200, 2000. Available at http://www.fda.gov/ohrms/dockets/00n1200.

Murray M. The Healing Power of Herbs (2nd edition), Prima Publishing 1995:228-239

Das SK, Gulati AK, and Singh VP. Deglycrryrhizinated Liquorice in Aphthous Ulcers, J Assoc Physicians India 1989;37:p647

Evans FQ. The Rational Use of Glycyrrhetinic Acid in Dermatology, Br J Clin Pract 1958;12:269-279

Sharaf A and Goma N. Phytoestrogens and Their Antagonism to Progesterone and Testosterone, J Endocrinol1965;31:289-290

Stormer FC, Reistad R, and Alexander J. Glycyrrhizic Acid in Liquorice – Evaluation of Health Hazard, Fd Chem Toxicol 1993;31303-312

Biglieri EG. My Engagement with Steroids: A Review-Steroids 1995;60(1):52-58

Schleimer RP. Potential Regulation of Inflammation in the Lung by Local Metabolism of Hydrocortisone, American Journal of Respiratory Cell and Molecular Biology 1991;4:166-173

Chandler RF. Glycyrrhiza Glabra In: De Smet PAGM, Keller K, Hansel R, Chandler RF, eds, Adverse Effects of Herbal Drugs, Volume 3 ed., New York:Springer 1997:67-87

Tyler V, The Honest Herbal (3rd edition), Binghampton, New York: Pharmaceutical Products Press 1993:p375

Spinks EA, Fenwick GR. The Determination of Glycyrrhizin in Selected UK Liquorice Products, Food Additives and Contaminants 1990;7:769-778

Dietary Supplement Information Bureau. www.content.intramedicine.com:Licorice

Healthnotes, Inc. 2001. www.healthnotes.com:Licorice

Natural Products Encyclopedia. www.consumerslab.com:Licorice

Rees, WD, Rhodes J, Wright JE et al. Effect of deglycyrrhizinated liquorice on gastric mucosal damage by aspirin. Scand J Gatroenterol 1979;14:605-7

Amer M, Metwalli M. Topical liquiritin improves melasma. Int J Dermatol 2000;39:299-301

Blumenthal M, Busse WR, Goldberg A et al. (eds.) The Complete Commission E Monographs: Therapeutic Guide to Herbal Medicines. Boston, MA: Integrative Medicine Communications 1998:161-2

Bardhan KD, Cumberland DC, Dixon RA, Holdsworth CD. Clinical trial of deglycyrrhizinised liquorice in gastric ulcer. Gut 1978;19:779-82

Das SK, Das V, Gulati AD, Singh VP. Deglycyrrhizinated licorice in aphthous ulcers. J Assoc Physicians India 1989;37:p647

Mills S, Bone K. 30 Principles and Practice of Phytotherapy. Churchill Livingstone:465 – 478

Armanini D, Palermo M. Reduction of serum testosterone in men by licorice. N Engl J Med 1999;341:p1158

Farese RV et al. Licorice-induced hyperminarlocorticoidism. New England J Med 1991;325:1223-7

DeSmet P et al. Adverse Effects Of Herbal Drugs I. Berlin, Springer-Verlag 1992:97-104

Epstein MT et al. Effect of eating liquorice on the rennin-angiotensin-aldosterone axis in normal subjects. Br Med J 1977;1:488-90

Takeda R et al. Prolonged pseudoaldosteronism induced by glycyrrhizin. Endocrinology Japan 1979;26(5):541-7

Gibson MR. Glycyrrhiza in Old and New Perspectives. Lloydia 1978;41(4):348-54

MacKenzie MA et al. The Influence of Glycyrrhetinic Acid on Plasma Cortisol and Cortisone in healthy Young Volunteers. J Clin Endocrin Metab 1990;70:1637-43

General References

Earl L. Mindell, R.Ph., Ph.D. and Virginia Hopkins, M.A. Prescription Alternatives, Hundreds of Safe, Natural, Presricption-Free Remedies to Restore & Maintain Your Health – 4th ED. McGraw Hill 1990

Edmunds – Mayhew et al. Pharmacology for the Primary Care Provider, Third Edition. Mosby Elsevier 2009.

Lyle MacWilliam MSc, FP for Nutrisearch Corporation. Nutrisearch Comparative Guide to Nutritional Supplements, A Compendeum of Products Available in the United States and Canada, 4th Edition. Northern Dementions Publishing 2007.

Well Being Journal Vol. 20, No. 6. Editors; Scott E. Miners et al. November/December 2011

Linus Pauling Institute. Soy Isoflavones.

The Weston A. Price Foundation. Mike Fitzpatrick PhD. Soy Isoflavaones: Panacea or Poison? 2009

James Meschino DC, MS, ND. Antioxidant Supplements May Reduce Cancer Risk: New Findings From the EPIC Study.

Kimberly Hayes Taylor, Reuters. Vitamin D Supplements Lower Death Risk : Study. www.nationalpost.com Nov. 29, 2011

Dr. Mercola. The Evidence Against Soy. www.mercola.com October 7, 2008

Dr. Mercola. Experts Finally Recognize The Dangers With Soy. www.mercola.com February 7, 2006

American Association for Cancer Research. "Soy isoflavones not a risk for breast cancer survivors, study finds." ScienceDaily, 5 Apr. 2011.Web. 19 Dec. 2011.

Dr. Mercola. "550 Times More Powerful Than Vitamin E- The Age-Defying Antioxidant You've Never Heard Of*"

Dr. Mercola. Soy: Is It Healthy or Harmful? www.mercola.com January 21, 2004

Dr. Mercola. This "Miracle Health Food" Has Been Linked to Brain Damage and Breast Cancer. September 18, 2010

Dr. Mercola. The Whole Soy Story: The Dark Side of America's Favorite Health Food. www.mercola.com July 17, 2008

Dr. Mercola. 10 Important Facts About Vitamin K That You Need to Know. www.mercola.com March 24, 2004

Dr. Mercola. Test Values and Treatment for Vitamin D Deficiency. www.mercola.com February 23, 2002

Dr. Mercola. Vitamin D is a Key Player in Your Overall Health. www.mercola.com November 1, 2008

Dr. Mercola. Valuble Insights Into the Importance of Vitamin D and Sun. www.mercola.com April 3, 2004

Dr. Mercola. Breakthrough Updates You Need to Know on Vitamin D. www.mercola.com February 23, 2002

Dr. Mercola. Vitamin D Update. www.mercola.com Dec 27, 2008

Dr. Mercola. "This Vitamin is So Extrodinary, It's Regulated by Government Agencies*" http://products.mercola.com

Chemotherapy, From Wikipedia, the free encyclopedia. http://en.wikipedia.org/wiki/chemotherapy November 15, 2011

Cancer Research UK. How Chemotherapy Works. http://cancerhelp.cancerresearchuk.org/about-cancer/treatment/chemotherapy November 8, 2011

HuffPost Living, the Canadian Press. 552 Million People Could Have Diabetes By 2030, Experts Say Many Cases Still Preventable. www.huffingtonpost.ca/2011/11/14/552-million-people-could... November 14, 2011

Soya- Information about Soy & Soya Products. Dr. Mercola is Anti-Soy http://www.soya.be/mercola.php .

Sally Fallon & Mary G. Enig PhD. Posted by Dr. Mercola. Newest Research on Why You Should Avoid Soy. April 9, 2010

Linus Pauling Intitiute. Soy Isoflavones. http://lpi.oregonstate.edu/infocenter/phytochemicals/soyiso/ Copyright 2004-2011

Dr. Mercola. Soy Can Damage Your Health; What Makes Soy Such a Risky Food to Eat? http://articles.mercola.com/sites/articles/archive/2010/09/18/soy-can-damage-your-health.aspx

Dr. John Zielonka Healthy Beliefs Deadly Choices

Dr. John Zielonka Nutrition Insanity

Dr. John Zielonka Human Performance Lecture Series

Dr. John Zielonka Sick Care vs. the Health & Wellness Paradigm

Part Three

The Role of Vitamin Supplementation in Disease

7

APPLE JUICE, STEWED MOSQUITOES, BAKING COOKIES AND CHEMICAL PATHWAYS

Now that you know that nutrition has an amazing role in your overall health, there's one more aspect that you may not have realized.

Understand that everything in your body is made from the nutrients that you have put into it. That knowledge gives you incredible power on how you can affect the workings of your body. Here's a silly example that illustrates the point. Imagine that you were a machine that was only capable of doing two functions. Your body was only capable of either producing apple juice or stewing mosquitoes. Obviously if all you consumed were apples, your machine would produce nothing but apple juice. On the other hand, if all you ate were mosquitoes, your machine would only be capable of stewing those same mosquitoes.

Understanding and appreciating this gives us incredible power over what happens in our body. Here's how. As stated before, since everything in our body is made up from the nutrients that we consume, we have the ability to modify or influence events in our body. For instance, the hormones made in our body are made from these same nutrients. Some hormones produce good reactions in our bodies and other produce bad reactions. If we ate nothing but the nutrients that produced good hormones, we would obviously influence our body to produce nothing but good hormones. On the other hand, if we continually consumed the nutrients that produced bad hormones (for lack of a better term), we would obviously produce more hormones that had adverse reactions in our body. One such hormone is a group known as prostaglandins which, among other things, are responsible for inflammation in our body. If we consume foods that are utilized by the body to produce chemicals that result in more inflammation, then obviously we would increase the inflammatory response in our body. On the other hand, if we minimized the constituents necessary to produce an inflammatory reaction, less inflammation would occur in our body. If we could accomplish this, there would be no need for anti-inflammatory drugs and the seriously adverse reactions that accompany them. This can also be said of many other reactions that occur in the body.

Now let's turn to baking cookies and chemical pathways. If I want to bake cookies, there are a number of steps and ingredients involved. If I miss a step or an ingredient, that will obviously change the outcome of my cookies. If it's a small step, i.e. I didn't put in enough salt, I'll still have my cookie – it just won't taste the same. If it's a bigger step, i.e. I forgot to turn the oven on or the butter was rancid, my cookies really won't be very good cookies.

Now apply this to the chemical pathways that are constantly happening in your body. One substance is added to another, which then may have something else added (known as a cofactor or enzyme) that converts it to another substance. By selectively choosing drugs or vitamins as cofactors and the types of nutrients we have in our body, we can ultimately influence what the final substance will be. In some cases, drugs or vitamins may even inhibit an enzyme and thus stop the conversion of one substance into another. This is how most drugs and vitamins work. Yes – that's right – there are many cases where a vitamin works exactly the same way that a drug does, minus the majority of the side effects, of course.

The following chapters will describe some of the most prominent illnesses known to mankind, and the science that shows the effectiveness of vitamin supplementation in both the management and prevention of those same conditions.

It's time to eat more apples, eat fewer mosquitoes, and consume the proper supplements that allow us to make only the best and healthiest cookies.

8

CARDIOVASCULAR DISEASE

Do you have a coin? Great. Now flip it. Heads – you'll die of cardiovascular disease – tails you won't. Worse yet, for approximately half of the population, the very first sign or symptom that they'll have in finding out that they have cardiovascular disease is having a heart attack. It gets worse. Forty percent of those people who have that first heart attack, not knowing there was a problem, will die from it.

One could argue that it gets even worse. You could consider that almost everyone has some form of heart disease. Your arteries might only be clogged ten or twenty percent, but in our sick care paradigm society we think that's normal. And worst of all, it's almost all preventable.

The next three chapters will cover the three key factors: cholesterol, heart disease, and high blood pressure.

9

HEART DISEASE
(MYOCARDIAL INFARCTION, STROKE, ANGINA AND CONGESTIVE HEART FAILURE)

Are you one of those above average health-wise people I spoke of earlier whose arteries are only clogged 10 to 20%? Well guess what? Comparing yourself to average is an incredibly low standard. And if you already suffer from one of the above, it's never too late to start getting healthier.

There is a substantial body of evidence that shows that anti-oxidants, especially vitamins C and E, can reduce your risk of heart disease.

VITAMIN E

A fourteen-year study of over five thousand men and women in Finland showed that those with the highest intake of vitamin E had the lowest rates of heart disease.

The nurses' health study followed over 87,000 female nurses aged 34 to 59 years old. After factoring in all other heart disease risk factors, those who consumed vitamin E supplementation at or above 100 I.U. daily showed a 41% reduction in the risk of heart disease.

The Health care professionals follow-up study of almost 40,000 men aged 40 to 75 showed the same results (46% reduction in risk) compared to non-supplementers or those who supplemented less than 100 I.U. per day.

Vitamin E reduces the risk of cardiovascular disease through three primary mechanisms.

1. As an anti-oxidant. Vitamin E travels in the bloodstream bonded to cholesterol. By acting as an anti-oxidant, it prevents free radicals from damaging cholesterol molecules. Cholesterol is far more likely to attach to arterial walls if it has been damaged.
2. It inhibits the proliferation of smooth muscle. This prevents the artery from narrowing.
3. It reduces platelet stickiness. This prevents platelets from clumping together in the artery and is the same principle mechanism through which aspirin reduces heart attack risk.

Numerous prominent researchers have shown that the level of vitamin E necessary to achieve these results can only be achieved through supplementation. 400 I.U. of dalpha-tocopherol and gamma-tocopherol is recommended daily.

VITAMIN C

The MONICA Study (Multinational **MONI**toring of Trends and Determinants in **CA**rdiovascular disease) was a project that was established in the early 1980s in many centres around the world to monitor trends in cardiovascular diseases over a ten year period. There were a total of 32 MONICA Collaborating Centres in 21 countries. The total population monitored was **ten million men and women** ages 25 to 64 years-old. This study showed that vitamin C blood levels above a certain level (50 mmol/litre) showed a 50% reduction in heart disease. The same study showed that **low levels of vitamin C and vitamin E were stronger predictors of future heart disease than were high cholesterol levels, smoking, or high blood pressure.**

Vitamin C also prevents free radical damage of cholesterol and, most importantly, is required to regenerate vitamin E.

Shockingly, 20 to 30% of the population don't even receive the daily amount of vitamin C necessary to prevent scurvy (60 mg/day), and most only 200-250 mg/day. Your total daily dose should be at least 1000 mg, preferably in an ascorbate form.

Vitamin E supplementation reduced the risk of all-cause death by 34% and the risk of death from heart disease by 47 to 63%. Simultaneous use of both vitamin C and vitamin E reduced the risk of all-cause death by 42%.

**Low levels of vitamin C and vitamin E
were stronger predictors of future heart disease
than were high cholesterol levels,
smoking, or high blood pressure**

It is of key importance to note that the use of a standard multi-vitamin showed no decrease in all-cause death. How can this be given the above? Simple. As we will discuss, the levels of vitamins C and E in many standard multi-vitamins simply "dabble" and do not provide the levels necessary to see the protective effects as shown by the science. This is the same reason why, although it's a nice thought, you'll never get the protective effects from food alone. That's why it's so important to supplement at optimal levels and ignore the ridiculous misleading "studies" that wrongly attempt to dissuade you from a lifetime of health.

Studies have also shown that it's never too late to start. Significant benefits have been shown in the elderly who sometimes wrongly believe it's too late to start or are scared that they may interfere with the multiple drugs that they are often taking.

B VITAMINS (Folic acid, B6, B12)

High levels of homocysteine are thought to increase our risk of heart disease through their toxic effects to the cells that line our blood vessels. A number of studies have shown that supplementing with folic acid, vitamin B6 and vitamin B12 can reduce homocysteine levels.

Folic acid is required to convert homocysteine to methionine, which is then converted to SAMe (s-adenosyl methionine), which is involved in the formation of DNA bases, neurotransmitter production and liver detoxification, before being converted back to homocysteine and the whole process starts all over again.

One significant study from the Journal of the American Medical Association showed that women who supplemented with a higher level of folic acid showed a 31% lower risk for heart disease, a 33% lower risk if they supplemented with B6, and a 45% reduced risk if they supplemented with both.

CO-ENZYME Q10 (CoQ10)

Also known as ubiquinone, CoQ10 is found in every cell of the body as it is an essential requirement for energy production. It enables your body to convert the food that you eat into ATP energy. This is the serious concern with cholesterol-lowering statin drugs as statins deplete your CoQ10 levels. When CoQ10 is in a deficiency state, there is a decline in energy production and cell function, which results in accelerated aging, heart disease, a decline in brain function, weakening of the immune system, and an increased risk of cancer. Given these facts, it's insane that we think statins are a rational way to lower cholesterol.

CoQ10 can be made in our body, but optimal levels are only made to age twenty and significant decreases are seen by age forty. It's a seventeen-step process that requires eight vitamins (mostly B) and several minerals (there's that synergy again).

The average intake in our diet is only 5 to 10 mg per day. You should supplement with 30 mg/day (you would need to eat half a pound of sardines or two and a half pounds of peanuts daily to get this level) although some experts recommend 60 mg/day, especially for seniors. It is not uncommon for those with heart disease to supplement as much as 100 to 300 mg per day. Of particular note is that scientists point out that CoQ10 not only addresses symptoms, it actually addresses the underlying biochemical cause of dysfunction.

HAWTHORN

Hawthorn is rich in flavinoids, such as Quercitin, which have been shown to improve coronary blood flow and strengthen contractions of the heart.

It also appears to act in a manner similar to cardiac glycoside drugs, such as digoxin and digitalis, enhancing ATP production.

Caution is warranted before supplementing with Hawthorn if you are taking cardiac glycoside drugs or ACE inhibitors.

CARNITINE

Carnitine transports fatty acids into the cell and helps the body burn fat. The heart requires L-carnitine as it uses fat as an energy source for heart contractions.

In cases of angina and congestive heart failure, doses of 1500 to 4000 mg have shown significant benefit in clinical trials. L-carnitine can also protect the heart against the damaging effects of the chemotherapy drug adriamycin.

Only L-carnitine (not D) should be used as a supplement but its use is restricted by Health Canada.

TAURINE

Taurine is a non-essential amino acid. It helps regulate the contractions and pumping action of the heart muscle. Studies have shown that it can even help to reverse the symptoms of congestive heart failure.

L-ARGININE

L-Arginine is an amino acid that has many purposes in the body. It, along with Ornithine, is used in high doses by some athletes as it increases the release of growth hormone.

L-Arginine is a precursor to the synthesis of nitric oxide, which causes vasodilation (opening up) of both the central and peripheral arteries, increasing blood flow. As such, it has been successfully used in the treatment of angina, congestive heart failure and even male impotence.

Care should be taken as L-Arginine can also act as a blood thinner in high doses. As such, it should not be used in conjunction with anti-coagulant drugs and other blood thinners without proper monitoring. It has also been reported to promote outbreaks of herpes lesions in afflicted individuals.

10

CHOLESTEROL

Our sick care paradigm has done a masterful job of warning society about the evils of cholesterol and the need to take statin drugs to keep cholesterol below a certain level.

Since this is a book on vitamins, I don't want to go off on what some may perceive as too much of a tangent, but this is key. If you appreciate the difference between a sick care paradigm and a health and wellness paradigm, and you also appreciate that either God of Mother Nature equipped you with something known as innate intelligence, you must ask yourself one question with respect to high cholesterol... Why?

Innate intelligence is your body's inborn intelligence to know what to do to survive. Your body is innately both self-healing and self-regulating. For example, you have trillions of red blood cells in your body, which last for about four months. Right now, red blood cell number 1,286,412,286,177 just died. It takes no conscious effort on your part to make another one. Cut your finger? Your body knows how to heal it.

This brings us back to why? If your body's innate intelligence is so great (it is – it's just that we as humans go out of our way to mess it up on a daily basis), then **why** does it lay down cholesterol to clog up our arteries?

Answering this question becomes key to your approach in dealing with high cholesterol. Of interest is the fact that it's a question most medical doctors and all drug companies will never ask. Their sick care paradigm assumes the body isn't intelligent and that any response your body has must be counteracted by drugs, side effects included, as there certainly couldn't be a reason for the body to react the way it is, could there?

So what's the reason? Well consider this; if we wiped out all of the cholesterol in your body, you would die. Cholesterol is necessary for many things, including the fact that it's what testosterone, estrogen, and vitamin D are made from, hence it's not in us by accident. It's also what half your brain's cerebral cortex is made of. Does cholesterol just randomly build in our arteries (the "we're innately stupid approach")? Or is that same build-up from cholesterol being laid down in our arteries as a way of cementing weaknesses in those same arteries to preserve their integrity (the innate intelligence approach)?

You can now appreciate why my tangent was important instead of just listing the natural alternatives to statin drugs. If you don't take steps to repair the underlying cause of a problem, then you'll be caught in a lifelong battle of your body trying to do one thing to save your life and your M.D. trying to defeat your body's innate intelligence thinking he's saving your life.

STATIN DRUGS

"nobody qualifies for statin therapy"
and
"statin drugs can best be described as toxins"
Dr. Stephanie Seneff, Ph.D.
Senior Research Scientist
Massachusetts Institute of Technology

Statin drugs (Lipitor, Crestor, Mevacor, Pravachol, Zocor, etc.) all function by blocking the enzyme in your liver (HMG-COA reductase) that makes cholesterol. The problem is that these drugs have serious side effects, the worst of which are rhabdomolysis (a life-threatening eating away of muscle – important since your heart is a muscle), heart failure, and dementia. Statins deplete your body of CoQ10, which is essential for heart function.

Statin drugs (Lipitor, Crestor, Mevacor, Zocor, etc.) all have serious side effects including death, heart failure and dementia

SO WHAT DO YOU DO?
To help repair damage to your arterial walls, two things are necessary; high doses of vitamin C for its collagen-building abilities, and high doses of essential fatty acids. These, along with each of the following will also help to lower cholesterol levels:

GUM GUGGUL (gugulipid)
Gum guggul, although completely natural, is widely prescribed in India as a drug that has been shown in human clinical trials to lower cholesterol by 14 to 27% and triglycerides by 22 to 33% within a four to twelve-week

period. It is very non-toxic with a proven safety record. It has also been shown to improve your HDL/LDL ratio, has anti-oxidant properties, and has been shown to reduce the stickiness of blood platelets. It increases the uptake of excess cholesterol out of the bloodstream and back into the liver.

One scientific study showed that gum guggul was equal to the cholesterol-lowering drug clofibrate in its ability to lower cholesterol, whereas another showed that gum guggul had the equivalent anti-inflammatory potency as both ibuprofen and phenylbutazone.

Dosage: To lower cholesterol and triglyceride blood levels, take 25 mg of guggulsterone three to four times per day. If taking a guggulsterone product standardized to five percent, you would take 500 mg three to four times daily.

POLICOSANOL

Policosonol, derived from natural sugar cane wax, had been shown in both human and animal studies to both lower bad cholesterol and raise good cholesterol in over 80 scientific studies. However, almost all of those studies have come under question as they were all done in Cuba by the same group who had a significant financial interest in sugar cane and policosanol. Although no significant adverse reactions have ever been shown with the use of policosanol, to err on the side of caution and to maintain a reasonable burden of proof, most other vitamin experts and I no longer recommend policosanol to manage high cholesterol until such findings can be independently verified as being scientifically valid.

PLANT STEROLS

Repeated scientific studies have shown that plant sterols have been able to lower LDL by 10%, lower triglycerides by 25% and raise "good" HDL cholesterol by 15 to 35%.

NIACIN

Numerous scientific studies have repeatedly demonstrated niacin's ability to lower LDL cholesterol by 10%.

"the best way to characterize statin therapy
is that it makes you grow old faster"
Dr. Stephanie Seneff, Ph.D.
Senior Research Scientist
Massachusetts Institute of Technology

11

HIGH BLOOD PRESSURE

High blood pressure affects 25% of the population, many of whom are not managing their condition properly or are suffering side effects of their prescribed drugs. In Canada, only 16% of those with hypertension are managing it properly – 84% are not! The most current scientific research states that all people with hypertension should receive intensive non-drug therapies to manage and improve their situation.

CALCIUM

A number of well-designed scientific studies have shown that calcium supplementation can effectively help lower blood pressure. Calcium encourages sodium excretion by the kidneys, especially so in sodium sensitive patients.

It also helps to relax the smooth muscle of arteries (with magnesium) to lower diastolic blood pressure.

The recommended dosage is 1000 to 1500 mg per day in 500 mg doses.

MAGNESIUM

Magnesium has also been shown to encourage sodium excretion by the kidneys and thus help lower blood pressure. The recommended dosage is 600 mg daily.

ESSENTIAL FATTY ACIDS

Over 60 scientific double-blind studies have shown that omega 3 fatty acids (either fish oil or flaxseed oil) can lower both systolic and diastolic blood pressure by up to 9mm. The recommended dose is 1000 mg twice daily.

CoQ10

A number of scientific studies have shown that CoQ10 can effectively and consistently lower blood pressure in hypertensive patients.

As previously discussed, CoQ10 is required for ATP energy production. Research has shown that 39% of patients with high blood pressure have a CoQ10 deficiency. Supplementation with CoQ10 corrects this underlying cause. Research also shows that this requires a minimum of 4 to 12 weeks to see results with ongoing supplementation warranted.

Studies have shown that, even in patients taking antihypertensive drugs, the addition of 60 mg of CoQ10 twice daily was able to markedly reduce both systolic and diastolic blood pressure. Therefore, CoQ10 can be taken safely with high blood pressure drugs to get even better results.

While 60 mg twice daily is recommended, dosages of 100 mg daily have been successful and amounts as little as 30 mg daily have been successful in mild cases.

HAWTHORN

In addition to bioflavinoids known as procyanidins that are helpful in congestive heart failure, hawthorn extract has also been shown to lower blood pressure.

These procyanidins act as cardiac glucoside agents (just as the drugs digitalis and digoxin as previously discussed) that increase energy (cyclic AMP) and they also act as vasodilators – in other words, they open up arteries, hence reducing pressure.

The dosage required is 100 to 250 mg up to three times daily if taken as your sole remedy. Again, the supplement should be standardized to 5% flavinoid content. At least 2 to 4 weeks is required to see a decline in blood pressure. Again, hawthorn should not be taken in patients taking digitalis or digoxin.

12

CANCER

As I write this chapter, the FDA just yesterday pulled the breast cancer drug Avastin in the United States. According to them, Avastin "does not appear to delay tumour growth, prolong life, or improve the quality of life for women with a form of breast cancer known as HER2 negative that has spread to other parts of the body". It was also stated that "the drug can also cause side effects that are potentially fatal, including high blood pressure, bleeding, haemorrhaging, heart attack, and development of perforations in the nose, stomach, intestines, and other parts of the body".

My question to you is – how did it ever get approved in the first place? More astonishing is the fact that FDA Commissioner Margaret Hamburg stated that "this was a difficult decision" (pulling the drug) and that it is still approved for use by Health Canada.

Cancer scares people. Even the word scares people. And if you've heard my lecture "Discover Wellness and Cancer" you'll know that way too many of my family are either living with it or have died from it.

"this was a difficult decision"
FDA Commissioner Margaret Hamburg on pulling the breast tumour drug Avastin which was unable to delay tumour growth, prolong life, or improve the quality of life for women yet had side effects that are potentially fatal, including high blood pressure, bleeding, haemorrhaging, and heart attack

Most chemotherapy acts by killing cells that divide rapidly as is the case with cancer cells. Unfortunately, it also harms cells that normally divide rapidly such as cells in the bone marrow, digestive tract, and hair follicles. Not surprisingly, side effects include a decreased production of blood cells, inflammation in the digestive tract, and hair loss. Newer cancer drugs attempt to attack abnormal proteins in cancer cells with a more targeted approach.

Chemotherapy can be considered highly successful in some cases, useless in others, and unnecessary in still others. Research has shown that, taking all forms of cancer together, patients who receive chemotherapy <u>on average</u> increase their five year survival rate by only 2%, from 61% to 63%. This average, however, varies greatly from 40% for testicular cancer, to only a 1.5% increased survival for breast and lung cancer, and 0% for prostate and pancreatic cancer.

There is a better way. While we're all waiting for scientists to come up with a "cure", the truth is that we already have a number of ways to prevent the majority of cancers – ways that have been scientifically proven with far, far fewer "side effects" than drugs such as Avastin. Please allow me to share them with you.

From the point of conception throughout your life, your cells are constantly dividing. To make a long story really short, as they divide replication of those cells is near perfect but not 100%. Eventually, your cells will exhaust their ability to replicate sufficiently and your physical body will die.

With each cell division, your telomeres (in Greek "telos" means end and "meros" means part – hence "end part") shorten. These "end parts" (telomeres) cap the ends of your chromosomes for protection. Telomerase is the enzyme responsible for the maintenance and elongation of telomere length. Telomere shortening is an early event in human tumour development and thus may contribute to both the mutation of the chromosome and the instability that speeds tumour progression.

Percentage of Cancers with Detectable Telomerase Activity

Bladder cancer	98%
Colorectal cancer	95%
Neuroblastoma	94%
Breast cancer	93%
Liver cancer	85%
Prostate cancer	84%

Therefore, increased risk of cancer, as well as cellular and tissue aging, are directly related to the shortening of telomeres with each cell division. Thus, any strategy that can slow the rate of cell division will clearly prolong the time that a cell will remain healthy and lower your risk of developing cancer. Certain nutritional factors have been clearly shown to either speed up or slow down the rate of cell division.

SPECIFIC SUPPLEMENTATION TO SIGNIFICANTLY LOWER YOUR RISK OF CANCER

VITAMIN D

As previously discussed, vitamin D (more specifically D3, known as cholecalciferol) is one of the "stars" of vitamin supplementation and one of the essential vitamins that is needed by everyone. Unfortunately, most people, especially Canadians and anyone north of the 42nd parallel (running through the middle of California and the tops of Arizona, New Mexico, Texas, and the Carolinas. Of interest is the fact that, the farther you get away from the equator, the more the rates of breast, prostate, and colon cancer increase) or south of the 42nd parallel in the southern hemisphere, are deficient especially during mid-fall to mid-spring. In fact, many experts advise supplementing beyond the 1000 I.U. daily limit set by Health Canada. Worse yet, at age 45 the enzyme in the kidney (alpha-hydroxylase) that converts vitamin D into its most active form (1,25-dihydroxyvitamin D or calcitriol) becomes less active. (Aside from cancer prevention, this is also a major factor for osteoporosis.)

Many organs (prostate, breast, brain, pancreas, skin, gonads, stomach, colon, kidney, connective tissue, parathyroid gland, activated T and B lymphocytes) actually have what are known as vitamin D receptors. This means that each of these organs is capable of extracting 25hydroxyvitamin D from the bloodstream and converting it into the much more potent 1,25-dihydroxyvitamin D (calcitriol). Studies show that this form of vitamin D exerts a number of anti-cancer effects on these tissues.

This conversion takes place via the kidney hydroxylase enzyme. As kidney function decreases, so does this conversion.

Anti-cancer benefits of 1,25-dihydroxyvitamin:

- slows down the rate of normal cell replication
- slows the rate of replication of prostate, breast, and colon cancer cells
- promotes newly formed normal cells to mature to their full adult potential
- enhances immune function
- has been shown to transform the appearance of prostate cancer cells back to healthy non-malignant looking and inhibit their replication (this effect was lost when 1,25-dihydroxyvitamin D was no longer present)

Very few foods, unfortunately, contain vitamin D in its natural form. Even milk has been shown in numerous studies to have far less vitamin D than stated on the label, which was already woefully inadequate. (One study showed that two-thirds of the samples had less than 80% and several samples had 0 to 50% of the amount stated on the label. Furthermore, many drugs deplete vitamin D levels.

Obviously, one should also decrease all lifestyle factors that speed up cell division (high animal fat diet, stress, alcohol use, drug use, and obesity).

VITAMIN D CONVERSION

Sunlight

⇓

7-dehydrocholesterol   ⇨

vitamin D3 (cholecalciferol)   ⇨

enters bloodstream   ⇨   enters liver

⇨   converted to 25-hydroxyvitamin D
(5x more potent than vitamin D3 cholecalciferol)

⇨   enters cells

⇨   converted to 1,25-hydroxyvitamin D calcitriol
(10x more potent than 25-hydroxvitamin D)

ANTI-OXIDANTS

As you know, we need oxygen to survive. But of that very same oxygen, approximately 5% of it is converted into very aggressive free radicals. These aggressive free radicals, which also come from smoking, pollution, pesticides, nitrosamines, and even exercise, attack the DNA of our cells causing cancerous mutations. (It is estimated that each cell in our body receives 10,000 free radical hits per day just from oxygen free radicals.)

It is obvious, then, that anything that can help quench these free radicals can help to reduce your risk of cancer. These include anti-oxidants such as vitamin E, vitamin C, beta-carotene, vitamin A, lycopene, lutein, zeaxanthin, bioflavinoids, and others. Your body is also capable of making its own anti-oxidants (that's how we're able to survive in an oxygen atmosphere), but the enzymes that make these anti-oxidants require very specific minerals for activation, namely magnesium, zinc, copper, manganese, and selenium.

Numerous scientific studies have shown that people who supplement with optimum levels of anti-oxidants and their appropriate required vitamins and minerals are able to substantially decrease their risk of cancer (not to mention their risk of other degenerative diseases and overall aging).

VITAMIN C

Ninety epidemiological studies have shown vitamin C to be effective in lowering the risk of breast, lung, cervical, rectal, stomach, pancreatic, and esophageal cancer. In addition to its anti-oxidant capabilities, vitamin C also blocks the formation of cancer-causing nitrosamines in the intestinal tract.

VITMAIN E

We have known for over 20 years that vitamin E is protective against colon, rectal, pancreatic, and stomach cancer. It also inhibits PG-2. PG-2 encourages the rapid growth and division of tumour cells and helps cancer cells escape surveillance by the body's immune system.

The Iowa Women's Health Study followed 35,000 women over the course of four years. Those in the top 20% of vitamin E supplementation had a 66% lower risk of developing colon cancer than those in the bottom 20%.

In the Alpha-Tocopherol, Beta-Carotene Cancer Prevention Study, long term supplementation (5 to 8 years) showed a 32% decrease in the incidence of prostate cancer and a 41% decrease in death due to prostate cancer than the non-supplemented group.

Vitamin E supplementation is also associated with reducing the spread and progression of breast cancer in women who already have the disease. A 25 to 35% decrease in mortality and recurrence was seen in supplementers vs. non-supplementers.

The same researchers conducted an 18 to 24 month study (ages 32 to 81) of high risk breast cancer patients whose tumour had spread to the lymph nodes in the axilla (underarm). They were put on a high dose of an anti-oxidant protocol containing the following:

Vitamin C	2850 mg
Vitamin E	2500 I.U.
Beta-carotene	32.5 I.U.
Selenium	387 mcg
CoQ10	90 to 390 mg

plus secondary vitamins, minerals, and essential fatty acids.

The following results were noted:
- none of the patients died (12.5% was expected)
- none of the patients showed further metastases
- quality of life was improved
- no weight loss occurred
- there was a reduced use of painkillers
- 19% showed partial remission

SELENIUM

Animal studies have shown that supplementation with selenium resulted in only a 3% tumour yield vs. 29% in the non-supplemented group. Areas in North America with low soil and crop selenium concentration show higher rates for colon and rectal cancer.

Human trials have shown that, in over 1300 subjects, those taking selenium (200 mcg) for five years showed a 58% reduction in colon and rectal cancer over the non-supplemented group.

Selenium reduces cancer risk in four ways:

1. It acts as an anti-oxidant.
2. It increases the anti-oxidant enzyme glutathione peroxidase, which is a strong anti-cancer agent.
3. It decreases the prostaglandin hormone PG-2.
4. It is an essential nutrient involved in 13 enzymes and proteins.

The average food intake is only 50 mcg, which is clearly not sufficient to maximize our cancer defenses.

In a five year study of over 30,000 men and women, supplementation with beta-carotene, vitamin E, and selenium showed:

- decrease in death rates from all cancers by 13%
- 21% decrease in stomach cancer
- 45% decrease in lung cancer

VITAMIN B

As previously discussed, folic acid is required to convert homocysteine to methionine, which is then converted to SAMe.

Homocysteine Methionine

↑

requires folic acid

⇨   S-adenosyl methionine (SAMe)

SAMe is necessary to synthesize DNA that makes up our genetic blueprint. Hence folic acid is essential to ensure that your DNA is properly duplicated from one cell to the next without genetic errors occurring. Fewer cell duplication errors results in longer normal cell life, fewer mutations, and thus less cancer.

ESSENTIAL FATTY ACIDS

The most unique function of essential fatty acids is that they are continually converted into prostaglandin hormones. As we will discuss thoroughly in chapter 15, a lack of essential fatty acids, specifically EPA and DHA, results in less production of what are known as the good prostaglandins (PG-1 and PG-3) and more of what is considered the bad prostaglandin (PG-2).

Unfortunately, deficiencies and imbalances of essential fatty acids are common due to modern day agricultural and food processing practices as well as our typical style of eating. Most experts agree it is virtually impossible to get optimal concentrations of essential fatty acids into your body unless you take an essential fatty acid supplement daily.

Both animal and human studies show that increased PG-2 is associated with increased cancer risk. It encourages more rapid cell division, which leads to increased genetic mistakes and less time to correct these errors, therefore, more cancerous mutations occur.

Higher PG-2 levels are associated with an increased risk of breast, colon, and prostate cancer whereas increased PG-3 is associated with a decreased risk of these cancers.

Supplementation with essential fatty acids (one of the five necessary supplements for everyone) can be accomplished through fish oil (EPA and DHA) and/or flaxseed.

Flaxseed (ground flaxseed powder) is an extremely rich source of a lignan precursor known as secoisolariciresinol diglucoside (SLD). Flaxseed contains 800 times more SLD than any other common food. The body takes this SLD and it is converted by bacteria in the large intestine into two powerful phytoestrogens. Phytoestrogens are estrogen-like compounds derived from plants (hence "phyto").

Flaxseed powder   ⇨   enterolactone

contains SLD   ⇨   enterodiol
                                 large intestine (phytoestrogens)

These two phytoestrogens (enterolactone and enterodiol) can then bind to estrogen receptor sites on breast tissue, the lining of the uterus, and cells of the cervix. By doing so, they tone down the overstimulation of the body's more powerful estrogens. This is extremely important because overstimulation of these tissues by the body's estrogen (or hormone replacement therapy or the birth control pill) leads to an increased risk of breast, uterine, and cervical cancer.

Flaxseed powder has also been shown to directly slow down the breast cell division rate (it is anti-proliferative).

In summary:
- lignans have been shown to inhibit the growth of estrogen-sensitive breast cancer cells;
- they inhibit the enzyme that produces the more dangerous estrogen hormone known as estrone;
- they slow down cell division and reduce colon cancer tumours;
- they inhibit the formation of blood vessels around cancer cells (this is known as anti-angiogenesis), which is a vital step in cancer prevention.

Prostate Cancer

In the U.S., over 200,000 men are diagnosed with prostate cancer every year, from which 30,000 die annually. In Canada, 1 in 8 men will be diagnosed with it in their lifetime and 1 in 4 will die from it. Survivors face difficult choices such as radiation, chemotherapy, and surgery with serious side effects including impotence and incontinence. Given this, men would be wise to do everything they can to prevent it in the first place.

These same phytoestrogens from flaxseed also help to prevent prostate cancer. Enterolactone and enterodiol block the overproduction of the estone hormone in fat cells. Estone hormone (especially seen with weight gain) causes prostate cells to make more DHT (dihydrotestosterone), which stimulates rapid cell division of prostate cells and promotes the growth of existing prostate cancer cells.

Flaxseed ⇨ Enterolactone ⇨ ↓Estrone

⇨ Enterodiol

Estrone ⇨ DHT ⇨ Prostate cancer

According to the journal of the National Cancer Institute, 75% of prostate cancer may be prevented if men improved their nutrition, which includes specific supplementation. Specific supplements block many of the steps in the chemical pathway that cause prostate enlargement and prostate cancer. In fact, many medical doctors in Europe prefer to use these supplements to treat prostate enlargement over prescription drugs.

75% of prostate cancer may be prevented
-National Cancer Institute

Especially after age 40, men experience a decline in testosterone production and an increase in other hormones (estrogen, prolactin, LH, FSH). This decrease actually leads to a build-up of testosterone in the prostate gland as there is decreased removal of testosterone. This testosterone build-up, combined with increased activity of the enzyme that converts testosterone, results in a build-up of DHT (dihydrotestosterone), which is largely responsible for prostate enlargement and prostate cancer.

Testosterone build-up in prostate ⇨ DHT
⇨ Prostate cancer

DHT in prostate cells:

- stimulates prostate cells to divide faster, therefore increased cells result in greater mass;
- more rapid cell division results in greater risk of cancer mutation;
- there is also less time for DHT to repair enzymes to correct these mutations;
- promotes the spread of existing prostate cancer cells;
- promotes the production of free radicals in the prostate.

Supplementation that blocks the build-up of DHT and/or aids in prevention of prostate cancer and enlargement include the following:
Saw Palmetto
Pygeum Africanum
Beta-sitosterol (inhibits the 5-alpha-redution enzyme)
Isoflavones
Stinging Nettle (inhibits DHT to bind the cell nucleus)
Indole-3-cerbinol (inhibits cell division)
Essential Fatty Acids
Zinc
Vitamin D
Lycopex
Flaxseed Powder

Keeping DHT levels in check is a critical step in preventing cancer cells from spreading and dividing throughout the prostate gland and metastasizing to other parts of the body. In fact, a small percentage of men are born with the genetic inability to make DHT. These men have been shown to be immune from prostate cancer over the course of their lifetime.

Men born with the genetic inability to make DHT have been shown to be immune from prostate cancer over the course of their lifetime

PSA TESTING

Just recently, PSA testing has come under significant fire where it has been shown to actually be detrimental to your health. To explain this, please understand that it is not so much that the test itself causes any adverse effects but rather that a positive finding in the test (which can't distinguish between non-fatal cases and serious life-threatening cases) leads to standard treatments with significant adverse effects and often in cases where aggressive treatment was not necessary. This of course is all the more reason to take the supplementation route in the first place.

What I found of most interest was an article in Men's Journal (Dec 2011/Jan 2012) discussing PSA testing, which quoted former Florida State University coach Bobby Bowden who said "when you have cancer, you'll do anything to get it fixed." My point would be if that's true, shouldn't you really do anything to make sure you don't get it in the first place?

Shouldn't you do everything to make sure you don't get cancer in the first place?

FLAXSEED POWDER VS. FLAXSEED OIL

Many, including health care professionals, are confused about the difference.

Flaxseed powder (ground flaxseed) is a rich source of the precursors to these phytoestrogens as well as soluble and insoluble fibre and has numerous health benefits. Flaxseed oil also has health benefits, but as a rich source of the omega 3 fatty acid known as alpha-linoleic acid that can be converted into PG-3. It is also associated with a reduced risk of breast and other cancers.

CoQ10

CoQ10 has been shown to reduce the risk of cancer in three ways:

1. it has anti-oxidant capability;
2. it has tumour suppressive ability;
3. it strengthens the immune system.

As previously mentioned, CoQ10 showed significant benefit in high-risk breast cancer patients. Of interest was the fact that those who supplemented with the highest amount of CoQ10 (300 mg daily) showed the greatest benefits.

CALCIUM

Studies have shown that higher calcium intake can reduce the risk of colo-rectal cancer by binding to bile acids and other sterols, thus blocking their conversion to cancer-causing secondary sterols.

It has also been shown, with vitamin D, to slow the rate of colon cell division.

DETOXIFICATION AND IMMUNE FUNCTION

As we age, (due to years of toxicity and deficiency – not the way it has to be), a decline in both our detoxification capacity and our immune function is evident. When this occurs, our bodies are less capable of identifying and destroying cancer cells. This is one of the reasons that we are more susceptible to disease as we age. Hence, it is essential to maximize the function of both these systems.

REISHI MUSHROOMS

Reishi mushrooms have been used for thousands of years in China and Japan.

Studies show Reishi mushroom extract can:

- boost the cancer cell killing capacity of certain immune cells, including macrophage cells and T-cells;
- increase the ability of immune cells to identify and kill many microorganisms;
- enhance the release of cytokines that signal the immune system to boost efficiency;
- increase the release of interferon, interleukin-1, macrophages, t-lymphocytes and more.

ASTRAGALUS

- Astragalus can increase the ability of natural killer cells to kill cancer cells

INDOLE-3-CARBINOL

- Indole-3-carbinol is one of the major anti-cancer substances found in cruciferous vegetables. It also acts as a phytoestrogen (as previously discussed).

Indole-3-carbinol has also been shown to convert some of the body's stronger, more powerful estrogens (estrone) into a safer, less cancer promoting form (2-OH-estrone). Studies have shown its benefits in reducing breast cancer risk.

PROBIOTICS AND PREBIOTICS

Studies have shown that supplementation with both probiotics and prebiotics reduces cancer risk, especially of colorectal cancer.

Supplementation of probiotics and prebiotics:

- improves detoxification processes;
- improves immune function;
- increases the proliferation of lactic acid bacteria (LAB);
- lowers the pH of the colon, which inhibits enzymes that produce bowel carcinogens;
- increases the proliferation of normal cells and decreases the proliferation of cancerous cells.

DETOXIFICATION PROGRAM

For all of the above reasons, a quality metabolic detoxification program, as will be discussed in chapters 44 and 45, is highly recommended.

GREEN TEA EXTRACT

Studies have shown compelling evidence that green tea extract may prevent cancer in the following ways:

- it increases anti-oxidant enzymes in the lungs, liver, and intestines;
- it increases detoxification enzymes in the lungs, liver, and intestines;
- it blocks the formation of cancer-causing nitrosamines;
- it suppresses activation of carcinogens in lung, breast, colon, and skin cancer cells;
- it blocks estrogen from attaching to estrogen receptors on breast cells.

ISOFLAVONES

Although controversial, as we will discuss thoroughly in chapter 28, isoflavones have been shown to be beneficial in the prevention of cancer.

13

DIABETES

Experts estimate that, by the year 2030, over half a billion people on the face of the planet will have diabetes.

While people are scared to death of cancer and consider heart disease to be the "silent killer", the truth is that diabetes is really the "silent killer" as it plays a huge role in cancer, heart disease, obesity and so much more. Most importantly, as I discuss in my lecture Discover Wellness and Diabetes, society's approach in thinking that they can be cured through drugs and insulin is an approach that will never work, but since this is a book on vitamins we'll save that discussion for another time.

By the same token, diabetes will never be "cured" solely through vitamins. Proper nutrition and exercise must come first, but the science shows that diabetes can be successfully managed with proper supplementation. In fact, if one led a lifetime of following all five of the keys to health, type 2 diabetes would be virtually non-existent.

Supplementation for diabetes would include all of the following:

- essential fatty acids (2,000-4,000mg)
- chromium (200mcg-1,000mcg)
- vitamin E (up to 900 I.U.)
- grape seed extract
- bilberry extract
- magnesium
- lipoic acid

(Many of these may be included in an optimal level comprehensive multi-vitamin/mineral)

CHROMIUM

Chromium is essential for normal glucose metabolism. It actually enhances the activity of insulin. Unlike other trace elements, once chromium is absorbed it is almost entirely excreted in the urine, hence, it must be supplied daily. Given that chromium from food and water only has about a 1% absorption rate, chromium supplementation with an absorption rate of 10-25% is required.

Numerous scientific studies have shown chromium's positive effects on potentiating the action of insulin and helping impaired glucose tolerance. Given that chromium supplementation may enhance the effects of diabetic drugs, you should consult your medical doctor before taking both.

MAGNESIUM

Magnesium deficiency may increase insulin resistance and supplementation in diabetes has been shown to increase insulin sensitivity.

VITAMIN E

Supplementation up to 900 I.U. daily has been shown to increase insulin sensitivity.

GRAPE SEED EXTRACT AND BILBERRY

Both have been shown to be beneficial in the management of diabetes.

ESSENTIAL FATTY ACIDS AND LIPOIC ACID

Both have been shown to be very beneficial in the treatment of diabetic neuropathy. Diabetics have a decreased ability to convert linolenic acid (LA) to gamma-linolenic acid, to help repair diabetic neuropathy and prevent nerve damage.

In Germany, lipoic acid is approved as a drug for the treatment of diabetic neuropathy. It improves insulin blood glucose metabolism, reduces glycosylation of amino acids, improves blood flow to the peripheral nerves, and stimulates regeneration of nerve fibres in diabetes.

14

OPTIMUM BRAIN FUNCTION

You've spent your entire life trying to stay healthy. You try to follow all of the five keys to health. You're confident that you've done the right things to help prevent heart disease and cancer so that you can live a long life. And then you start to forget things. Your memory isn't quite what it used to be and where did your car keys go? In Asia, you're the revered old wise one. In North America you're the senile old person. Then you realize a startling (frightening for some) conclusion. You spent all this time trying to extend the life of your body only to realize that your mind may not be what it should for the last five, ten, or twenty years of your life.

There are two key components of the process that results in the decline of optimal mental function and memory loss that is common as we age.

1. Brain cells are damaged by free radicals over the course of our lifetime.
2. There is a decrease in the production of brain chemicals known as neurotransmitters.

FREE RADICAL DAMAGE

Obviously, our brains need oxygen. Over time, unfortunately, the cumulative effects of this oxygen include oxygen free radicals. Not only does this damage brain cells, but it may even encourage the formation of what is known as amyloid protein. Amyloid protein is the key substance that promotes the development and progression of Alzheimer's disease. As free radical damage continues, not only will brain cells cease to function normally, some will be destroyed.

NEUROTRANSMITTERS

The brain chemical responsible for memory and recall is known as acetylcholine. It is formed through the following chemical pathway:

Choline + acetyl coenzyme A $\Rightarrow$ acetylcholine

This addition requires an enzyme known as choline acetyl- transferase.

As we age (especially after age 60), there is a significant drop in the production of this enzyme (choline acetyl-transferase) and hence we lose our ability to retrieve memories, learn new things, and process information at an optimal level.

WHAT SHOULD YOU DO?

Knowing the above, the answer becomes obvious. Provide your brain with the antioxidants necessary to slow or prevent free radical damage and supplement with the appropriate nutrients to boost the production of acetylcholine and/or slow down its breakdown. There is nothing graceful about aging when it involves neurological decline, especially if there's something that you can do about it. The following supplements have been proven to help with the above:

VITAMIN E (antioxidant)

Studies have shown that people with higher levels of vitamin E scored higher in cognitive tests than those with lower levels of vitamin E. 400 I.U of vitamin E is the recommended daily dose.

The Alzheimer's Disease Co-operative study showed that, in moderately advanced cases of Alzheimer's, vitamin E supplementation of 2,000 I.U. daily resulted in a significant slowing of the functional deterioration of the brain. Studies have also shown it to be beneficial for Parkinson's disease.

VITAMIN C (antioxidant)

While not as effective as vitamin E, vitamin C has also been shown to be effective in helping to prevent free radical attacks on brain cells. Given that vitamin C is necessary for optimum vitamin E function, it is wise to supplement with it for optimal brain function.

CHOLINE

Supplementation with choline has been shown to increase the brain's level of choline, from which the neurotransmitter acetylcholine is made. Choline supplementation has been shown to be very effective in the management of Alzheimer's, Parkinson's and senile dementia. Lecithin is a rich source of choline, however, studies to date have not shown as good a response solely to lecithin, hence, specific choline supplementation is recommended, especially CDP-choline. It has been shown to cross the blood-brain barrier and also to increase adrenaline and dopamine levels.

PHOSPHATIDYLSERINE

This is the major phospholipid in the brain and helps to maintain the membrane of brain cells. In many parts of Europe (especially Italy and Scandinavia), phosphatidylserine supplementation is widely used to restore declining mental function and depression in the elderly. The serine portion of phosphatidylserine can also be converted into choline in the brain.

Numerous studies have shown improvement in memory, behaviour, mood, and cognitive function in the elderly with moderate to severe senility and in Alzheimer's patients. Be aware that phosphatidylserine used to be derived from cows but, due to the scare of Mad Cow disease, is now derived from soy. The recommended dose is 100 mg three times per day.

HUPERZINE A

Huperzine A has been used in Chinese medicine for centuries. It has been shown to improve memory and in cases of Alzheimer's and dementia it has actually been shown to out-perform certain prescription drugs in its ability to preserve acetylcholine. It does this by inhibiting the enzyme that breaks down acetylcholine in the brain (acetylcholine esterase). Huperzine has been shown to have a longer lasting effect than the prescription drugs tactrine and doneprizil.

BACOPA MONNIER

For years, ayurvedic practitioners (traditional medicine native to India) have recommended this supplement, which has even been shown to increase intellectual activity in children.

ACETYL-L-CARNITINE

The acetyl portion provides one of the building blocks to make acetylcholine. Acetyl-l-carnitine also increases energy production of brain cells and enhances the production of cardiolipin, required by brain cells for energy production. Although it has been shown to be very effective, safe, and non-toxic, Health Canada still disapproves of its use in Canada.

IF YOU'RE TAKING PRESCRIPTION DRUGS. . .

You must check with your medical doctor if you're taking any prescription drugs for Alzheimer's, Parkinson's, or dementia before taking any of the above five acetylcholine enhancers. Since these five supplements enhance acetylcholine similar to what your prescription drug is meant to do, the effects will be compounded where too much acetylcholine production can actually cause a serious toxic level (known as cholinergic syndrome).

ALSO AVOID

Ginkgo Biloba, vinpocetine, and DMAE. Although all three have been shown to be beneficial to some degree, they have side effects that could cause problems. Ginkgo biloba and vinpocetine increase blood flow to the brain (usually a good thing), but have the potential in rare cases to cause internal bleeding.

THE VITAMIN B FAMILY

B vitamins are essential for proper neurological function as clearly demonstrated in many scientific studies. Of interest is the fact that different B vitamin deficiencies showed different neurological deficiencies. Low levels of B12 and folic acid were associated with spatial copying whereas B6 was more involved with memory.

B12 and folic acid act as co-enzymes in the production of neurotransmitters as well as the production of SAMe, which has anti-depressant properties. B6 is a co-factor for brain chemicals such as dopamine, norepinephrine, and serotonin.

Low blood levels of B6, B12, and folic acid have also been shown to result in higher levels of Homocysteine, which is associated with a higher risk of cerebrovascular (stroke), cardiovascular and peripheral vascular (narrowed arteries in the legs and arms) disease. Some studies have shown that patients with high homocysteine levels functioned at the same cognitive level as those with mild Alzheimer's disease.

This is yet one more reason why a comprehensive multi-vitamin multi-mineral supplement is mandatory for all individuals.

CoQ10

Parkinson's is a progressive disease that affects the part of the brain (substantia nigra) that produces dopamine. Dopamine is one of the brain chemicals responsible for controlling body movement.

A study of significant importance appeared in the Archives of Neurology (Oct. 2002) and showed when early stage Parkinson's patients supplemented with either 300 mg, 600 mg, or 1200 mg of CoQ10 per day for sixteen months they showed significantly less impairment. Patients given the highest dosages showed the best improvement with results apparent at the eight-month mark.

Numerous researchers have shown that Parkinson's patients have a defect in their ability to produce adequate amounts of CoQ10, which is necessary to generate ATP (energy) and dopamine. CoQ10 also acts as an anti-oxidant.

ESSENTIAL FATTY ACIDS

As we will discuss thoroughly in the next chapter, essential fatty acid supplementation reduces PG-2, thus reducing inflammation, and is involved in neurodegenerative diseases.

DHA (docosahexaenoic acid) has been shown to increase brain function and intelligence.

EFA and DHA have also been shown to be of significant benefit in children's learning disorders (attention deficit disorder, (ADD), and attention deficit hyperactivity disorder, (ADHD)).

Again, this is another reason why essential fatty acids are one of the five key supplements required by everyone.

ST. JOHN'S WORT

St. John's Wort is a plant that derives its name from old English where wort is a plant which usually flowers around the feast of St. John.

There is an abundance of scientific evidence to support the use of St. John's Wort in cases of mild to moderate depression. St. John's Wort has been found to be effective in 55% of cases after 4 to 6 weeks of use. If this figure still seems low to you (just over 1 in 2), bear in mind that it has been found to be equally or more effective than Prozac with far fewer side effects after 2 months of use and just as effective as the prescription drug Zoloft, again with far fewer side effects.

Caution is warranted here as it is not effective in the treatment of severe depression and it is extremely unsafe to take if you are currently taking other anti-depressant drugs.

15

CHRONIC PAIN, INFLAMMATION, AND ARTHRITIS

Nearly 1 in 5 North Americans live with chronic pain. Not temporary pain, but rather constant, chronic pain for which most have no solution.

Most attempt to "manage" their pain through a variety of drugs as recommended by both their medical doctor and the drug companies. What price do you pay for this approach? According to the National Institute of Health and the American Medical Association, 100,000 Americans die each and every year from the "side effects" of so-called properly prescribed drugs. Talk about being caught between a rock and a hard place.

What they (including foundations and associations dedicated to chronic pain) don't talk about is the science that shows significant improvement with the use of natural supplementation, often equalling or even surpassing the effects of drugs, yet without the side effects. As such, arthritis sufferers, back pain, neck pain, and headache sufferers cost North Americans billions of dollars in disability, not to mention the fact that they have a significantly lower quality of life. Eighty-five percent of the population will suffer back pain at some point in their life and fifty million Americans suffer from arthritis. Suffering or turning to drugs is not the answer.

"But hey – I've tried some of this stuff before and it didn't work!"

What does "tried" mean? Did you dabble in amounts that were too small, take it for too short a duration, take the wrong supplement, or not take a comprehensive approach? What would happen if you took the same approach with drugs? You'd also get less than optimal results and, of course, more adverse reactions.

The science says there are basically four different approaches:

1. Remember chapter 7, "Apple Juice, Stewed Mosquitoes, Baking Cookies, and Chemical Pathways"? By taking specific supplements that decrease your body's ability to produce inflammation, your body will produce less inflammation. (ESSENTIAL FATTY ACIDS)
2. Take natural anti-inflammatories. Get the same positive effects with far fewer negative effects. (i.e. bromelain, curcumin, etc.)
3. Rebuild joint and cartilage. (i.e. glucosamine, MSM, etc.)
4. Take anti-oxidants (vitamin E, vitamin C, selenium) to prevent further free radical damage.

1. ESSENTIAL FATTY ACIDS

Prostaglandins are hormones in our body that are made from the different types of unsaturated fats (essential fatty acids) that we either consume in our diet or get from supplements. The three main types of prostaglandin hormones are PG-1, PG-2, and PG-3 (PG = prostaglandin). PG-1 and PG-3 produce positive effects on our health whereas PG-2 produces significant negative effects on our health. Not surprisingly, most North Americans have dietary habits that produce far too much PG-2 and not enough PG-1 and PG-3.

PG-2 is made from an unsaturated fat known as arachidonic acid, which is found in fatty meats and high-fat dairy products. PG-2 encourages inflammation. It worsens joint, muscle and tendon conditions, including arthritis as well as other inflammatory conditions.

Arachidonic acid also comes from linoleic acid (an unsaturated fat found in vegetable oil including corn oil, sunflower oil and safflower oil). Since these oils are grossly over consumed in North America from processed and deep-fried foods, the body produces far too much PG-2 and not enough PG-1 and PG-3. PG-2 isn't just responsible for increased inflammation and pain; it also plays a role in cancer development, cardiovascular disease, and even bad skin. (You would get far better skin from spending your money on essential fatty acid supplementation from the inside than all the expensive creams in the world applied from the outside.)

In addition to preventing the formation of PG-2, supplementing with essential fatty acids will also promote the production of PG-1 and PG-3. PG-1 and PG-3 provide a number of health benefits, including suppressing inflammation and pain.

The building block for PG-1 is an unsaturated fat known as gamma-linolenic acid (GLA). Its highest concentration is actually found in borage oil (22% yield) whereas most people tend to know evening primrose oil better, which only has a 9% yield of GLA.

GLA can also be formed in the body from linoleic acid but people with diabetes, PMS and eczema have been shown to have a defect in the enzyme that converts linoleic acid to GLA. This conversion is also affected by the consumption of alcohol, refined sugars, hydrogenated fats and the aging process. Not surprisingly, almost everyone has less than optimal levels of GLA. Studies have shown that supplementation with GLA can reduce pain and swelling in arthritis patients, including rheumatoid arthritis. Even without these health conditions, optimizing your PG-1 levels each day through supplementation with borage oil is a wise decision.

PG-3 is produced in the body from the omega-3 fatty acid known as eicosapentaenoic acid (EPA). It is found in cold-water fish (salmon, mackerel, anchovies, sardines, and tuna) and of course EPA supplements. EPA can also be produced in the body from DHA (docosahexaenoic acid) and from alpha-linolenic acid (ALA) found in flaxseed oil. PG-3 is also known to reduce inflammation.

Unfortunately, as I discussed in *Nutrition Insanity*, most individuals unknowingly suffer from an essential fatty acid deficiency or imbalance, which contributes to numerous health conditions, including cancer, heart disease, stroke, accelerated aging, poor skin and of course inflammation.

That is why essential fatty acids (EFAs) are one of the five essential supplements required by everyone. Ideally, your EFA supplement should be high quality, high potency omega 3 and 6 fatty acids derived from flaxseed oil, borage oil and fish oil (EPA and DHA). Also remember that all supplements work synergistically. There are certain vitamins and minerals that are required as co-factors in the enzyme reactions that convert healthy essential fatty acids (flaxseed, borage and fish oils) into PG-1 and PG-3. These include vitamins B3, B6, C, and E, zinc, magnesium and selenium. This is why an overall optimal multi-vitamin-mineral is also one of the five essential supplements required by all.

2. NATURAL ANTI-INFLAMMATORIES (Please be sure to read chapter 40)

Bromelain – contains anti-inflammatory enzymes that science has proven have the ability to suppress pain and inflammation from sports injuries, both rheumatoid and osteoarthritis and other joint conditions. Bromelain has been shown to inhibit the enzyme (cyclooxygenase), which inhibits the synthesis of PG-2 just as most anti-inflammatory drugs attempt to do. Bromelain is also fibrinolytic (it breaks down fibrin), which minimizes local swelling. Best of all, unlike all anti-inflammatory drugs (Celebrex, Voltaren, Naprosyn, Ibuprofen, Advil, etc.) which are nasty on the stomach and can cause internal bleeding and death, Bromelain doubles as a digestive aid, which actually benefits the stomach.

Curcumin – is the active anti-inflammatory agent found in the spice turmeric. It has been shown to inhibit the activity of enzymes (5-lipoxygenase and cyclooxygenase) thus blocking the production of pro-inflammatory eicosanoids (again PG-2 and what is known as LTB-4). One large scientific double-blind study showed that curcumin was as effective as the powerful anti-inflammatory drug phenylbutazone in reducing pain, swelling and stiffness in rheumatoid arthritis patients. It has also been shown to be effective in the treatment of post-surgical inflammation, lowering histamine levels and is a potent antioxidant.

Boswellia – has been shown to improve symptoms in patients with osteoarthritis and rheumatoid arthritis by inhibiting the 5-lipoxygenase enzyme in white blood cells.

White Willow Bark Extract – provides anti-inflammatory phenolic glycosides, which have been shown to be effective in the treatment of arthritis, back pain, and other joint conditions. These phenolic glycosides are known to inhibit the enzyme cyclooxygenase, which blocks the production of PG-2 and also exerts a mild analgesic effect. While it has been shown to be slower acting than ASA, it is of longer duration in effectiveness and, unlike ASA, is unlikely to cause any bleeding disorders.

Ginger Root Extract – contains compounds that have shown clinical benefit in the management of various arthritic and muscle inflammation problems, including rheumatoid arthritis, osteoarthritis and myalgias. The active constituents (gingerols or oleo-resins) inhibit the cyclooxygenase and lipoxygenase enzymes. (It should not be given to patients with gallstones or those taking warfarin or coumadin.)

Quercetin – is a bioflavonoid that blocks the release of histamine and other inflammatory enzymes.

3. REBUILDING JOINT AND CARTILAGE

Many times throughout the writing of this book, I have come to the conclusion that, regardless of people's awareness of the science, most people's health decisions really come down to what I described in one of my first books, *Healthy Beliefs, Deadly Choices*. Most people make their health decisions based on what they believe. One of those incorrect beliefs is the belief perpetuated by most medical doctors and all drug companies that we're all supposed to get arthritis as we age.

Osteoarthritis (the most common type of arthritis) affects 40 million Americans. While one of the contributing causes of osteoarthritis is the age-related decline in the body's production of glucosamine starting at age 45, does this mean that age causes osteoarthritis, or does it simply mean that we should begin supplementing with glucosamine?

Chondrocytes → Glucosamine sulfate → N-acetyl-galactosamine sulfate + Glucuronic acid → Chondroitin sulfate + hyaluronic acid

Hyaluronic acid increases the viscosity of synovial fluid, helping to reduce joint wear and tear. As such, glucosamine sulfate is essential to the synthesis of both chondroitin sulfate and hyaluronic acid.

Chondroitin sulfate forms what is known as the ground substance of joint cartilage (glycosaminoglycans, proteoglycans or mucopolysaccharides). Ground substance fills in the gaps between collagen fibers within cartilage similar to the mortar between bricks. Again, any decrease in glucosamine sulfate results in a decline in this ground substance and joint cartilage with subsequent joint space narrowing and arthritic degeneration.

Glucosamine sulfate has been the subject of more than 300 scientific investigations and over 20 double-blind clinical studies. Researchers indicated that glucosamine supplementation was shown to be highly effective in the treatment of osteoarthritis in all of the double-blind clinical trials that met their inclusion criteria.

Glucosamine is easily absorbed in the gastrointestinal tract (90 to 98%) whereas less than 13% of chondroitin sulfate is absorbed, making it significantly less effective.

Therefore, glucosamine sulfate supplementation:
1. stimulates the synthesis of ground substance;
2. stimulates the synthesis of collagen;
3. is required for the production of hyaluronic acid.

Glucosamine sulfate also delivers the mineral sulfur (hence the name) which is a vital nutrient for the maintenance of joint cartilage.

Glucosamine sulfate supplementation has also been investigated in head-to-head studies against non-steroidal anti-inflammatory drugs (NSAIDs) in the treatment of osteoarthritis. In a number of these trials, glucosamine supplementation was shown to produce better results than ibuprofen and other NSAIDs in relieving the pain and inflammation of osteoarthritis. Unlike many NSAIDs, glucosamine has not been shown to produce any of the adverse side effects that are frequently encountered with the use of NSAIDs.

Chondroitin sulfate supplementation, on the other hand, is not warranted. Its molecule size is too large to be properly absorbed and as such is of little or no benefit. It is far better to supplement with glucosamine sulfate, which the body can then convert to chondroitin sulfate.

MSM is a naturally occurring sulfur compound where supplementation, at levels that exceed those attainable from food alone, has potent anti-inflammatory properties and can help to halt the further destruction of joint cartilage in osteoarthritis as well as improvement in joint mobility.

4. ANTI-OXIDANTS

Numerous scientific studies have shown that supplementation with anti-oxidants can reduce any perceived need for NSAIDs via the same chemical pathways.

One randomized, double-blind study pitted vitamin E supplementation against the anti-inflammatory drug diclofenac sodium in hospitalized rheumatoid arthritis patients. Patients were either given 400 mg of natural vitamin E three times daily, or the standard anti-inflammatory dosage of diclofenac sodium. After three weeks of treatment, both groups showed the same significant degree of improvement with respect to joint stiffness, improved grip strength, and pain reduction. Vitamin C and selenium have also shown benefits.

Fibromyalgia

Of all the chronic pain syndromes, fibromyalgia is often considered one of the worst where often the diagnosis alone becomes debilitating. It needn't be.

Supplementation including 5-HTP, SAMe and melatonin as well as magnesium (300-600 mg per day) and malic acid (1,200-1,400 mg per day) showed significant improvement. A quality multi-vitamin including high levels of vitamin B is also beneficial for energy production and stress relief.

Part Four

Not All Vitamins
Are Created Equally

16

DON'T DABBLE

By now you have either confirmed once and for all that you made the right choice in taking vitamins or if you weren't a vitamin taker hopefully you finally realize the importance of taking multivitamin supplements on a daily basis regardless of your beliefs. If you're still unsure, appreciate that spinach stored at room temperature loses 70% of its vitamin C content within just 24 hours after picking and even if refrigerated still loses 50% of its vitamin C content within 48 hours.

Now here comes the even bigger challenge. Which ones do you take? Vitamins are like everything else; some are simply much better than others. Better quality, better dissolution, better source ingredients, better processing and manufacturing methods, better binders and fillers and so on and so on. But how do you know?

The average person dabbles in vitamins. They may believe they are knowledgeable, but much of that information has come from marketers with their own motives. A common site I see is when a person holds up two different brands of vitamins and says "This one has 500 mg of calcium and this one has 500 mg of calcium". "This one has 500 mg of vitamin C and so does this one, so they must be the same." They are not. What is the source of the calcium? Is it a calcium carbonate or calcium citrate? There's a huge difference where calcium citrate (more expensive) is a highly absorbable source of calcium, whereas calcium carbonate (the cheapest form of calcium) is actually a risk factor **for** osteoporosis. Was it cold processed (good) or heat processed (not good)? What are the binders and fillers, which may cause upset stomach? Was the vitamin C an ester C or ascorbate (highly absorbable and more expensive) or ascorbic acid (much cheaper but not as well absorbed and hard on your enamel if it's in a chewable form)?

This is why really good vitamins are more expensive than cheaper ones. You're really not getting a deal if you pay 50% less for something that is 95% less absorbed. To complicate matters, while you typically get what you pay for, there are of course some expensive vitamins that are of poor quality but also have slick marketing. So how do you know? I recommend two ways:

1. Consider purchasing your vitamins from a qualified health care professional whom you trust and knows their nutrition well. This could be a chiropractor, a naturopath, a homeopath, or an advanced nutritionist who specializes in optimum health. Typically we will have access to the best labs in North America (and the world), which will include supplements that are not available in drug stores or most nutrition stores. Your health care professional will go far beyond just comparing quantities. They will look for labs with superior methods and practices, which include sources, ratios, combinations, dissolution, fillers and so much more.

2. Any good health care professional will have done this already but you can also go to "The Comparative Guide to Nutritional Supplements", which ranks over 1,500 vitamins and supplements with a "Health Support Profile". This ranking is based on 18 criteria:

    1. Completeness
    2. Potency
    3. Mineral forms
    4. Bioactivity of vitamin E
    5. Gammatocopherol
    6. Anti-oxidant support
    7. Bone health
    8. Heart health
    9. Liver health
    10. Metabolic health
    11. Ocular health
    12. Methylation support
    13. Lipotrophic factors
    14. Inflammation control
    15. Glycation control
    16. Bioflavinoid profile
    17. Phenolic compound profile
    18. Potential toxicities

    Guess what? You are not expected to know this. Unless you have a chemistry degree - as I do -most of this would sound like Latin to you. Leave it to an expert you trust (hence recommendation #1). Vitamins are ranked from 0 to 5 stars with some well-known daily vitamins receiving 0.5 stars – yes, that's one half of a star.

Vitamin Ratings from "The Comparative Guide to Nutritional Supplements" (by Lyle MacWilliam) for some common supplements. (Rating out of 5.0)

Centrum Performance 0.5
GNC Multi Ultra Mega 1.5
GNC Multi Prevention 1.0
Life Daily – one 50+ 0.5
Melaleuca Vitality for Men 1.0
Melaleuca Vitality for Women 1.0
Natural Factors Super Multi Iron Free 1.5
Jamieson Super VitaVim 1.5
One a Day Active 0.5
Quest Extra Once a Day 1.0
Shaklee Advanced Formula Vita-Lea 1.0
SISU Multi-Vi-Min 1.0
Swiss Super Adult 1.5
Weil Daily Multivitamin Optimum Health 2.0

It shouldn't surprise you that the two supplement brands that I carry in my office are tied for #1 out of 1,500 vitamins with 5 stars and a Gold Medal winner: Douglas Laboratories and Core Science (www.corescience.ca), which is actually produced by Douglas Laboratories. Just to let you know how well-educated and impressive a chiropractor's expertise is when it comes to nutrition, three of the top five vitamin brands in North America were either invented by or run by chiropractors in either Canada or the United States.

Another important factor to re-iterate is that vitamin supplementation is all about optimum health – not about treating a disease or symptom only after you've allowed it to happen. For example, seniors are told that they need more calcium for their osteoporosis (good bone health requires far more than just calcium). As such, some marketers have vitamins "for those over 60" with more calcium, leading buyers to believe that this is better suited for them. Well, let's once again ask a common sense question to show this marketing tactic for what it is. If you have osteoporosis at age 65, wouldn't it have made sense to take just as much of a bone mineral supplement at age 50 to have helped prevent it in the first place? And since peak bone mass occurs at ages 25 to 30, shouldn't that be the time when we're maximizing our nutrition? In fact, many researchers believe osteoporosis should be viewed as a pediatric disease. Again, think the true definition of health and the health continuum and it's hard to go wrong.

On the same note, don't listen to the silly health care professional who tells you not to take glucosamine sulphate for osteoarthritis because the "glucose" is bad for your diabetes. The amount of glucose is far less than any one piece of fruit you'll eat that day, yet has significant benefits in helping to prevent degeneration.

Last but not least, most vitamins are best taken with food as fat soluble vitamins require fat to dissolve but then again, your qualified health care professional would tell you that.

17

18 HEALTH CRITERIA FOR THE OPTIMUM SUPPLEMENT

The most comprehensive independent review of nutritional supplements in North America is conducted by well-known scientist Lyle MacWilliam and detailed in "NutriSearch Comparative Guide to Nutritional Supplements". The eighteen health criteria used to evaluate a product are as follows.

1. Completeness

Quite simply, how complete is the product? Does it contain each of the 47 nutrient categories that based on scientific research are necessary for optimal physiological function and that must be ingested as they cannot be made by the body? These 47 nutrient categories include vitamins, plant-based antioxidants, trace elements and minerals, and essential fatty acids.

2. Potency

How much of each nutrient does a product contain compared to a "blended standard" derived from 12 leading scientists based on the latest scientific information?

3. Mineral Forms

Minerals are bound with other substances to help them cross into the bloodstream. Good mineral forms include what are known as amino acid chelates and organic acid complexes. They tend to:

- mimic the natural form during the digestive process;
- make the mineral more bioavailable and more likely to be absorbed;
- be easier on your stomach and less likely to cause irritation (this becomes more of a problem as you age due to a decrease in stomach acidity);
- not block other minerals.

Good Mineral Forms
- chelated to amino acids or
- joined to organic acids
- citrate
- malate
- succinate
- alpha-ketogluterols
- aspartate

Poor mineral forms are not surprisingly much cheaper to produce but offer poor absorption, stomach intolerance, and may even block other minerals.

Poor Mineral Forms
- carbonate
- oxides
- sulphates
- phosphates

4. Vitamin E Bioactivity

Vitamin E exists in eight different forms. The most active and the only form actively maintained in humans is alpha-tocopherol. Furthermore, this form should always be in its natural form (d-alpha-tocopherol) vs. the synthetic form (dl-alpha-tocopherol) as it is more bioavailable and twice as potent.

5. Gamma-Tocopherol

Although vitamin E is essential in the alpha-tocopherol form, high doses of it can actually decrease the gamma form which is essential for improving cardiovascular function, reducing inflammation, and preventing cancer. As such, gamma-tocopherol should also be present in a 2:1 alpha to gamma ratio.

6. Anti-oxidant support

There is substantial scientific evidence to support the need for the key anti-oxidants (vitamin C, vitamin E, and beta-carotene) as well as vitamin A, alpha-lipoic acid, lycopene, CoQ10, and selenium that help prevent or repair damage caused by oxidative stress.

7. Bone Health

Healthy bones require 24 bone-building minerals. These include vitamins D, C, K, B6, B12, folic acid, calcium, magnesium, boron, silicon, and zinc.

8. Heart Health

Nutrients that help protect the heart and cardiovascular system must be present must be present – specifically vitamin E (alpha and gamma forms), beta-carotene, CoQ10, calcium, magnesium, l-carnitine or acetyl-l-carnitine, lycopene, phenolic compounds, and procyanidolic compounds (PCOs).

9. Liver Health and Detoxification

Are the nutrients present that support and preserve glutathione which is necessary for cellular health and liver function? These include vitamin C, cysteine and n-acetyl-cysteine, selenium, B2, and B3.

10. Metabolic Health

Are nutrients present that are essential for proper metabolic support and the regulation of glucose metabolism to help prevent diabetes? These include vitamins B3, B6, B12, C, E, CoQ10, biotin, magnesium, chromium, manganese, and zinc.

11. Ocular Health

Are nutrients present that are essential for proper vision including the prevention of cataracts and macular degeneration? These include vitamin C, E, A, beta-carotene, and the carotenoids lutein and zeaxanthin.

12. Methylation Support

Homocysteine is a powerful oxidizing agent believed to be responsible for the initial damage to the inner walls of the arteries and subsequent plaque formation. Vitamins B2, B6, B12, folic acid, and trimethylglycine are required by the body to produce methyl donors that reduce homocysteine.

13. Lipotropic Factors

Are nutrients present that help the liver eliminate toxins that we are subjected to on a daily basis and that accumulate in both the liver and brain? These include choline, lecithin, and inositol.

14. Inflammation Control

Are nutrients present that help prevent inflammation at the cellular level? These include the essential fatty acids EPA and DHA, vitamin C, alpha-lipoic acid, gamma-tocopherol, flavinoids, PCO, and phenolic compounds.

15. Glycation Control

Are nutrients present that help slow the progress of many degenerative diseases, including Alzheimer's, Parkinson's, and cancer?

16. Bioflavinoid Profile

Is the bioflavinoid family that attacks free radicals throughout the body and supports many bodily functions present? This includes citrus flavinoids, soy isoflavones, quercetin, hesperidin, rutin, bilberry, resveratrol, grape seed extract, and pine bark extract.

17. Phenolic Compound Profile

Are phenolic compounds (derived from green tea, curcumin, and olives) that are potent defenders against free radicals present?

18. Potential Toxicity

Are any of the nutrients present at levels that could build in the body to levels that could actually become toxic with prolonged intake? Specific examples include iron toxicity or vitamin A toxicity in high prolonged use, hence the preferred form of beta-carotene.

18

READING YOUR VITAMIN LABEL

Now that you have a much better understanding of what the experts look for in a vitamin, let's test that new-found knowledge.

First and foremost, you must read the label. I know that sounds obvious, but many don't do this for a number of reasons:

a) it could be that they're not sure what they're looking for;
b) it could be that they just assume it will be as good as the glitzy marketing hype says it is;
c) it may even be that the print is simply too small to read.

If you're serious about your health, as everyone should be, then either invest the time to investigate your supplement or buy from a health care professional whom you trust. Ideally you should do both.

Multi-vitamin Sample Label #1

Vitamin A	50,000 I.U.
Vitamin B	2 mg
Vitamin C	50 mg
Calcium	15 mg
Ma Huang	100 mg

Would you consider this a good product to take and what can you tell me about it based on the eighteen criteria in the previous chapter?

Your obvious answer should be that this would be a terrible supplement to take and in fact dangerous for a number of reasons:

1. As a multi-vitamin it is nowhere even close to being complete or comprehensive.
2. Its vitamin A content, unless under the direct supervision of a qualified health care professional, is excessive (in fact it would be disallowed by Health Canada). Over time, given that vitamin A is a fat-soluble vitamin, this level would be considered toxic.
3. Not only is the vitamin B content incredibly low, the B vitamins are a family of vitamins: B1, B2, B3, B5, B6, B2, and folic acid. While it is highly unlikely that you would see this on a vitamin label, many flyers and marketing materials are indeed this misleading.
4. The vitamin C level doesn't even meet RDA levels to prevent scurvy. Secondly, what form of vitamin C is it?
5. What is the calcium bound to? Is it calcium carbonate, calcium citrate, or some other form? Not only is it also an incredibly low amount, is it the amount of the actual calcium (elemental calcium) or the calcium and its bound substance (i.e. carbonate)?

6. Just because you don't know what a substance is, don't simply ignore it. Ma Huang is ephreda. It's dangerous enough, (it can cause sudden death), let alone at such a high level.

Multi-vitamin Sample Label #2

Vitamin A	5,000 I.U.
Beta-carotene	15,000 I.U.
Vitamin B1	75 mg
B2	75 mg
B3 (niacinamide)	100 mg
(niacin)	20 mg
B5	150 mg
B6	100 mg
B12	100 mcg
Folic Acid (Folate:L-methylfolate, Metafolin®)	800 mcg
Biotin	300 mcg
Vitamin C (calcium ascorbate)	1,000 mg
Vitamin D3 (cholecalciferol)	1,000 I.U.
Vitamin E (d-alpha tocopherol succinate with mixed tocopherols)	600 I.U.
Vitamin K2 MK-7 (menaquinone-7)	50 mcg
Calcium (citrate/ascorbate)	500 mg
Magnesium (citrate)	500 mg
Potassium (chloride)	100 mg
Iodine (kelp)	200 mcg
Zinc (citrate)	15 mg
Copper (chelate)	2 mg
Manganese (sulfate)	9 mg
Chromium (chelate)	200 mcg
Selenium (citrate)	200 mcg
Bioflavinoids	100 mg
Betaine	100 mg
PABA	50 mg
Molybdenum (citrate/gluterate/malate/fumerate)	50 mcg
Vanadium (citrate)	25 mcg
Continued on next page	

Choline (bitartrate)	200 mg
Lycopene	6 mg
Co-enzyme Q10 (ubiquinone)	25 mg
Garlic (deodorized)	50 mg
Ginseng (Siberian)	10 mg
Alpha-Lipoic Acid	6 mg
Glutathione	6 mg
Inositol	100 mg
N-Acetyl-Cysteine	50 mg
Lutein	5 mg
Astaxanthan	4 mg
Zeaxanthin	1 mg

Now let's use the eighteen point criteria in a chart form to make our analysis easier. Does Sample Label #2 meet all of the necessary criteria?

1. COMPLETENESS – Does it have a significant number of the 47 nutrient categories necessary for optimal health or will you be combining it with another product that will complement it?	YES
2. POTENCY – Are the amounts of each supplement at an optimal level?	YES
3. MINERAL FORMS – Are the minerals (i.e. calcium, magnesium, etc.) bound to good forms (amino acid chelate or organic acid complexes like citrate, malate, succinate, aspartate, alpha-ketogluterate) or not as good forms (carbonate, oxides, sulphates, and phosphates)?	YES

4. VITAMIN E BIOACTIVITY – Is the vitamin E in a d-alpha-tocopherol form?	YES
5. GAMMA-TOCOPHEROL – Is there additional vitamin E in a gamma-tocopherol form?	YES
6. ANTI-OXIDANT SUPPORT – Does it contain key anti-oxidants, namely vitamins A, C, E, beta-carotene, CoQ10, alpha-lipoic acid, lycopene, and selenium?	YES
7. BONE HEALTH – Does it contain the main bone building substances, namely vitamins D, C, K, B6, B12, folic acid, calcium, magnesium, boron, silicon, and zinc in their preferred forms and adequate quantities?	YES
8. HEART HEALTH – Does it contain heart-beneficial compounds, namely vitamin E (both alpha and gamma forms), beta-carotene, CoQ10, calcium, magnesium, l-carnitine or acetyl-l-carnitine, lycopene, phenolic compounds and PCOs (procyanidolic compounds)?	YES

9. LIVER HEALTH AND DETOXIFICATION – Does it contain glutathione, vitamin B2, B3, C, selenium, and cysteine or n-acetyl-cysteine?	YES
10. METABOLIC HEALTH – Are the nutrients present that are essential for normal glucose metabolism, namely B3, B6, B12, C, E, CoQ10, biotin, magnesium, chromium, manganese, and zinc?	YES
11. OCULAR HEALTH – Are nutrients present for proper vision and to help prevent cataracts and macular degeneration? These include vitamins A, C, E, beta-carotene, and the carotenoids lutein and zeaxanthin.	YES
12. METHYLATION SUPPORT – Are vitamins B2, B6, B12, folic acid, and glycine present to reduce homocysteine levels?	YES
13. LIPOTROPIC FACTORS – Are choline, lecithin, and inositol present to assist in toxin removal from the brain and liver?	YES

14. INFLAMMATION – Are nutrients present that assist in preventing inflammation at the cellular level? These include EPA, DHA, vitamin C, alpha-lipoic acid, gamma-tocopherol, flavinoids, PCO, and phenolic compounds.	YES
15. GLYCATION CONTROL – Are nutrients present that help prevent degenerative diseases including Alzheimer's, Parkinson's, and cancer?	YES
16. BIOFLAVINOID PROFILE – Are bioflavinoids present?	YES
17. PHENOLIC COMPOUNDS – Are phenolic compounds present (i.e. green tea, curcumin)?	YES
18. POTENTIAL TOXICITY – Are any quantities well beyond optimal levels that would be considered toxic?	There are no toxicity concerns

The above of course applies to wanting a comprehensive overall supplement. If you were looking for a supplement specific to a particular disease or condition, it may contain far fewer than the 47 nutrient categories. However, you should ensure that the nutrients that it does contain have been shown to be beneficial to your condition and you should still be supplementing with a quality overall wellness formula.

19

WHAT'S NOT ON THE LABEL

Now that you have a much better understanding of what's on a vitamin label, guess what? There's just as much important information that's NOT on the label.

How is the vitamin manufactured? Where do the raw materials come from? Who oversees their quality? How sanitized is their equipment? Is their expertise really in producing a quality vitamin or in marketing just any vitamin? How are their products formulated? Who are their experts?

Suddenly, choosing the best quality vitamin becomes a much more involved task. As you've now discovered, some of the best known brand names are clearly not the best quality vitamins.

Fortunately, there are well established North American and international protocols, certifications, and accreditations that are held by the best labs.

The best labs will comply with ALL of the following:

- Their focus will be on elevating the science, expertise, and art of creating nutritional supplements to achieve unparalleled quality.

- Their team includes a number of PhDs, scientists, researchers, other doctors, and advanced nutritionists who are experts in their field.
- There is continual re-investment of substantial resources to improve and upgrade education, training, manufacturing equipment, and laboratory processes.
- Rigorous manufacturing practices and procedures are designed to monitor and verify quality throughout every step of the production process.

Certification should include:

1. CGMPs (current Good Manufacturing Practices) for nutritional supplements in accordance with USP31. Good manufacturing practices are practices and the systems required to be adapted in manufacturing and quality control. Although there are many, all guidelines follow a few basic principles.

   - Manufacturing processes are clearly defined and controlled. All critical processes are validated to ensure consistency and compliance with specifications.
   - Manufacturing processes are controlled, and any changes to the process are evaluated.
   - Instructions and procedures are written in clear and unambiguous language (good documentation practices).
   - Operators are trained to carry out and document procedures.
   - Records are made, manually or by instruments, during manufacture. These records demonstrate that all of the steps required by the defined procedures

and instructions were in fact taken and that the quantity and quality was as expected. Deviations are investigated and documented.

- Records of manufacture (including distribution) that enable the complete history of a batch to be traced are retained in a comprehensible and accessible form.
- The distribution minimizes any risk to quality.
- A system is available for recalling any batch from sale or supply.

2. Manufacturing facilities have received registration from NSF International.

3. ISO 9001 and ISO 17025 accreditation/in-house laboratory certification. These standards mean that they are compliant with one of the highest and most recognized standards of quality in the world. When comparing supplement suppliers, ask them for verification of their laboratories ISO certification.

4. NutriSearch* Gold Medal of Achievement Winner. *NutriSearch is the publisher of the independent NutriSearch Comparative Guide to Nutritional Supplements.

5. Veri-Match – electronic label match to formula system to ensure content accuracy.

6. SOPs (written Standard Operating Procedures) in accordance with cGMPs.

7. VCP (Vendor Certification Program) ensuring raw material quality.

8. Their on-site laboratories, under the supervision of staff PhDs, should constantly monitor quality. From raw materials entering the facility through testing dosage potency and tablet/capsule disintegration, in-house labs must ensure product quality and consistency.

> **Chemical Analysis Laboratory** ensuring potency of formula components using ICP, GF/AA, HPLC, and FT-NIR
> **Physical Analysis Laboratory** ensuring dosage weight, hardness, disintegration, and overall consistency and appearance
> **Microbiology Laboratory** testing all raw materials and products for yeast, mold, and bacterial purity in accordance with USP31.

9. Ingredients are sourced only from trusted industry leaders.

10. All ingredients are tested for purity and potency by independent certified laboratories.

11. Supplements are hypo-allergenic.

12. Supplements are free of wheat, yeast, gluten, corn, sugar, starch, soy (unless noted), preservatives, and hydrogenated oils.

13. Supplements are made with vegetable capsules when possible.

While taking an average vitamin is usually better than taking nothing, I personally would only want the very best going into my body. Many people who have been dissatisfied with vitamins in the past don't realize that any negative reaction (i.e. upset stomach, etc) is usually due to the cheap binders and fillers in that product.

By obtaining your vitamins from health care professionals and the very best labs that follow all of the above protocols, you can rest assured that you are obtaining what's best for your health.

Part Five

When Vitamins and Drugs Do and Don't Mix

20

CONTRAINDICATIONS: WHEN VITAMINS AND DRUGS DON'T MIX

Let's be perfectly blunt. If you're one of these people who avoids vitamins because you believe they have just as many adverse reactions as drugs, then you're out to lunch. Both the American Medical Association and the National Institute of Health have confirmed that 100,000 people die in the United States each and every year from so-called properly prescribed drugs. That's a large commercial airplane full of people each every day, whereas adverse reactions from vitamin supplementation pale in comparison.

Having said that, you'd also be out to lunch if you didn't appreciate that the taking of drugs and vitamins at the same time requires proper supervision, but not necessarily for the reasons you might think.

Many medical doctors incorrectly tell you to get off all your vitamins when taking any drug simply "to be on the safe side". The truth is that this is incredibly dangerous advice as vitamin supplementation is beneficial to your health and why would you want to stop doing something beneficial for your health, especially in a time of need? Often this advice is given because your medical doctor may not know what specific combinations are inadvisable. By the same token, you may be just as responsible as you may not have told your medical doctor that you are taking vitamins.

In most cases it's not so much that a vitamin causes a serious or deadly interaction, as many people believe. Rather, it potentiates the action of the drug. What this means is that if you're on a blood thinner such as coumadin or warfarin and at the same time you're taking vitamin E, which acts as a natural blood thinner, then the compound effect of being essentially on two blood thinners (one drug, one natural) may thin the blood more than desired. As with other drugs, the risk of unexpected results may be influenced by your age, gender, genetics, nutritional status, and concurrent disease states and treatments.

The biggest areas of concern for drug-vitamin interactions are bleeding disorders, brain chemistry imbalances, heart muscle dysfunction, and internal organ dysfunction or toxicity. To prevent or minimize the risk of any drug-vitamin interaction you must observe all of the following:

1. While the following chart is a great overview, always consult with your medical doctor if you are on any type of prescription drug or non-prescription (over the counter) drug and taking vitamins. Be sure to inform your medical doctor of the exact amounts/dosages of all drugs and supplements.

2. Ensure that your medical doctor has a thorough understanding of vitamin supplementation and drug interaction. Many don't. There are numerous cases

where natural vitamin supplementation combined with a prescription drug actually makes the drug more effective to your benefit. There are many other instances where a natural vitamin can lessen the adverse reactions created by a drug (i.e. probiotic supplementation with antibiotics, CoQ10 with statin drugs, or glutathione with Tylenol use).

3. Stick to what I refer to as the core vitamins, as noted in chapter 3. Serious adverse reactions are highly unlikely when taking vitamins B, C, D, or E in their recommended dosages. Of all adverse reactions reported to the FDA in 1998, 17% were related to ephedra. You should never take ephedra. Magazines such as Newsweek and Consumer Reports make great cover headlines when they tell you of deadly vitamins to avoid but they often list supplements that are anything but core or mainstream. (If I want to learn about which lawnmower I should buy I may use Consumer Reports. I'm certainly not going to them for advice on health.)

4. Too much of anything can create a problem. While most people don't drink enough water, it is possible (although rare) to die from drinking too much water. The same applies to vitamins. While you want to take optimal levels of vitamins well beyond RDA levels, ensure that you do not take toxic levels, especially of those which are fat soluble.

5. Ensure that your vitamins come from the best quality labs as described in chapter 19.

Potential Drug-Vitamin Interactions/Contra-Indications that You Must Take Into Consideration and Discuss with a Qualified Health Care professional Prior to Taking

If you are taking this prescription drug or have this condition...	...then supplementation with this should be monitored by the appropriate health specialist.
Anti-coagulants/blood thinners (i.e. warfarin, Coumadin, aspirin, Plavix)	Vitamin E above 400 I.U. Ginkgo Biloba Garlic Ginseng CoQ10 St. John's Wort Gum Guggul Policosanol High doses of EFA High doses of Reishi mushrooms
Diabetic on insulin	EFA above 900 mg Ginseng Chromium Glucosamine sulphate (blood glucose should be monitored during 1st month of use)
High blood pressure drugs	Policosanol High doses of Reishi mushrooms
Digitalis or Digoxin	Licorice root St. John's Wort Hawthorn Indole-3-carbinol
Anti-arrhythmic drugs	Hawthorn Ginseng
Corticosteroids	Echinacea
Kidney failure or on dialysis	Horse chestnut

Kidney removed	Check with specialist
Received any organ transplant	Check with specialist
Previous breast cancer	Read chapter 28 (chapter on Soy)
Sickle Cell Anemia	Multi-vitamin
Hemolytic anemia	Horse chestnut Multi-vitamin
Hemochromatosis (iron storage disease)	Avoid iron
Liver disorder	Horse chestnut, 5HTP
Hemophilic	Multi-vitamin
Wilson's Disease (copper storage disease)	Avoid copper
Pregnant or breast feeding	Avoid vitamin A above 5000 I.U. and herbal supplements
History of allergic reaction or intolerance to particular supplements	Obviously avoid that particular supplement. However, consider that it might also be a particular form or inclusion of poor binders or fillers. Exercise caution.
Barbituates Sedatives Hypnotic drugs Anti-anxiety drugs	St. John's Wort Valerian Kava Ginseng Melatonin 5HTP
Anti-seizure	GLA Indole-3-carbinol
Alzheimer's drugs	Huperzine A COP-choline Phosphatidylserine Ginkgo Biloba
Gingivitis	Iron

Additional Notes:

If you are taking a supplement containing beneficial liver detoxification substances such as glutathione, milk thistle, or indole-3-carbinol, the increased function of your liver may actually speed up the clearing of drugs from your liver. While this is generally not a problem, your medical doctor may need to alter the dosage of your drugs.

Please note that this list may not cover all drugs or conditions.

21

TAKING THESE DRUGS?
THEN YOU MUST TAKE THESE
VITAMINS

I've just told you which drugs you need to be careful about if you're taking vitamins (or is that which vitamins to be careful about if you're taking drugs – it all depends on your paradigm).

Many MDs warn you of this for your safety and many drug companies wish to put the fear of God into you for other reasons.

However, what most drug companies and MDs aren't telling you is that there are a number of well known drugs that not only shouldn't scare you off vitamins, it's essential that you actually take vitamin supplementation.

If you're taking this drug...	...then be sure to supplement with this vitamin as it is being depleted.
Acetaminophen (main ingredient in Tylenol)	Glutathione and Milk Thistle

If you're taking this drug...	Be sure to take this...
Ace inhibitors	Zinc
Acid or H2 blockers	Vitamin B, D, and multi-minerals
Antibiotics	Probiotics, Prebiotics, Vit. B
Antacids	Calcium and Vitamin D
Aspirin	Vitamin C, folic acid
Beta Blockers	CoQ10
Bisphosphonates (osteoporosis)	Calcium and Vitamin D
Celebrex	Folic acid
Diabetes drugs	B vitamins
Digoxin	Vitamin B1, calcium, magnesium, phosphorous
Diuretics	Vitamin B, C, and multi-minerals
Laxatives	Multi-minerals
NSAIDs (non-steroidal anti-inflammatories) i.e. ibuprofen, naproxen, etc.	Folic acid, Vitamin C
Statins (cholesterol) i.e. Lipitor, Zocor, etc.	CoQ10
Steroids	Multi-minerals

Why is it essential that you supplement with these nutrients if you're taking these drugs? Because some of these drugs are doing more harm than good. Which are the worst offenders?

1. Acetaminophen (Tylenol)

Acetaminophen consumption is actually the number one cause of acute liver failure. Acetaminophen depletes the liver of glutathione which is essential for proper liver function. Acetaminophen is also very hard on the liver in terms of detoxification. Supplementing with glutathione will obviously replenish the liver whereas milk thistle can help the detoxification process.

2. Antibiotics

Whereas antibiotics may have been considered the magic bullet decades ago, all of the problems that have come about due to their gross overuse and overprescribing it is now common knowledge.

Antibiotic resistant bacteria are now prevalent, gastro-intestinal disorders such as Crohn's, diverticulitis, and irritable bowel syndrome are widespread, and millions of prescriptions were given for viral infections on which antibiotics had no positive effect.

Antibiotics don't just kill off bad bacteria, they kill off all bacteria. Given that good bacteria are essential for proper gastro-intestinal (GI) function and more importantly proper immune function, supplementation with both probiotics and prebiotics is essential.

3. Antacids

Antacid use is recognized as a risk factor for osteoporosis, hence the need for calcium and vitamin D supplementation. What makes this so insane is that the best known antacid, Tums, actually markets itself as a calcium supplement claiming to aid in osteoporosis. What's even scarier is that Tums is recommended by doctors and by the National Osteoporosis Foundation.

4. Bisphosphonates

Following the insanity of Tums, bisphosphonates prescribed for osteoporosis can actually deplete the body of calcium and vitamin D.

5. Statins

The most widely prescribed drug in North America is Lipitor, a statin drug used to lower cholesterol in the hopes of helping prevent a heart attack. What statin drugs also do is deplete co-enzyme Q10 (CoQ10), which is essential for energy production in the heart muscle. That's right – what they've prescribed in the belief they're preventing a heart attack may actually cause one.

Finally. . .

A great number of drugs either impair zinc absorption or deplete zinc status. The most common drugs that may increase zinc requirements include:

1. Anticonvulsants (e.g. sodium valproate)
2. Caffeine
3. Alcohol
4. Hormone Replacement therapy
5. H-2 Receptor Antagonists (antacids)
6. Tetracyclines
7. ACE Inhibitors
   a. Clofibrate
   b. Corticosteroid drugs: increase zinc excretion
   c. Ethambutol (animal study)
   d. Loop diuretics: increase urinary excretion of zinc
   e. Oral contraceptives

f. Penicillamine
g. Thiazide diuretics: increase urinary excretion of zinc
h. Valproic acid
i. Zidovudine (AZT)

Given that zinc is involved in more chemical reactions in the body than any other mineral (from prostate support to immune function and so much more), additional zinc supplementation is advised.

22

WHICH WOULD YOU TAKE?

Given the knowledge that you now have, I'd like you to use your common sense and tell me which of the two drugs you would rather take in each of the following scenarios:

Scenario 1

CONDITION
Drug A and Drug B are both used in the treatment of high cholesterol.

Mode of Action
Drug A blocks the synthesis of cholesterol in the liver by inhibiting the HMG-CoA Reductase enzyme.

Drug B lowers cholesterol by increasing the uptake of LDL cholesterol from the blood, reducing oxidation of LDL cholesterol, and reducing the stickiness of blood platelets.

Effectiveness Based on Scientific Studies

Scientific studies indicate that Drug A and Drug B were equal in their ability to lower cholesterol levels and improve blood lipid profiles.

Adverse Reactions

Drug A can cause liver damage, fatigue, upset stomach, gas, constipation, abdominal pain, cramps, and in rare cases a life-threatening condition known as rhabdomyolysis.

On rare occasions Drug B may cause minor gastrointestinal distress, diarrhea, nausea, and skin rash. Drug B has no apparent risk of liver damage, no risk of rhabdomyolysis, and no risk of kidney damage.

Which would you take – Drug A or Drug B?

Scenario 2

CONDITION

Used for reducing the pain and inflammation of osteoarthritis.

Effectiveness Based on Scientific Studies

Randomized controlled studies showed that Drug B was superior to Drug A in relieving pain and inflammation.

Adverse Reactions

Drug A adverse reactions include gastritis, peptic ulcer, GI bleeding, erosion of the intestinal lining, liver and kidney toxicity, tinnitus, and death.

Drug B adverse reactions are mild and infrequent. They may include mild GI upset, drowsiness, skin reactions, and occasional headache.

Which would you take – Drug A or Drug B?

Scenario 3

CONDITION
Arthritis.

Effectiveness Based on Scientific Studies
Scientific studies show that both Drug A and Drug B are equally effective.

Adverse Reactions
Drug A adverse reactions include gastritis, peptic ulcer, GI bleeding, erosion of the intestinal lining, liver and kidney toxicity, tinnitus, and death.

Drug B adverse reactions may include gastric upset or diarrhea at high doses.

Which would you take – Drug A or Drug B?

Scenario 4

CONDITION
Rheumatoid arthritis, joint inflammation, and chronic pain.

Mode of Action
Both drugs essentially reduce or prevent the production of prostaglandin series 2.

Effectiveness Based on Scientific Studies
Drug A and Drug B had equivalent effectiveness in reducing pain, swelling, and stiffness in patients with rheumatoid arthritis.

Adverse Reactions

Drug A: Intestinal tract ulcers with potential internal bleeding in 10 to 30% of long term users, erosion of the stomach lining and intestinal tract in 30 to 50% of users and associated with 10,000 to 20,000 deaths in the U.S. each year. May also cause severe bone marrow toxicity and dangerously low white blood cell counts. Now used in horses.

Drug B has rare side effects including heartburn and reflux. Good "side effects" include that it can help lower histamine levels and is a potent anti-oxidant.

Which would you take – Drug A or Drug B?

Scenario 5

CONDITION

Rheumatoid arthritis

Mode of Action

Both reduce the synthesis of pro-inflammatory prostaglandins and leukotrienes.

Effectiveness Based on Scientific Studies

One randomized double blind study of hospital patients showed equivalent results in reduction of joint stiffness and pain after three weeks.

Adverse Reactions

Drug A: Intestinal tract ulcers with potential internal bleeding in 10 to 30% of long term users, erosion of the stomach lining and intestinal tract in 30 to 50% of users and associated with 10,000 to 20,000 deaths in the U.S. each year. It may also cause severe bone marrow toxicity and dangerously low white blood cell counts. Now used in horses.

Drug B: No significant concerns other than its effectiveness may potentiate other drugs.

Which would you take – Drug A or Drug B?

Scenario 6

CONDITION
Menopausal symptoms and PMS.

Effectiveness Based on Scientific Studies
Both Drug A and Drug B were effective at reducing the symptoms of the above conditions.

Adverse Reactions
Millions of women have stopped using Drug A due to the significant risk of increased breast cancer and ovarian cancer.

Drug B has no significant side effects and has been used in Germany by millions of women.

Which would you take – Drug A or Drug B?

ANSWERS

Did you choose Drug B each time? Read below...

Scenario 1

Drug A is the drug clofibrate – a statin drug.

Drug B as you may have guessed is a natural supplement. It is known as Gum Guggul (or Gugulipid or guggulsterone)

The points to be made are important. Number one, people have been so brainwashed to believe that while vitamins are nice for the concept of health, when things get serious it's time to take drugs. This is a belief that isn't based on fact, as in this case both A and B are just as effective based on the science. To discover if you're stuck in this belief system you simply need to honestly answer whether your choice would be different now that you know one is a drug and the other a natural supplement.

Now ask yourself this same question again if I were to tell you that while gum guggul is a natural substance, it is actually classified as a drug in India where it has been widely prescribed with great success for the past twenty-five years.

Lastly, gum guggul has the equivalent anti-inflammatory potency as the drug phenylbutazone and ibuprofen.

Scenario 2

Drug A is ibuprofen and other NSAIDs (non-steroidal anti-inflammatory drugs).

"Drug B" is the non-drug, natural supplement glucosamine sulphate.

Scenario 3

Drug A is Motrin.

Drug B is the non-drug, natural supplement MSM. Studies show it works even better when combined with glucosamine sulphate.

Scenario 4

Drug A is the powerful anti-inflammatory phenylbutazone.

Drug B is the non-drug, natural supplement curcumin.

Scenario 5

Drug A is diclofenac sodium.

"Drug" B is actually vitamin E.

Scenario 6

Drug A is hormone replacement therapy.

Drug B is the non-drug natural supplement black cohosh.

The whole idea is to understand that contrary to many people's beliefs, the choice of using a natural supplement over a drug does not mean that you are reducing adverse side effects at the cost of less effectiveness. Many supplements are just as effective and in some cases far more effective, they work in the same manner, and they almost always (if not always) have significantly fewer and much less harmful adverse reactions.

Please also note that studies show that vitamin supplementation can be superior to other devices, not just drugs. Numerous studies have shown horse chestnut seed to be superior to compression stockings in the management of chronic venous insufficiency.

Lastly, again contrary to many people's beliefs, being on a drug is not the time to avoid all natural supplementation. Scientific studies have shown that the drug Tamoxifen (used in the treatment of breast cancer) actually works better when used in conjunction with the natural supplement melatonin. If your medical doctor is not aware of this, it may be time to seek a second opinion.

Vitamins are your friend. The only thing you have to do to make them work in your favour is to actually take them.

Part Six

Analyzing Your Health

23

THE OPTIMUM HEALTH PARADIGM

One of the key components in choosing the appropriate vitamin supplementation is to determine your reasons for taking vitamin supplementation.

If you are someone who truly understands the health and wellness paradigm and wishes to achieve an optimal level of health, then this answer is easy. You should supplement at optimal levels on a daily basis with each of the supplements discussed in chapter 3, namely a comprehensive multivitamin/ mineral, essential fatty acids, vitamin D, probiotics, and phytonutrients. This should be done throughout the course of your lifetime from childhood onward. The goal goes beyond disease prevention and strives to allow you to achieve optimum function, optimum performance, and optimum health.

If, on the other hand, you supplement with vitamin C or zinc lozenges only when you have a cold or you supplement with calcium only after you find out you have osteoporosis, (osteoporosis requires so much more than just calcium) then you are living, as is most of society, in a sick care paradigm.

Many people falsely believe that if your approach is natural vs. drug oriented then you must be in a wellness paradigm. This is incorrect. While I do believe that a natural approach is far superior to a drug approach, both are still trying to ease symptoms after the problem has arisen.

The reason this becomes important is that the sick care paradigm motivates people to take vitamin B to increase their energy or vitamin D to help with their osteoporosis or calcium for their high blood pressure. The optimal health or health and wellness paradigm has people taking all of their essential nutrients regardless of any symptoms they may or may not have, knowing that all of these nutrients work hand in hand in a synergistic fashion.

24

INVESTING IN AND
TESTING YOUR HEALTH

Canadians supposedly pride themselves on their health. If that were true, why do we have so many sick Canadians?

Americans? It's the same thing, but for different reasons. Americans pride themselves on their technological and scientific advances, yet why does the U.S. rank 37th for overall health in the world? (Try naming 36 other countries, let alone 36 with better healthcare.)

By now you should realize that you need to invest in your health, both time and effort as well as financially. What many Canadians really pride themselves on is the belief that their healthcare is free. It's nice that you may have an insurance plan, but insurance is meant for emergencies and while you should never waste a benefit if someone else is willing to pay for your health, you are ultimately the person who pays for your health one way or another. You're allowed to spend a dollar of your own money on your own health and quite frankly there's no better investment. For what many spend at Starbuck's on a daily basis you could easily have a top quality nutritional supplement.

Given that the science has shown (although most medical doctors are unaware of this) that low levels of vitamin C and vitamin E were stronger predictors of future heart disease than were high cholesterol levels, smoking, or high blood pressure, why have we been so brainwashed into thinking that the gold standard for testing is the typical medical blood test panel?

Standard Blood Tests

- Total Cholesterol
- HDL-Cholesterol
- LDL-Cholesterol
- Fibrinogen
- Triglycerides
- Glucose
- Fructosamine
- Hemoglobin AIC
- Homocysteine
- Hemoglobin
- Hematocrit
- Albumin
- Platelet Count
- Prothrombin Time (INR)
- C-Reactive Protein
- Total Cholesterol / HDL Ratio
- Erythrocyte Sedimentation Rate
- White Blood Cell Count (WBC)
- Creatinine
- Uric Acid
- Blood Urea Nitrogen (BUN)
- Total Protein
- Red Blood Cell Count (RBC)
- Globulin
- Albumin/Globulin Ratio
- Bilirubin
- Alkaline Phosphatase
- HIV 1 and 2
- Serum Ferretin

You could choose to simply invest in quality supplements for a lifetime of better health. You could also invest (beyond your insurance in most cases) in finding out if you have any additional deficiencies in these key substances:

Key Vitamin and Anti-Oxidant Tests

- Vitamin E
- Vitamin C
- Carotene
- Selenium

- Vitamin D (25hydroxy cholecalciferol)
- Folic Acid
- Vitamin B12
- Holotranscobalamin II

Key Hormone Tests

- DHEA
- Total Estrogens
- Free T3
- Free T4
- Cortisol
- Total Progesterone
- DHEA/Cortisol Ratio
- Total Testosterone
- Thyroid Stimulating Hormone
- Progesterone/Estrogen Ratio
- Total Testosterone/Estrogen Ratio
- IGF-1 – males and females 50+

Vitamin Profile

Vitamin E Above 27.5 umol/L or 1.18 mg/dL
Studies show that blood levels in the optimal range are associated with decreased risk of heart attack and other vascular diseases.

Vitamin C Above 50 umol/L or 0.88 mg/dL
Studies show that blood levels in the optimal range are associated with decreased risk of heart attack and other vascular diseases.

Selenium Above 120 ug/L
Blood levels in the optimal range are associated with a significant decreased risk of colon cancer.

Vitamin D (25-hydroxy cholecalciferol) 85 to 120 nmol/L or 0.68 to 1.43 mg/dL
Vitamin D levels in the optimal range are associated with a decreased risk of osteoporosis, colon, breast and prostate cancers and multiple sclerosis.

Vitamin B12 Above 300 pg/mL
Low levels of vitamin B12 are associated with an increased risk of cancer. This is especially true for breast cancer where a low level of vitamin B12 has been linked to a 2.5 to 4.0 times greater risk.

Holotranscobalamin II Range: 70 to 130 pg/mL
This is the most active form of vitamin B12 in the human body. Low levels are associated with an increased risk of cancer.

Folic Acid Above 4 ng/mL or 10 nmol/L
Folic acid and vitamin B12 are required to make DNA in our cells as our cells replace themselves from one generation to the next. Folic acid levels below 4 ng/mL (10 nmol/L) is the level at which chromosomes break within our DNA allowing cancerous mutations to occur more easily. Low levels of folic acid are strongly associated with colon, cervical and other cancers.

CoQ10   At or above 2.0 mcg/ml

Low levels of coenzyme Q10 are associated with an increased risk of congestive heart failure and lowered immune function. Maintaining a minimum blood level of 2.0 mcg/ml is associated with reducing mild to moderate high blood pressure and improving early stage congestive heart failure when coenzyme Q10 has been administered via supplementation. Coenzyme Q10 deficiency is also a primary underlying cause of Parkinson's disease and supplementation has been shown to slow the progression of the disease. The body makes coenzyme Q10, which is required for energy production within our cells. By age 40-45 there is a significant decline in coenzyme Q10 synthesis, which creates a need for coenzyme Q10 supplementation to compensate for what the body no longer produces for itself.

Hormone Profile

DHEA   Men: 250 to 450 mcg/dL Women: 150 to 350 mcg/dL

DHEA is a hormone made in the adrenal glands and is the raw material from which the body makes many other steroid hormones (e.g. estrogen, testosterone, progesterone, cortisol). DHEA also helps to maintain bone density, slows skin aging by maintaining collagen levels, improves fat burning, enhances mood, sexual virility and responsiveness, boosts immune function, and helps to combat the undesirable effects of high cortisone levels (which accompany chronic or acute stress). Chronic stress tends to depress DHEA levels. Men with a history of prostate cancer and women with any previous reproductive cancer should not take DHEA supplements.

Cortisol   9 to 14 mcg/dL

Cortisol is a hormone made in the adrenal glands from DHEA. Stress and aging increase the production and secretion of cortisol into the blood stream. High levels of cortisol promote heart disease, diabetes and obesity by raising blood sugar and insulin, which increases and aggravates diabetic tendencies. This also leads to increased blood triglycerides, fat storage and weight gain - all of which increase heart disease risk. Chronic high cortisol levels weaken the immune system and decrease cognitive performance by the brain, adversely affecting memory, reaction time and problem solving.

DHEA/Cortisol Ratio   15:25

As we age the body makes more cortisol and less DHEA. The same is true in regards to chronic stress. As such, stress can speed up aging by creating an imbalance in the DHEA/Cortisol ratio.

Thyroid Stimulating Hormone (TSH)   1.0 - 2.0 mU/L or 1-2 uU/mL

TSH is a hormone released from the pituitary gland that instructs the thyroid gland to secrete more thyroid hormone into the blood stream. Thyroid hormone (T3 and T4) sets the metabolic rate for virtually all tissues of the body. High TSH levels indicate low thyroid function, whereas low TSH levels indicate an overactive thyroid. A TSH level between 0.2 mU/L and 1.0 mU/L indicates thyroid dysfunction, which often occurs with aging (between ages 40-50) and usually responds to specific thyroid supplementation whereas levels below 0.2 uM/L may require a prescription of thyroid hormone. Low thyroid function slows metabolism and results in weight gain, cold hands and feet, physical and mental lethargy and weakened immune function.

Free T4 (Thyroid hormone - Thyroxine)
1.2 - 1.4 ng/dL (15.4-18.0 pmol/L)
Most thyroid hormone (thyroxine) made in the thyroid gland is in the form of T4. However, before thyroxine can be used by the tissues of the body it has to be converted to T3. If Free T3 levels are below 2.6Â pg/mL or the T4 level is below 0.70ng/dL, then thyroid hormone replacement therapy may be required.

Free T3 (Thyroid hormone)
Men:2.90-3.20Â pg/mL   Women:2.80 -3.20Â pg/mL
T3 is the most active form of thyroxine hormone. Some individuals have a difficult time converting T4 into T3. In these cases supplementation with thyroid support nutrients is recommended.

Total Estrogens
Men: Less than 100Â pg/mL
Women:180-200Â pg/mL(under 50) 60-120Â pg/mL(over 50)
Estrogen is a dominant female hormone that contributes to many physical female characteristics. It affects mood, brain function, bone density, skin, cholesterol levels and other functions. High levels of estrogen contribute to increased risk of breast cancer, and possibly prostate cancer in men.

Total Progesterone   Men: 1500 - 2500Â pg/mL
Women: 2000 - 14,000Â pg/mL (under 50 years old)
2000 - 8000Â pg/mL (over 50 years old)
Progesterone is a dominant female hormone that supports brain function, bone density, skin and female reproductive tissues. Supplementation with a combination of black cohosh, soy isoflavones and gamma-oryzanol is beneficial.

Total Testosterone
Men: 6000 - 9000Â pg/mL   Women: 120 - 900Â pg/mL
Testosterone is a dominant male hormone. It helps to maintain lean mass, metabolic rate, strength, sexual virility, bone density and other functions. Men and women with low levels may benefit from testosterone replacement therapy or DHEA supplementation. However, testosterone replacement therapy may increase the risk of prostate cancer in men. Men with a history of prostate cancer and women with a history of any reproductive cancer should not supplement with DHEA. In men, DHEA supplementation requires semi-annual PSA testing.

Progesterone/Estrogen Ratio
Men: 15 to 20:1 Women: 10 to 20:1
This is the optimal ratio for these hormones for longevity and total well-being.

Total Testosterone/Estrogen Ratio
Men: 80 to 120:1   Women: 2 to 5:1
This is the optimal ratio for these hormones for longevity and total well being.

IGF-1 (after age 40)   Above 250Â mcg/L or ng/mL
IGF-1 is an indicator for levels of growth hormone. As we age, growth hormone levels decline, which speed many aspects of the aging process. The ingestion of natural growth hormone releasing agents can often increase IGF-1 to more youthful levels and provide significant anti-aging benefits. If you have a history of cancer you are advised to not supplement with growth hormone releasing agents.

It's worth the small investment in your health to know your blood levels of the key vitamins, minerals and hormones as they are truly your most important health indicators.

25

12 HEALTH BELIEFS THAT YOU MAY NEED TO CHANGE FOR THE SAKE OF YOUR HEALTH

Although all of the following have been covered elsewhere in this book, they bear repeating here due to their importance.

1. The biggest factor in your health is your beliefs about your health.

I write about this at length in my book *Healthy Beliefs Deadly Choices*, but to be succinct, appreciate this example:

After reading this book some people will come to the logical conclusion that they need to take vitamin supplementation for the rest of their life whereas others, having been presented the exact same facts, will not. It all comes down to your beliefs. Please appreciate two things:

1. You're allowed to change your beliefs, and

2. You're entitled to have any belief you want but that belief will have a consequence, good or bad, whether you believe it or not.

2. Someone else is responsible for your health.

Whoever this someone else is I hope that they really care about you if you actually believe this one. Are they a really, really good friend or your closest relative who actually truly likes you? If on the other hand you believe that the government has your best interests at heart then good luck – you'll need it. Your health is your life and your most valuable asset. Don't ever entrust it to anyone else and appreciate that the decisions that you make over your lifetime will impact your health over that same lifetime.

3. Healthcare is free and/or I'm entitled to it.

As I first said in my last book *Healthellaneous*;

"Good health is not a right that you're entitled to; rather it's your obligation that you achieve and maintain it over the course of your lifetime."

As for the free part, if you're a resident of the U.S., you're wondering what on earth I'm talking about. If you're a Canadian you may have this belief that healthcare is free. You couldn't be more wrong. Half of your tax dollars go to healthcare and it is estimated that for residents of the U.S., by the year 2043 100% of your tax dollars will go to healthcare. You're allowed to spend a dollar of your own money on your most valuable asset and you should.

4. Are you living in a sick care paradigm or a health and wellness paradigm?

Just because you've gone natural doesn't mean that you're a health and wellness person. While I would almost always choose natural and while it almost always has far fewer side effects, if I pop my vitamins only to treat a condition or mask a symptom, I'm still in the sick care paradigm. The health and wellness paradigm is all about a lifetime of optimal health regardless of any pain, symptom, or disease.

5. Vitamins are nice but when it gets serious it's time to turn to drugs.

If I had to take a drug to immediately save my life of course I would. But after reading this book you should realize that there are many cases where a natural supplement works just as effectively, often in the same manner, and almost always with far fewer adverse reactions. Always check with your doctor but let common sense and facts dictate your choice, not fear and emotion.

6. I don't need to take vitamins – I can get everything I need from food.

After reading this book there's no way that you can rationally have that belief, hence you and I must have a different definition of the word "need".

If a man were pointing a gun directly at you and starting to squeeze the trigger would you "need" to move out of the way? By not taking vitamin supplements, the result is the same – it just takes longer.

7. It's always better to get your vitamins from food.

Contrary to most experts, this is both right and wrong. Of course the word is "supplement" which means "in addition to", so supplements never replace the need for good eating, and almost always getting vitamins and minerals from your food is ideal because they work synergistically with one another. However, you might be surprised as to how a case-controlled study reported in Nutrition and Cancer, Volume 40, 2001 showed that women who consumed adequate amounts of vitamin C and vitamin E supplements demonstrated a 63% reduced risk of ovarian cancer whereas anti-oxidant consumption from food alone was not associated with a reduction in risk – only users of vitamin supplements derived the risk reduction benefit.

8. "I hear of people dying from natural supplements all the time – they're just as dangerous as drugs."

Not even close. Rare deaths make the news because they're so rare, unlike the 100,000+ who die every year from drugs in the U.S. alone. The sad thing is that we've become so used to them (and accepting of them) that they're no longer "news". These rare deaths also occur from "non-core" supplements or gross misuse or serious drug reactions.

Any good health care professional or vitamin supplier not only has absolutely no problem with strict guidelines and quality control, they insist upon it. The only problem is we're not sure the same guys who approved thalidomide, celebrex, hormone replacement therapy, and statin drugs are the ones who are best qualified to set the standards.

9. The studies aren't clear.

Only if you're looking through fogged glasses. If you're still **choosing** to **believe** the rare poorly-designed study against the countless positive ones then you'll have to accept the consequences of your belief system. Are you consciously or subconsciously choosing to only believe the few studies that support your beliefs while ignoring all the others? Do you only hang around people with your same beliefs thus re-enforcing your bias? Have you read a handful of newspaper headlines or magazine articles and think you're an expert? Did you try taking a less than optimal amount and/or for a less that optimal length of time, not "feel" any change, and then conclude they don't work?

We're not even close to knowing everything there is to know about health but we know more than enough to be a lot healthier – we just need to act. Take your vitamins.

10. If I'm taking drugs I can't take vitamins.

In some cases, this might be true. In other cases, you certainly can – it just needs to be monitored, and in other cases, it's even more important and actually essential that you do supplement if you're taking drugs. Read chapters 20 and 21 thoroughly and talk to your doctor. Better yet, supplement all your life and you may never need to go on drugs in the first place.

11. I can't take glucosamine sulphate because…

1. Because you're allergic to sulphur? Not possible. Sulphate refers to sulphur, which is contained in every cell in your body and thus it's impossible to be allergic to sulphur. You might be allergic to sulfa used in sulfa drugs and sulfate-containing food additives, which is different from glucosamine sulphate.

2. Because you're a diabetic? The impact of the glucose component of glucosamine sulphate to a diabetic is usually not of great concern, especially given the great benefits of glucosamine sulphate, but if you are a diabetic then you should simply have your medical doctor monitor your glucose levels over your first month of glucosamine sulphate use.

3. Because you're allergic to shellfish? If you have a severe allergy to shellfish then it is conceivable that you may be sensitive to the use of glucosamine and caution should be exercised. However, top quality

pharmaceutical grade glucosamine is generally devoid of shellfish contaminants.

12. Lycopene has to be cooked to be effective.

If that were true lycopene supplements would have no effect. The reason you're told that lycopene is more absorbed in tomato sauce than it is in a raw tomato is that, being a fat-soluble substance, it needs fat. Take your supplement or use olive oil on your tomato.

And an extra bonus

Time release formulas work – don't work.

Why not simply be your own time release formula? Take your vitamins throughout the day with each meal and your problem is solved.

26

WOULD YOU LIKE TO LIVE LONGER OR DIE EARLIER?

Will you see the occasional newspaper headline that says taking a multivitamin has no benefit in saving or extending your life? Of course you will. Is it accurate? Of course it isn't.

As we've discussed, if you:

- dabble in vitamins
- use too low an amount
- use the wrong form
- use the wrong combination or
- ask the wrong question

. . . then you can get a study to say anything. What do the good studies show?

The European Journal of Nutrition in July 2011 showed that people who took anti-oxidant supplementation at the beginning of an 11-year study period had a 48% reduction in the risk of death from cancer and a 42% reduction in the risk of death from all causes. To prove my previous points, the same study showed that taking only a basic multivitamin/ mineral without meaningful doses of anti-oxidants showed no benefit in reducing risk of death from cancer or all causes.

Another important study reported in the National Post on November 29, 2011, from the American Journal of Cardiology found similar substantial benefits from vitamin D supplementation. Analyzing data on over 10,000 patients, researchers at the University of Kansas found that 70% were deficient in vitamin D. This deficiency nearly doubled a person's chance of dying while correcting this deficiency with supplements resulted in a lower risk of death by 60%.

The lead researcher, Dr. James L. Vacek, a professor of cardiology at the University of Kansas Hospital and Medical Center stated;

"We expected to see that there was a relationship between heart disease and vitamin D deficiency; we were surprised at how strong it was. . . it was so much more profound than we expected."

The cardiologists found that those who were vitamin D deficient were:

- more than twice as likely to have diabetes;
- 40% more likely to have high blood pressure;
- 30% more likely to have cardiomyopathy; and
- **three times as likely to die from any cause.**

The same is true of lifelong supplementation with essential fatty acids. Numerous quality scientific studies have proven that supplementation with omega-3 fatty acids resulted in the following:

- 20 to 29% fewer deaths from cardiac causes;
- 13 to 57% lower risk of sudden cardiac death;
- 71 to 85% reduction in all-cause mortality in previous heart attack survivors;
- 41% reduction in all-cause mortality in breast cancer survivors;
- 44% reduction in inflammatory disease mortality in healthy women 49 years of age and older.

What about an aspirin a day? Used long term it does more harm than good. While it decreases the risk of some types of stroke, it increases the risk of others. It works by blocking the formation of prostaglandins 2 just as essential fatty acids do but aspirin, unlike essential fatty acids, also blocks the formation of the good prostaglandins (PG-1 and PG-3). Hence, why take it when you can get the same benefits from EFAs without the risks?

Worse yet, long term aspirin use causes gastric bleeding and ulcers, suppresses the immune system, and promotes macular degeneration, the leading cause of blindness in the U.S. The British Medical Journal found that the risk of G.I. bleeding/hemorrhage didn't change whether you were taking 50 mg or 1500 mg – in other words, going lower dose aspirin still had the same adverse risk of intestinal bleeding.

The science is clear. Pass on the aspirin, take the right supplements in the right amounts, and you'll live longer.

**Pass on the aspirin,
take the right supplements in the right amounts
and you'll live longer**

27

WHO SHOULD REGULATE VITAMINS?

Since this book is on the science of vitamins, this chapter will be incredibly short as I don't want to waste any time discussing the politics of vitamins.

At the extremes of this debate are two groups. The anti-vitamin group (or pro-drug group) who believes that vitamins are just as deadly as drugs and must be regulated by Health Canada and the FDA. At the other end are the pro-vitamin group who have no interest in the government interference (or control) of their natural approach to health.

The truth lies in the middle. I'm fully in favour of reasonable controls to ensure that natural supplementation is actually based on science, that products are safe and that they actually contain what they're supposed to .

What I'm against is having this done by governmental agencies with incestuous ties to drug companies that are blinded by politics, red tape and hidden agendas, not to mention lacking in common sense. I actually had to decrease the amount of vitamin D in my multi-vitamin because Health Canada limits your daily intake to 1,000 I.U.

contrary to all the current evidence. It also limits vitamin K from all sources to a maximum of 120mcg after which it is available only by drug prescription. Digestive enzymes can only be taken for 3 days after which medical supervision is necessary.

In November 2011, the Canadian Medical Association Journal published an editorial that supplements should be held to the same standard as drugs. Dr. Matthew Stanbrook, one of the article's authors and the deputy editor for scientific content at the journal, believes that most vitamin studies are flawed and that supplements have not been proven to the same standard for effectiveness and safety as drugs. Dr. Stanbrook should be reminded that this comes from the people who brought you thalidomide, vioxx, celebrex, Lipitor, hormone replacement therapy, Avastin and all the other drugs that kill over 100,000 Americans each and every year from "properly prescribed" drugs. Dr. Stanbrook, as well as all other medical doctors and drug reps who have the same beliefs, should also be reminded that this article is an editorial based on beliefs and not the small percentage of medicine that has actually been scientifically proven. The time has well past that people no longer give in to the fear mongering and turf protection from those who believe they have all the answers while living in their glass houses. The truth is that those who strive for optimal health would actually want to be held to a much higher standard than the drug approval process.

Taking well-known core vitamin supplementation from reputable sources over the course of your lifetime while limiting (or eliminating) the use of prescription drugs is almost always likely to result in a far better quality and quantity of life with far fewer adverse effects. We can't afford to wait for the government to come to this conclusion and we certainly don't need them to interfere with our ability to do so.

28

THE TRUTH ABOUT SOY
HEALTHY OR HARMFUL?

Some of the world's foremost experts state that the science unequivocally shows that compounds found in soy are able to significantly reduce your risk of both breast cancer and prostate cancer and that soy has a wide array of health benefits. Some of the world's other foremost experts believe that soy can actually cause breast cancer and that it is an "endocrine disrupter", actually causing many harmful effects.

How can they both be right?

I don't have the unequivocal answer but let's review the facts and try to apply some common sense.

In case you haven't noticed, health, aside from being essential for life, is also big business. Drug companies make money. Lots of it. That is their primary goal and anyone who disagrees is probably suffering the side effects of too many drugs.

Health-related companies (food, products and supplements) also strive to make money.

Enter soy. In 1999 the U.S. FDA approved a health claim for soy that it may reduce the risk of heart disease. Following that approval, soy quickly found its way into thousands of health products and sales went from millions to billions of dollars in North America. As such, to be kind, it's not surprising that anyone who is pro-soy or involved in the soy industry would be likely to focus on the benefits and downplay the negatives.

Re-enter dairy. Soy milk and soybean take away from the dairy farmers, which is also big business. Naturally, anyone who is pro-dairy or involved in the dairy industry is likely to focus on the perceived benefits of dairy and downplay the negatives, while highlighting the negatives of soy and downplaying the benefits. (Reminds you of drug companies vs. vitamin companies, doesn't it?) Some of these people might actually be sincerely convinced that they're right. Let's look at what we know to be true.

There are parts of soy that are definitely not good for you.

Is the average soy product healthy? No. Why? Because we've gone out of our way to mess it up. Like so many other foods, current North American processing methods have ripped out nutrients or added toxins.

- 91% of soy grown in the United States is genetically modified (GM). This is done mainly so that the soy grown will be resistant to a toxic herbicide known as "Roundup". While this may increase farming efficiency, it certainly results in a more toxic product.
- Soy contains natural toxins known as "anti-nutrients" (saponins, soyatoxin, phytates, oxalates, protease inhibitors, goitrogens and estrogens).
- Soy contains hemagglutinin, which is a clot-forming substance that causes red blood cells to clump together.

- Soy contains goitrogens, which block the synthesis of thyroid hormones and interfere with thyroid function.
- Soy contains phytates which prevent the absorption of certain minerals including calcium, magnesium, iron and zinc.
- Soy may contain toxic levels of aluminum and manganese as soybeans are processed by acid washing in aluminum tanks.

Hence, most soy products are really not healthy. To be fair, however, a lot of fruits and vegetables have been genetically modified. Wheat certainly contains phytates. And let's not forget the world of processed foods, on which the average consumer spends 80% of their grocery bill. Does this mean that I'm defending soy? Of course not. It means that most of our food is crap (all the more need to supplement) and that soy is not the devil food, it's just like a lot of other foods – not very healthy.

So what type of soy is healthy?

The fermented ones. After a long fermentation process, the phytic acid and anti-nutrient levels of the soybeans are reduced, and their beneficial properties -- such as the creation of natural probiotics -- become available for benefit to your digestive system.

1. Natto which are fermented soybeans with a sticky texture and strong, cheese-like flavor. Natto has high concentrations of nattokinase, which acts as a very powerful blood thinner. It is also the highest source of vitamin K2 of any food and has very powerful beneficial bacteria known as bacillus subtilis.
2. Tempeh is a fermented soybean cake with a firm texture and nutty, mushroom-like flavour.

3. Miso is a fermented soybean paste with a salty, buttery texture.
4. Some consider Soy sauce to actually be healthy as it is traditionally made by fermenting soybeans, salt, and enzymes, however, be very careful because many store bought varieties are artificially made using various chemical processes.

Unfermented soy, which includes soy proteins, soy oils (soybean oil), and soy milk, would not be considered healthy for all the reasons previously described.

Now for the biggest controversy. Soy contains isoflavones.

- Isoflavones are a class of what is known as phytoestrogens. "Phyto" means that they are plant-derived; hence they are plant-derived compounds that can have estrogen-like effects. While soybeans and soy products are typically believed to be the richest sources of isoflavones in the human diet, they are actually most abundant in the Asian herb kudzu. They are also found in small amounts in certain legumes, grains, and vegetables.
- The average intake of isoflavones in many Asian countries, including China and Japan, is 25 to 50 mg/day, whereas in most Western countries the average daily isoflavone intake can be as little as 2 mg.
- In soybeans, isoflavones are present as glycosides, which means that they are bound to a sugar molecule. When soy is digested or fermented this sugar molecule is released, leaving what is then known as an isoflavone aglycone. The best-known isoflavone aglycones are known as genistein and daidzein.

- Soy isoflavones and other phytoestrogens can bind to estrogen receptors in the body where they exert weak estrogenic activity. They mimic the effects of estrogen in some tissue and block the effects of estrogen in others. When they block the effects of estrogen in reproductive tissue, they may help reduce the risk of hormone-associated cancer in the breast, uterus, and prostate.

So what's the problem? Some scientists believe isoflavones prevent breast and other forms of cancer and are incredibly good for you while other scientists believe that these same isoflavones may cause breast cancer. Here's where the confusion begins:

- The Linus Pauling Institute states that epidemiological studies of dietary soy and breast cancer have shown conflicting results. Breast cancer incidence in Asia, where average isoflavone intake from soy foods is 25 to 50 mg/day, is lower than breast cancer rates in Western countries where average isoflavone intake is less than 2 mg/day. However, they state that many other hereditary and lifestyle factors may contribute to this difference.
- They further state that some studies suggest that a higher soy intake during adolescence may lower the risk of developing breast cancer later in life, but they also state that there is little evidence that taking soy isoflavone supplements decreases your risk of breast cancer.
- Dr. Joseph Mercola, well-known web health expert, states that isoflavones may promote breast cancer, yet the Science News reports that soy isoflavones are not a risk for breast cancer survivors in a study of 18,312 women between the ages of 20 and 83, reported in April

2011. The same study (which combined four National Cancer Institute studies, namely the Shanghai Breast Cancer Survival Study, the Life After Cancer Epidemiological Study, the Women's Healthy Eating and Living Study, and the Nurses' Health Study) actually showed that women who consumed the highest amount of soy isoflavones (more than 23 mg/day) had a 9% reduced risk of mortality and a 15% reduced risk of recurrence compared to those who had the lowest isoflavone intake. To continue the confusion, however, these percentages were not found to be statistically significant.

- The same Dr. Mercola who is extremely anti-soybean oil and anti-soy protein admits that he uses soybean oil ("bad soy" to use his term) in the CoQ10 supplements that he sells.

- Dr. Mike Fitzpatrick Ph.D. and phytoestrogen expert, in reporting for the Weston A. Price Foundation states that "under some conditions genistein has been found to inhibit breast cancer cell growth" yet it also states "there is no consensus amongst scientists that isoflavone ingestion reduces breast cancer risk".

- The same Weston A. Price Foundation is quite anti-soy. It states that it is a non-profit education centre yet it receives significant funding from dairy farmers.

- The same Weston A. Price Foundation quotes Dr. Daniel Sheehan at the FDA in their anti-soy position where Dr. Sheehan "likens soy products to herbal medicine", where "the confidence that soy products are safe is clearly based more on belief than hard data".

- The Nutrition Committee of the American Heart Association states that it has found little evidence that soy-based foods and supplements significantly lower cholesterol, yet they admit that a large amount of soy protein might lower bad cholesterol (LDL) by 3%. It is of interest to note that the American Heart Association is quick to point out that soy apparently has no positive benefits on good cholesterol (HDL), yet I've never heard them point out that cholesterol drugs (statins) also have no positive benefits on HDL cholesterol.

- The Linus Pauling Institute states that epidemiological studies do not provide consistent evidence that high intakes of soy foods are associated with reduced prostate cancer risk.
- Yet world renowned nutrition expert Dr. James Meschino states that research in this area reveals that there are at least eight modes of action through which soy isoflavones (genistein and diadzein) may defend against prostate cancer:

1. Anti-proliferative-soy isoflavones have been shown to inhibit two key enzymes within prostate cancer cells that trigger cell division and growth. By blocking their activity soy isoflavones have demonstrated an impressive ability to greatly inhibit the growth and division of prostate cancer cells under experimental conditions.
2. Soy isoflavones stimulate the synthesis of sex hormone-binding globulin in vivo, thus reducing the plasma concentration of free, unbound sex hormones. As a result there is less available (unbound) testosterone and other steroid compounds that are free to bind to prostate receptors and exert their potentially hyperproliferative effects. It is well established that certain androgens and estrogens are linked to the progression and promotion of prostate cancer and higher serum levels of sex hormonebinding globulin is associated with a reduced risk of many hormone dependent cancers.

3. Soy isoflavones have demonstrated the ability to help block the over production of certain steroid hormones that influence the promotion and progression of prostate cancer.

4. The over production of estrogen hormone from adipose tissue is also associated with increased prostate cell proliferation and prostate cancer.

5. Genistein, the most intensively researched soy isoflavoinoid, also acts as a cellular antioxidant. As soy isoflavones are known to concentrate within prostatic fluids they are considered to be an important defense against free radical damage and the cancerous mutations that are known to arise from free radical damage to prostate cells.

6. Soy isoflavones have also been shown to selectively encourage prostate cancer cells to undergo programmed cell death (apoptosis).

7. Soy isoflavones demonstrate an ability to hinder the ability of cancer cells from growing the necessary capillaries that feed their growth as they attempt to spread (metastasize) to adjacent tissues. It appears that genistein, in particular, blocks the synthesis and/or release of growth factors required to form the extensive network of blood vessels necessary to aid the spread of the malignancy.

8. Soy isoflavones bind to androgen and estrogen receptors on the prostate gland, partially blocking access to the cell of testosterone, estrone and related hormone modulators of prostate cell (and prostate cancer cell) growth. The net effect appears to be a down-regulation influence whereby the growth and cell division rate of prostate cells is slowed.

According to Dr. Meschino, "by all accounts sufficient evidence now exists to encourage the more frequent consumption of foods, supplements and nutraceuticals that are a rich source of soy isoflavones as a means to help prevent prostate cancer".

- Dr. Meschino also states that phytoestrogens demonstrate a number of properties that are considered to be important in the prevention and possibly treatment of breast cancer. These compounds, which are structurally similar to estrogen made by the body, bind to the estrogen receptors on breast tissue, toning down the influence of the body's more dangerous estrogens. The body's estrogens and estrogen replacement therapy are known to increase the risk of breast cancer. By competing with estrogen for binding to receptors on breast tissue, phytoestrogens have been shown to minimize some of estrogen's more undesirable effects.

Finally, from a purely scientific mechanism, it is known that there are two receptor sites for estrogen on breast tissue (alpha and beta). When phytoestrogens (plant-based estrogens) bind to estrogen receptors in the breast, they reduce the ability of stronger estrogens from over stimulating these cells. The same is true of other reproductive tissues such as the cervix, uterus, and in males, the prostate gland. The body's estrogens (estradiol, estrone and estriol), estrogen replacement therapy and the estrogen in oral contraceptives primarily stimulate the alpha-receptors, which encourage breast cells (and breast cancer cells), to rapidly divide and proliferate resulting in more cancerous mutations.

Phytoestrogens, on the other hand, are known to primarily stimulate the beta receptors on breast cells, which in turn encourages a slower, more controlled cell division rate which is associated with reducing the risk of breast cancer. Phytoestrogens can bind to alpha receptors but have only 1/1000 to 1/10,000 the estrogen effect as estradiol. As such, phytoestrogens are capable of toning down the estrogen influence of more powerful estrogens on reproductive tissues. Studies repeatedly show that a higher ingestion of phytoestrogens results in the prevention of reproductive cancers in women and men.

Genistein can also exert an estrogen-like effect on bone metabolism by specifically binding to the same nuclear receptors to which estrogen binds. However, unlike estrogen, genistein does not bind with an equal affinity to both the alpha and beta estrogen receptors. Genistein has a relative affinity for receptor site B that is approximately 7 to 30 times greater than its affinity for receptor site A, and compared with estrogen, genistein is 500 times weaker in its binding to receptor site A. This is important, as reproductive tissues such as the breast and uterus are rich in A type receptor sites, whereas bone contains greater amounts of the B type receptor sites. When genistein binds with the estrogen receptor it has the ability to alter gene expression in ways that favor the maintenance of healthy bone formation.

What does all this mean?

It means that the scientific community at large has different opinions and different biases on soy isoflavones.

What should you do?

Given the fact that there are different receptor sites, the mechanisms described by Dr. Meschino, and the recently published study in Science News, I have little concern over any adverse affects of soy isoflavones, rather I recognize the benefits of genistein provided I'm sure that I'm taking a good quality source. I would not, however, take soy protein or soy oils.

If you're still concerned, you can choose to err on what you believe is the "side of caution". However, be aware that everything has a risk-benefit ratio. What you believe to be the side of caution means that while you're avoiding a potential perceived risk, you're also avoiding a potential benefit, which also carries a risk.

Finally, let me approach this confusion (are soy isoflavones healthy or harmful?) in a way that I haven't seen discussed anywhere else. Please answer one question for me:

Do you consider broccoli and flaxseed powder healthy?

The obvious answer (please admit this to yourself) is yes, of course they're healthy. Why is this important and what does it have to do with soy isoflavones? Both flaxseed powder and indole-3-carbinol, one of the main ingredients in cruciferous vegetables such as broccoli that makes them so healthy, act as phytoestrogens just as isoflavones do. You would certainly never stop eating broccoli, would you?

You'll discover in chapters 31 and 33 that I've taken the approach in Core Science products that attempts to combine both science and patient choice. Vitamin K is present in both the multi-vitamin and bone health product – it's just not from soy. Genistein (an isoflavone) is also present in the bone health product but again, it's not from soy – just to make you feel more at ease even though I have no concerns as I have discussed .

Either way, if you focus on every other nutrient, you're likely to be much healthier.

29

STARS AND UPCOMING STARS

One of the key themes that you should realize by now is that nutritional supplementation works best synergistically. In other words, 1+1+1=12. Calcium has far superior effects on bone health if it's combined with vitamin D and other minerals. Vitamin E works far better if you have enough vitamin C. That's one of the reasons why the sick care paradigm is so inferior to the health and wellness approach. Your health requires all the components for optimum function, not simply single specific substances for symptom relief.

Having said that, you may find it strange that I'm now going to single out these three particular nutrients. I do so because the first one is so beneficial and so backed by science that even the biggest naysayers would find it difficult to disagree. By accepting even one supplement, it may open the door for other naysayers to finally come over from the dark side. The other two have been around for a while but their potential emergence as rising stars is finally being noticed.

VITAMIN D

The scientific benefits of vitamin D have been incredibly well documented and hence it is one of the five key supplements that everyone is required to take as an essential component of optimal health.

How important is vitamin D? Dr. William Grant, Ph.D., research scientist, and vitamin D expert, found that 30% of cancer deaths could be prevented simply by supplementing with higher levels of vitamin D. In fact, 18 different scientific studies have shown that supplementing with vitamin D significantly reduces mortality from all causes. What was once seen as only preventing rickets, vitamin D now goes well beyond osteoporosis. It has been shown to help prevent cancer, bolster the immune system, help regulate insulin levels, maintain muscle strength, optimize brain activity, improve heart function, and help regulate blood pressure.

Given its vast benefits, it's actually sad that the vast majority of U.S. residents and Canadians are grossly deficient in this vitamin. It is estimated that 85% of Americans are deficient, even higher for Canadians, and 95% for seniors. Having darker skin pigmentation (African American, Indian, or Middle East ancestry), limiting your outdoor activities or always wearing significant sun protection just makes it worse. And of course there's this thing called winter. Average vitamin D levels are 15 to 18 mg/ml. Optimal is 50 to 70 mg/ml.

Vitamin D, made from cholesterol and from UVB sunlight is technically a fat-soluble vitamin that acts like a hormone. It is present in cold water fish but more so in the fat and skin. It is also found in smaller amounts in fortified milk and orange juice but this has been added back into these liquids, hence you're required to consume extra fat or sugar simply to get what is essentially a poorer quality supplement. It is far better just to take a good quality supplement.

Adding to the problem is that most people aren't even aware that they're deficient in this essential nutrient. The best way to determine your need is with a blood test. If we were a rational society, we would realize that it makes far more sense to be testing for vitamin D levels in a health and wellness paradigm than it does to be doing most of the routine blood tests that we currently do in our sick care paradigm. However, waiting for the government to both recognize and pay for this is just as unreasonable. It is not a valid excuse to wait for someone else to pay for your health.

When I speak of vitamin D what I always mean is specifically vitamin D3, known as cholecalciferol. The absolute minimum dosage is 1000 I.U. and in fact should probably be much more. Unfortunately, most government agencies and medical doctors still believe that they're being prudent and erring on the side of caution by setting this as a maximum limit. (Health Canada limits the amount in multi-vitamins to a daily dose of 1000 I.U.) In my opinion this is not prudent, rather it's just a way of ensuring that the public will never reach optimal health, decided upon by a group of individuals who have limited knowledge in the field and are living in the sick care paradigm. While it's true that vitamin D is fat soluble and thus has the potential to become toxic, this would usually take significantly higher doses. Many experts recommend 2000, 3000, 5000 I.U. and more where even the American Academy of Pediatrics has recently doubled its recommendation for young children to 400 I.U. per day. Again, get your blood tested.

VITAMIN K

Referred to by some as "the forgotten vitamin", and by others as "the new vitamin D", vitamin K was discovered in 1929 by a Danish scientist and hence named because of its role in "Koagulation" (blood coagulation). However, this fat-soluble vitamin's role goes well beyond blood clotting.

It is essential for building strong bones, where scientific studies have shown it to be equivalent to the biphosphorate drug Didronel and other Fosamax-type drugs.

Other studies have shown that it slowed the growth of cancer cells in lung cancer patients and has shown benefit in treating leukemia. It's deficiency may be a contributing factor in Alzheimer's and normal insulin function. It promotes heart function, memory, skin function, immune function, and is "anti-aging".

Vitamin K is really in three forms; K1, K2, and K3. K1 (phylloquinone) is found naturally in plants. K2 (menaquilone) is made by bacteria in the gastrointestinal tract and K3 (menadione) is a synthetic form which is not recommended.

K1 is found in dark green vegetables, but you would need to eat a pound of spinach daily to get optimal levels. K2 is found in fermented soybean products such as natto as well as fermented cheeses such as cheese curds. Vitamin K deficiency is made worse by taking antibiotics, cholesterol drugs, and aspirin. Hence, again the need to supplement. Caution should be taken by those who take anticoagulants, are pregnant, have had past stroke occurrences, and those prone to blood clotting.

My highest recommendation goes specifically to vitamin K2-7 (K2 as many forms) from a non-soy source. It is usually safe at doses even 100 times the RDA.

ASTAXANTHIN

This anti-oxidant is in the carotenoid family (such as beta-carotene) but is considered far more powerful. It helps protect your eyes, brain, and nervous system from oxidative stress, promotes skeletal and joint health, is "anti-aging", and is great for your skin (reduces wrinkly dry skin and age spots).

Athletes find it can increase strength, stamina, endurance, and recovery from exercise as well as reduce joint and muscle soreness.

It's even responsible for a salmon's colour and increases its ability to swim upstream and gives flamingos their colour.

What makes it special is that it is many times more potent at free radical scavenging than vitamin C, E, and beta-carotene, and hundreds of times more powerful at singlet oxygen quenching than vitamin E, vitamin C, CoQ10, and green tea.

Part Seven

My Best Recommendations And Why

30

CONFLICT OF INTEREST?
I DON'T THINK SO

I strongly considered ending this book at this point. After all, I believe it has provided a wealth of information that could not only change your life, but save it. What more could you ask for from a book?

More to the point I strongly considered not including the remaining chapters because I didn't want to be perceived by some people as trying to sell you anything. As I'm sure you know, there are some people who believe that everyone has an ulterior motive. I didn't want those people to have any additional excuse to not follow through on my health advice and the vast amount of science that supports it.

But the three things happened:

1. The realization that those people already have enough excuses to not follow through on their health and one more from me wasn't going to make a difference. Besides, when I'm speaking of optimal health I'm not going to lower my standards to their level.

2. There is additional information in the following chapters that not only gives specific recommendations but explains why I've made them.
3. My patients asked me to. Why? Because they trust me, they know my expertise, and they know I have their best interests at heart.

Remember chapter 1? I sell vitamins. I sell those that I believe are the very best in the world. Why on earth would I not? They're the ones that my family and I take and they're only available through qualified health care professionals. They're an essential part of health and I can make recommendations in the best interests of your health. If you follow through on my recommendations, great. If you don't, I sincerely hope that this book has been of benefit to you. And if you can find other nutritional supplements that are equal in every way, then good for you.

But after a few years, even with access to the best labs in North America, I still found that there wasn't a product that had everything that I wanted in a nutritional product. So what did I do? I designed my own. I played a key role in the design of the original Core Science and today I now own the company.

Not surprisingly then, most of the following recommendations are for Core Science products. Not necessarily because they're mine, but rather why on earth would I have designed them if it wasn't to be the best? In fact, that's how the original was designed. We looked at what was considered the best product at that time (already a five-star) and then how this could be improved upon.

Now let's not be naïve. Of course there are many other products that are big on hype and to be kind shall I say are misleading on the science. I noticed this firsthand when Core Science was first designed. I thought I knew a lot back then but upon taking a closer look at numerous other products, even I found it amazing at the poor quality of some in the interests of lowering costs. Core Science, on the other hand, was easy. It was going into my body.

You should know if the person giving you advice has a financial interest in any product that they're recommending. This applies to far more than just vitamins and that's why I'm making my connection very clear here. But the fact that I do doesn't make the recommendation any less valid. If I want an opinion on dentistry I'm not going to ask my plumber.

Please read each of the following chapters to discover not only my specific recommendations but also to discover some of the key elements in their design and what you should be looking for in any product that you're currently taking.

31

MULTI-VITAMIN / MINERAL #1

Recommendation:

Core Science Ultimate Health Pack (available in Men's or Women's)

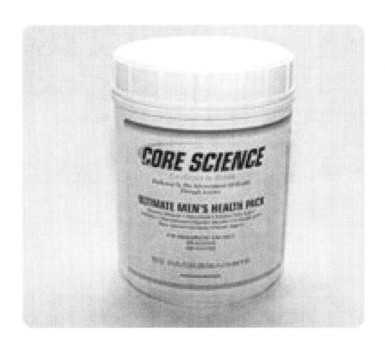

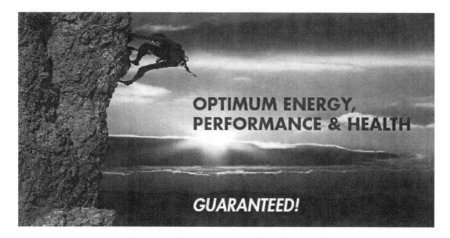

OPTIMUM ENERGY,
PERFORMANCE & HEALTH

GUARANTEED!

ALL NATURAL CORE SCIENCE
Dedicated to the Advancement of Health Through Science

Core Science was originally developed by Doctors, Scientists and Nutritionists for them and their families. It is the most potent and comprehensive supplement available today and is based on the latest scientific evidence and research. Approved by Health Canada and surpassing all requirements of the FDA in the United States, it combines the ultimate blend of science and optimum health. It is a single, easy to take optimum nutritional supplement of unsurpassed quality, effectiveness and value containing optimum levels to maximize your health.

- Elite Athletic Performance
- More Energy and Vitality
- Improved Neurological Function
- Superior Cardiovascular Function
- Prevent Pre-mature Aging
- Strong Healthy Bones
- Less Stress, Enjoy Life More
- Improved Insulin Response
- Improved Digestion & Metabolism
- Stronger Immune System
- Better Organ Function
- Improved Cholesterol Levels
- Hormonal Balance, Smoother Skin
- Feel Stronger and Healthier

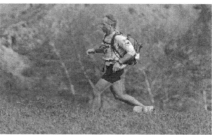

"It's amazing what my body can withstand now that I take Core Science"

Pat ran a marathon everyday for 20 days across the Sahara Desert in 131 degrees fahrenheit weather.

PROTECT YOUR HEALTH WITH
THE WORLD'S BEST NUTRITIONAL SUPPLEMENT

NOT ALL VITAMINS ARE CREATED EQUALLY

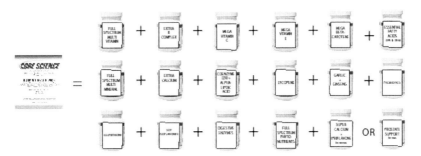

* The Highest Quality Vitamins and Minerals from the Purest All Natural Sources
* Essential Energy Producers, Neural Accelerators, Metabolism Boosters
* The World's Best Bone Mineral Complex * Molecular Distilled Essential Fatty Acids
* Pure Digestive Enzymes, Pro-Biotics, Phyto-nutrients and so much more
* Dissolution times which meet or exceed the highest standards in the world

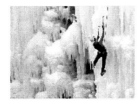
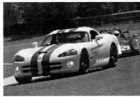
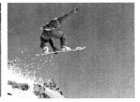

REAL TESTIMONIALS FROM REAL PEOPLE

"In 4 months I have lost an additional 31 pounds above and beyond my exercise and nutrition just from taking my Core Science" -Darren

"As a Mixed Martial Artist my training and recovery requires the very best nutrients. Core Science is the answer" - Matt

I have increased mental clarity & focus, increased energy, improved metabolism and a sharper memory. Supplementation is necessary. I strongly recommend Core Science!" - Kevin

"I feel smarter. I can focus better and actually pay more attention in conversations." -Sarah

" I have tried all the best known vitamins that claimed to be the best. None of them can compare to what Core Science has done for me." - Jamie

"As the main founder of Core Science, I practice what I preach. I've flown jet fighters and been on zero gravity flights. My patients will tell you I have unlimited energy and health as you should too." - Dr. Z

Please visit www.CoreScience.ca to order
Also available at OCNHC, World Exchange Plaza, Ottawa, Canada

CORE SCIENCE

ULTIMATE HEALTH PACKS DATA SHEET DAILY DOSE (As of Feb 2012)

Both the Men's and Women's Packs contain all of the following (Daily dose = 1 pack 2 times daily)

Vitamin A	5,000 I.U.
Beta-carotene	15,000 I.U.
Vitamin B1	75 mg
B2	75 mg
B3 (niacinamide)	100 mg
(niacin)	20 mg
B5	150 mg
B6	100 mg
B12	100 mcg
Folic Acid (Folate:L-methylfolate, Metafolin®)	800 mcg
Biotin	300 mcg
Vitamin C (calcium ascorbate)	1,000 mg
Vitamin D3 (cholecalciferol)	1,000 I.U.
Vitamin E (d-alpha tocopherol succinate with mixed tocopherols)	600 I.U.
Vitamin K2 MK-7 (menaquinone-7)	50 mcg
Calcium (citrate/ascorbate)	500 mg
Magnesium (citrate)	500 mg
Potassium (chloride)	100 mg
Iodine (kelp)	200 mcg
Zinc (citrate)	15 mg
Copper (chelate)	2 mg
Manganese (sulfate)	9 mg
Chromium (chelate)	200 mcg
Selenium (citrate)	200 mcg
Bioflavinoids	100 mg
Betaine	100 mg
PABA	50 mg
Molybdenum (citrate/gluterate/malate/fumerate)	50 mcg
Vanadium (citrate)	25 mcg
Choline (bitartrate)	200 mg
Lycopene	6 mg
Co-enzyme Q10 (ubiquinone)	25 mg
Garlic (deodorized)	50 mg
Ginseng (Siberian)	10 mg
Alpha-Lipoic Acid	6 mg
Glutathione	6 mg
Inositol	100 mg
N-Acetyl-Cysteine	50 mg
Lutein	5 mg
Astaxanthin	4 mg
Zeaxanthin	1 mg

PLUS (Both Men's & Women's)
OPTI-EPA Essential Fatty Acids EPA & DHA (Enteric coated)

Opti-EPA™ enteric-coated softgels supply significant amounts of essential omega-3 fatty acids, derived from marine lipid concentrate. Processed by molecular distillation, Opti-EPA is an excellent source of these fatty acids, providing 660 mg of eicosapentaenoic acid (EPA) and 340 mg docosahexaenoic acid (DHA) per daily dose. Omega-3 fatty acids are intimately involved in the control of inflammation, cardiovascular health, myelin sheath development, allergic reactivity, immune response, hormone modulation, intelligence, brain development, memory loss and behavior.

Daily Dose (2 capsules) contains:
Pure Eicosapentenoic Acid (EPA)..............660 mg   Pure Docosahexaenoic Acid (DHA)..............340 mg
with Rosemary extract, Ascorbyl palmitate and mixed vitamin E tocopherols

PLUS the following on the next page...

PLUS (Both Men's & Women's)
GFS 2000 SUPER GREEN FOOD

GFS 2000 Super Green Food Capsules provide a wide variety of vitamins, minerals, enzymes, antioxidants, essential amino acids, and other important phytonutrients.

Daily Dose (2 capsules) contains:

Green Food Supplement....................1,056 mg
Providing:
Wheat Grass Juice Powder..................44.5 mg
Barley Grass Juice Powder..................44.5 mg
Alfalfa Grass Juice Powder..................44.5 mg
Green Papaya.....................................44.5 mg
Blue Green Algae:
Spirulina..89 mg
Chlorella (cracked cell)...........................89 mg
Broccoli (freeze-dried powder)..................89 mg
Cauliflower (freeze-dried powder)............89 mg
Lecithin (with Phosphatidylcholine).........222 mg
Wheat Sprout Powder (gluten-free).........44.5mg mg
Acerola Berry Juice Powder.....................33 mg
Beet Juice Powder................................22 mg
Spinach/Octacosanol Powder..................56 mg
Dunaliella salina....................................6 mg

Green Tea Extract (60% catechins)................. 6 mg
Milk Thistle...6 mg
 (Silybum marianum, 80% silymarin)
Ginkgo Biloba..4.5 mg
Bilberry (25% anthocyanidins)........................ 4.5 mg
Proanthocyanidins.. 4.5 mg
(as Grape Seed Extract and Pine Bark Extract OPC 85)
Probiotic Cultures (dairy free)............1.1 Billion C.F.U
(as lactobacillus Acidophilus (DDS-1), L. Rhamnosus,
L. bifidus, Bifidobacterium lactis, B. longum, B.bifidum
and Streptococcus thermophilus.

Fructooligosaccharides (FOS) 111

NutraFlora
In a base of Apple Pectin, Bromelain (flower stem pineapple plants), Parsley, Celery and Watercress

PLUS (Women only)
CAL-6 + MG™

Cal-6 + Mg™ is a special proprietary chelate complex of 6 sources of calcium including citrate and microcrystalline hydroxyapatite concentrate. This unique formula has several advantages compared to other calcium supplements. It contains glutamic acid and lysine to ensure pH balanced calcium and magnesium in an optimal 2:1 ratio. It is a highly soluble form with added vitamin D and vitamin C that achieves proper transport and absorption by the body.

Daily Dose (2 tablets) contains:

Calcium (from calcium citrate, gluconate, lactate, carbonate, ascorbate and microcrystalline hydroxyapatite .... 500 mg
Magnesium (Magnesium HVP Chelate)... 250 mg   Boron (citrate)... 2mg   Glutamic acid... 50 mg   Lysine HCL... 24 mg
Vitamin D.... 267 IU   Vitamin C (ascorbic acid)... 34 mg

PLUS (Men only)
URO-PRO *Enhance prostate function *Cancer risk reduction *Antioxidant support

Uro-Pro is a synergistic and comprehensive combination of vitamins, minerals, amino acids, herbals, and other nutrients, carefully formulated and specifically designed to support the healthy structure and function of the prostate. It may significantly improve several aspects of prostate function, including nocturnal frequency, maximum flow and volume, decrease cholesterol levels in the prostate, have a positive effect on urine flow and frequency of urination, provide potent antioxidant protection from oxidative damage to the prostate and may also decrease prostate specific antigen (PSA) levels.

Daily Dose (2 capsules) contains:

Saw Palmetto (standardized extract).....................320 mg
Pygeum Africanum (standardized extract)............100 mg
Pumpkin Seed Powder.......................................200 mg
L-Glycine...100 mg
L-Alanine..100 mg
L-Glutamic Acid...100 mg

Proanthocyanidins (OPC 85+)..................20 mg
Vitamin A..5,000mg
Vitamin E (d-alpha Tocopheryl Succinate) 60 mg
Vitamin B-6.. 50 mg
(Pyridoxine HCL/Pyridoxal-5-Phosphate)
Zinc (elemental, picolinate)....................30 mg

Directions: Take 1 ultimate health pack with breakfast and 1 with lunch or dinner.
This product does not contain yeast, wheat gluten, soy protein, milk/dairy, corn, sodium, sugar, starch, artificial colouring, preservatives or flavouring.

CORE SCIENCE'S DISSOLUTION AND DISENTIGRATION TIMES MEET
OR EXCEED THE HIGHEST STANDARDS IN THE INDUSTRY
for maximum absorption and optimum bio-availability .

WHY I RECOMMEND IT

When we refer to a "multi-vitamin", times have changed. A "multi-vitamin" used to be vitamins A through E with maybe a few minerals added. Today, a "multi-vitamin" is really a comprehensive nutritional supplement containing optimal levels of vitamins, minerals, anti-oxidants, phytonutrients, and much more.

I recommend it because:

- It is produced by one of only four labs that received a five-star rating and is a Gold Medal ribbon winner (Douglas Labs). The five star labs are Douglas Labs, TrueStar Health, Usana and Creating Wellness Alliance.
- It's original formula was based on an original five-star supplement and then improved upon.
- It contains numerous unique formulations such as Metafolin®, not found in most multi-vitamins, which is a patented natural form of (6S) 5-methyltetrahydrofolate (5-MTHF). It contains only the S isomer of 5-MTHF and has been shown to be the only form of folate to be able to cross the blood brain barrier. It also contains intrinsic factor which is necessary to allow the intestines to properly absorb vitamin B12. Without intrinsic factor, B12 deficiency can occur even with B12 supplementation.
- It stays on the cutting edge of research by including substances such as superior quality soy-free vitamin K2 (M-7) and Astaxanthin.
- Its quality , source of raw materials, processing methods, and expertise are second to none.
- Remember the second example in chapter 18 "Reading Your Vitamin Label"? That was just half of the Core Science Ultimate Health Pack (and all of the Core Science Daily Wellness Pack discussed in the next

chapter). It meets or exceeds all eighteen criteria for an optimal nutritional supplement.

- Remember chapter 3, "Which Vitamins Are Necessary For Everyone?" The Core Science Ultimate Health Packs have all five and infact, to my knowledge, are the only packs on the market that contain all five essential components. They contain:

1. Comprehensive, high potency multi-vitamin / mineral
2. Vitamin D
3. Essential fatty acids
4. Probiotics
5. Phytonutrients

- The Ultimate Health Packs not only contain probiotics, they also contain prebiotics (more in chapter 41).
- It used to be one of the few vitamins that I know of that contained a full spectrum of digestive enzymes to enable you to obtain even more nutrients from the foods you eat until Health Canada decided to limit the use of enzymes beyond 3 days unless under the direct supervision of a health care professional.
- Core Science has the unique ability to change its formulas should new advances in science dictate it.
- The Core Science Ultimate Health Packs replace 17 different bottles of vitamins in convenient packs for compliance and ease of use.
- Dissolution times meet or exceed the highest standards.
- The men's formula contains additional nutrients proven to support optimal prostate health.
- The women's formula contains additional bone mineral support in its best and most absorbable form.

MULTI-VITAMIN / MINERAL #2

Recommendation:

Core Science Daily Wellness Pack

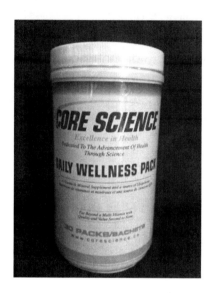

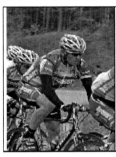 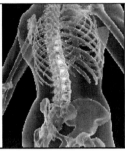 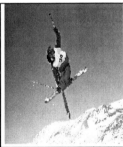

DAILY WELLNESS PACKS

(Daily dose = 1 pack per meal 3 times daily)

Vitamin A	5,000 I.U.
Beta-carotene	15,000 I.U.
Vitamin B1	75 mg
B2	75 mg
B3 (niacinamide)	100 mg
(niacin)	20 mg
B5	150 mg
B6	100 mg
B12	100 mcg
Folic Acid (Folate:L-methylfolate, Metafolin®)	800 mcg
Biotin	300 mcg
Vitamin C (calcium ascorbate)	1,000 mg
Vitamin D3 (cholecalciferol)	1,000 I.U.
Vitamin E (d-alpha tocopherol succinate with mixed tocopherols)	600 I.U.
Vitamin K2 MK-7 (menaquinone-7)	50 mcg
Calcium (citrate/ascorbate)	500 mg
Magnesium (citrate)	500 mg
Potassium (chloride)	100 mg
Iodine (kelp)	200 mcg
Zinc (citrate)	15 mg
Copper (chelate)	2 mg
Manganese (sulfate)	9 mg
Chromium (chelate)	200 mcg
Selenium (citrate)	200 mcg
Bioflavinoids	100 mg
Betaine	100 mg
PABA	50 mg
Molybdenum (citrate/gluterate/malate/fumerate)	50 mcg
Vanadium (citrate)	25 mcg
Choline (bitartrate)	200 mg
Lycopene	6 mg
Co-enzyme Q10 (ubiquinone)	25 mg
Garlic (deodorized)	50 mg
Continued on next page	

Ginseng (Siberian)	10 mg
Alpha-Lipoic Acid	6 mg
Glutathione	6 mg
Inositol	100 mg
N-Acetyl-Cysteine	50 mg
Lutein	5 mg
Astaxanthan	4 mg
Zeaxanthin	1 mg

This product does not contain yeast, wheat gluten, soy protein, milk/dairy, corn, sodium, sugar,
starch, artificial colouring, preservatives or flavouring. If seal around cap is broken, do not use. For optimal storage conditions, store in a cool, dry place. (15-20C/59-68F)

WHY I RECOMMEND IT

The Core Science Daily Wellness Packs were designed, for lack of a better term, to be a "step down" from the Ultimate Health Packs. I hate to use the term "step down" as they're still essentially a better supplement than almost anything else on the market, but they were designed for people where finances may be a concern or who aren't willing to make as much of an investment in their health as the Ultimate Health Packs.

They are in fact the exact same pills that you will find in the Ultimate Health Packs except that in the Ultimate Health Packs you also get the additional EFA capsule, the phytonutrient capsule, and the additional prostate or bone health support depending on your gender.

- It is produced by one of only four labs that received a five-star rating and is a Gold Medal ribbon winner (Douglas Labs).
- It's original formula was based on a five-star supplement and then improved upon.

- Its quality , source of raw materials, processing methods, and expertise are second to none.
- It used to be one of the few vitamins that I know of that contained a full spectrum of digestive enzymes to enable you to obtain even more nutrients from the foods you eat until Health Canada decided to limit the use of enzymes beyond 3 days unless under the direct supervision of a health care professional.
- Core Science has the unique ability to change its formulas should new advances in science dictate it.
- The Core Science Ultimate Health Packs replace 17 different bottles of vitamins in convenient packs for compliance and ease of use.
- Dissolution times meet or exceed the highest standards.

If taking the Daily Wellness Packs it is recommended that you take an additional EFA and probiotic supplement to achieve optimal health.

32

LIQUID VITAMINS AND KIDS' FORMULAS

LIQUID VITAMINS AND KIDS FORMULAS

Why do I include both of these in the same category? Because the solution solves both problems.

Informed parents want the best for their children, and there's no better way to achieve that than by having your child take natural supplementation. The level of health issues that could be solved by doing so would be incredible.

However, reality also sets in where most kids don't want to take quality supplements and hence we feel we're stuck with Flintstone's chewables.

By the same token, while most have no problem swallowing pills, capsules, and tablets, there are some who see vitamins as "horse pills" that they simply can't swallow or are uncomfortable doing so which clearly affects compliance and the benefits to your health.

The answer for both groups? Liquids. This way, children can often take the same supplement but, depending on their age, just a smaller amount and adults can be far more compliant with their health and daily supplementation.

Some people also suggest that liquids are more easily absorbable, however, any quality vitamin pill should have excellent dissolution and disintegration in which case absorbability of either should not be an issue.

Recommendation:
Core Science Ultimate Liquid Vitamin

The Difficulty in Designing a Liquid Vitamin
Remember where I described how the original formula of Core Science was designed. Well, as we speak, the exact same thing is happening with liquid Core Science. Even with access to the best labs and nutritional companies in North America, I've yet to find a liquid multi-vitamin that has everything that I would want in a supplement. Hence, as I'm writing this book I'm also designing a new liquid Core Science for use by adults and children.

But there's a catch. There are two difficulties:

1. To take everything in a Core Science Ultimate Health Pack and liquefy it a) isn't possible and b) would end up being a cup of liquid as a daily dose if it were.
2. Since there are no cheap binders, fillers, sweeteners, or other things that I don't want in Core Science, making it taste good is also a challenge. The purer a vitamin, the worse it usually tastes. (That's why I don't recommend that you chew the Core Science Ultimate Health Packs.)

I'm hoping to have the new formula available shortly after this book appears in print, hopefully in February 2012.

Why do I recommend it? Obviously it has as many of the benefits of the Core Science Ultimate Health Packs as reasonably possible.

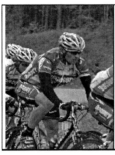 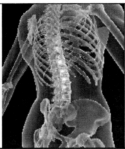 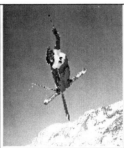

Core Science Ultimate Liquid Vitamin
Data Sheet

Directions: Optimal daily dose - take one tbsp.(15ml) with each meal (3 meals per day).

Ingredients per optimal daily dose (45 ml):

Natural Beta carotene 5 000 IU
Vitamin C (Ascorbic Acid) 1 000 mg
Vitamin D3 (Cholecalciferol) 1 000 IU
Vitamin E (d-alpha tocopherol acetate) 400 IU
Vitamin B1 (Thiamine mono) 50 mg
Vitamin B2 (Riboflavin) 25 mg
Vitamin B3 (Niacinamide) 50 mg
Vitamin B3 (Niacin) 20 mg
Vitamin B5 (Pantothenic Acid) 50 mg
Vitamin B6 (Pyridoxine HCl) 50 mg
Folic Acid 1 000 mcg
B12 methylcobalamin 500 mcg
Vitamin K2 (MK-7) 100 mcg
Biotin 250 mcg
Calcium (citrate) 500 mg
Iodine (Potassium iodide) 100 mcg
Magnesium (citrate) 250 mg
Zinc (Gluconate) 15 mg
Selenium (citrate) 200 mcg
Manganese (citrate) 5 mg
Chromium (picolinate) 200 mcg
Potassium (gluconate) 25 mg
Chloline bitartrate 50 mg
Inositol 25 mg
Molybdenum (citrate) 25 mcg
Boron (citrate) 500 mcg
Citrus bioflavonoid Blend 25 mg
Quercetin dehydrate 10 mg
Green tea extract 10 mg
Co-enzyme Q10 10 mg
Grape seed extract 5 mg
Lutein 5 mg
Lycopene 5 mg
Betaine 10 mg
L-Glutathione 5 mg
Alpha Lipoic Acid 5 mg

Other ingredients: Purified water, Natural Glycerine, Natural flavours, Xanthan, Gum, Citric Acid, Potassium Sorbate, Sodium Citrate and Purified Stevia extract.

Store in a cool, dry place. Refrigerate after opening.

33

BONE HEALTH and OSTEOPOROSIS
BONE HEALTH EXTREME

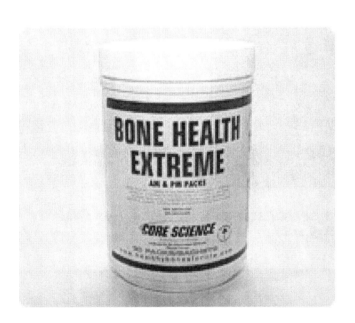

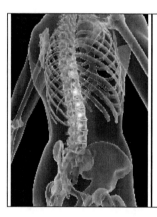

Which of these people should be concerned about Osteoporosis?

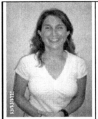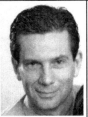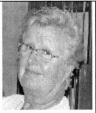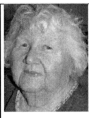

Answer: All of them.

Osteoporosis is not something that only women in their 60's, 70's and 80's should be concerned about. What you don't know (and don't do) could kill you. If you think milk is the answer, think again. Take our quiz to see what you know and how to achieve healthy bones for life.

Please answer the following TRUE or FALSE.

T F 1. Osteoporosis is mostly an older women's disease.
T F 2. Milk products provide all the bone mineral support you need.
T F 3. Osteoporosis is not a killer disease.
T F 4. Genetics is the biggest factor in achieving healthy bones.
T F 5. The only mineral necessary for healthy bones is calcium.
T F 6. All calcium found in nutritional supplements is the same.
T F 7. Ideally, calcium should be "locked" into your bones to prevent degeneration.
T F 8. Women should only be concerned about osteoporosis after menopause.
T F 9. X-ray is a good way to determine bone loss.
T F 10. Bone mineral supplements are not necessary if you have good nutrition.
T F 11. Bones naturally become brittle as you get older and there's absolutely nothing you can do about it.
T F 12. Vitamin C is necessary for optimum bone health.

For the correct answers obtain a copy of Dr. Zielonka's
"Healthy Bones for Life" workshop on CD and DVD.

BONE HEALTH EXTREME from Core Science
"The World's Best Bone Nutritional Supplement"

................over please

DATA SHEET

CORE SCIENCE BONE HEALTH EXTREME

Directions: Daily Dose - Take 2 packs per day, one with breakfast and one with lunch or dinner or as directed by your healthcare professional.

Daily dose of 1,000mg of the best forms of elemental calcium,
over 3,000 IU vitamin D, the best vitamin K, the best essential fatty acids,
magnesium, boron, trace minerals, protein, cutting edge Genestein and so much more!

Each pack contains:

Cal-6 + MG™
Each tablet contains: Calcium 250 mg (from calcium citrate, gluconate, lactate, carbonate, ascorbate and microcrystalline hydroxyapatite)
Magnesium (Magnesium HVP Chelate)... 125 mg
Boron (citrate)...1mg
Glutamic acid... 25 mg
Lysine HCL... 12 mg
Vitamin D....133 IU
Vitamin C (ascorbic acid)... 17 mg
In a base of silica

Vitamin D 1000 IU
Uncoated, bisected, round, white tablet
Each tablet contains: Vitamin D (vitamin D-3/Cholecalciferol) 25mcg (1000 IU)
Non-medicinal ingredients: Cellulose, silica, and vegetable magnesium stearate.

Calcium Microcrystalline
Hydroxyapatite 1000mg
Coated, oblong shaped, white tablet
Each tablet contains: Calcium Microcrystalline Hydroxyapatite 1000mg
(yielding Calcium 250mg, Phosphorus 130mg)
Boron (aspartate) 2.5mg
Non-medicinal ingredients: Cellulose, vegetable stearate and silica.

Vitamin K2
(as Meniaquinone-7)
Each capsule contains: Vitamin K2 – M7 90 mcg (NOT FROM SOY)
Non-medicinal ingredients: Cellulose, vegetable stearate, calcium citrate and silica.

Bonistein-Max™
Oblong clear soft gel with a yellowish-white opaque liquid fill
Each capsule contains: Vitamin D3 (Cholecalciferol) 10mcg (400 IU)
Vitamin K1 (phytonadione) 50mcg
Genistein 15mcg
Fish Oil (sardine) 730mcg
(EPA 267.5mg, DHA 130mg, Total Omega-3 fatty Acids 500mg)
Non-medicinal ingredients: Medium chain triglycerides, vegetable glycerine, SeaGel* carrageenan
(from red seaweed extract), beeswax, vegetable starch and water.
Contra-Indications: Do not take if you are pregnant or breastfeeding. This product contains vitamin K,
which interferes with either the prescription drugs Coumadin and Warfarin.
Do not take this product if taking either of these drugs.
This product contains Bonistein. Bonistein-Max contains a patent-pending blend
of ingredients. Bonistein is a trademark of DSM Nutritional Products.
*SeaGel is a registered trademark of FMC BioPolymer. Patent Pending.

Bone Health Extreme is distributed exclusively by Core Science, Ottawa, Canada

More women die from the related effects and complications of osteoporosis than breast cancer, uterine cancer, and cervical cancer combined. As such, proper bone health is essential beginning in your teenage years (if not sooner as some researchers suggest) to maximize peak bone mass which occurs between age 25 and 30. Beginning supplementation with calcium when you're in your sixties is not the best answer.

Even with the best supplementation, proper eating habits are mandatory to achieve an appropriate acid-alkaline balance. Finally, bone health goes way beyond calcium, and dairy is not the answer. (So as to not tangent off into another book, please view my lecture "Healthy Bones for Life".)

WHY I RECOMMEND IT

- It is produced by one of only four labs that received a five-star rating and is a Gold Medal ribbon winner (Douglas Labs).
- Its quality , source of raw materials, processing methods, and expertise are second to none.
- Core Science has the unique ability to change its formulas should new advances in science dictate it.
- Dissolution times meet or exceed the highest standards.
- Calcium is available in a complete bone mineral form known as microcrystalline hydroxyapatite (MCHC), which contains all the constituents of bone.
- It also contains calcium in its citrate form, which is highly absorbable.
- It contains optimal levels of vitamin D3 (cholecalciferol), essential for bone health.
- Essential fatty acids are required for bone health.

- Vitamin K in its best form for bone health is present and is not from soy.
- It contains isoflavones that are NOT derived from soy.
- It contains a wide spectrum of trace minerals and protein, essential for bone health.
- Many doctors and vitamin brands don't know or don't take into account that your body is only capable of absorbing 500 to 600 mg of calcium at a time. Core Science Bone Health Extreme takes this into account.

In the bone health category I also recommend:

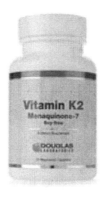

Why do I choose to single out Vitamin K2 for optimal bone health when there are so many other constituents that are also necessary for essential bone health? I do so for two reasons:

1) Because most people do not recognize the importance of Vitamin K2 in bone health (you certainly should after reading chapter 29);

2) Because many people seem to have difficulty in getting the right form of Vitamin K from the right source or as previously discussed, even getting the right information.

If you're taking Core Science Bone Health Extreme the above Vitamin K2 is the exact source already used in it. However, should you not be, very few multi-vitamins or bone health products, other than Core Science, even include this important nutrient, let alone in its proper source and type.

What makes this type so superior? As discussed on the Douglas Labs' data sheet:

"Vitamin K2 (as MK-7) is more bioactive and has proven more effective than vitamin K1 and other menaquinones. MK-7 showed eight times the half-life of vitamin K1 in a 24-hour serum concentration level after 1 mg of each form was ingested. Thus, MK-7 can be administered in low dosages only once a day, typically 1/1000 that of a MK-4 dose. Furthermore, the study showed better utilization and improved osteocalcin carboxylation for MK-7 after 6 weeks. Numerous studies reveal long-chain menaquinones, such as MK-7 are more effective in supporting arterial health than vitamin K1 menaquinones. Douglas Labs' Vitamin K2 as menaquinone-7. (MK-7) is derived from geraniol and farnesol. Geraniol is the primary part of rose oil, palmarosa oil, and citronella oil. Farnesol is present in many essential oils such as citronella, lemon grass, rose, and musk. This natural form of MK-7 has been extensively tested for molecular identity and bioequivalence when compared to MK-7 from fermented soybeans (natto). It is the all-trans form, thus providing a significantly higher purity of the only biologically active form."

34

OPTIMUM IMMUNE SYSTEM FUNCTION
IMMUNE BOOST MAX

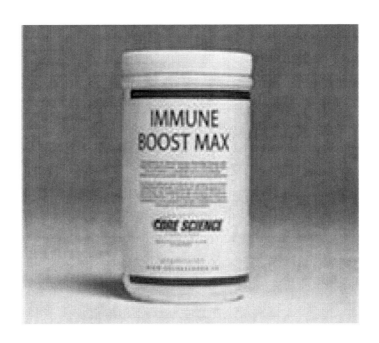

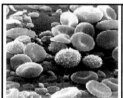

CORE SCIENCE IMMUNE BOOST MAX – 30 packs

Each Core Science Immune Boost Max pack contains;
   1 Mycoceutics capsule + 1 Ascorbplex 1000 Buffered tablet + 1 DL-Winter Formula capsule +
   1 Basic Anti-Oxidant tablet + 1 Garlic (odourless) tablet + 1 American Ginseng capsule.

Suggested Usage:	Take one pack with each meal for a total of 3 packs per day or as prescribed by your healthcare practitioner.
Mycoceutics: **Each capsule contains:**	Tan, hard, gelatine capsule. **Beta-1, 3-Glucan (purified yeast) 7.5mg** **Organic Mushroom Combination 600mg** (Cordyceps (Mycelium), Reishi (Mycelium), Maitake (Mycelium), Shiitake (Mycelium), Coriolus (Mycelium), Polyporus (Mycelium), Wood Ear (Mycelium), Tremella (Mycelium), Poria (Mycelium), Hericium (Mycelium).
Non-medicinal ingredients:	Gelatin (capsule), water, magnesium stearate and silica.
Ascorbplex 1000 Buffered: **Each tablet contains:**	Coated, oblong, white tablet with specks. **Vitamin C 1000mg,** Calcium 90mg, Potassium 60mg, Pectin 100mg, Bioflavonoids 100mg, Magnesium 400mcg
DL-Winter Formula: **Each capsule contains:**	Natural gelatin capsule containing green powder. **Echinacea (entire plant) 175mg** **Goldenseal (leaf and root) 175mg** **Red Clover (flower) 100mg** **Proanthocyanidins (from Grape Seed Extract) 5mg** **Elderberry (flower and berry, standardized extract) 200mcg**
Non-medicinal ingredients:	Gelatin (capsule) and vegetable stearate.
Basic Anti-Oxidant: **Each tablet contains:**	Coated, oblong, white tablet with dark specks. **Vitamin A (5 % Beta-Carotene) 10,000 I.U.** **Vitamin C (Ascorbic Acid) 1000mg** **Vitamin E (d-alpha Tocopheryl) 100 I.U.** **Magnesium (Magnesium Oxide) 100mg** **Zinc (Krebs*) 15mg** **Selenium 50mcg**
Non-medicinal ingredients: *Krebs:	Cellulose, vegetable stearate and silica. Citrate, Fumarate, Malate, Glutarate and Succinate Complex
Garlic (Odourless): **Each tablet contains:**	Coated, round, off-white tablet with specks. **Allium sativum (Garlic(bulb))(deodorized, Pure-Gar®) 500mg**
Non-medicinal ingredients:	Cellulose, vegetable stearate and silica.
American Ginseng-V: **Each capsule contains:**	Natural vegetable capsule containing off-white powder. **Panax quinquefolius L. American Ginseng 200mg** **Herbal Extract (root)/ Standardized to provide 10mg ginsenosides**
Non-medicinal ingredients:	Cellulose and vegetable stearate.

This product does not contain yeast, wheat gluten, soy protein, milk/dairy, sodium, sugar, starch, or artificial colouring. If seal around cap is broken, do not use. For optimal storage conditions, store in a cool, dry place. (15-25C)

Imported in Canada by Douglas Laboratories   **Distributed by Core Science**   www.corescience.ca

Many people still think that your immune system is only involved in preventing or recovering from colds and the flu.

Your immune system plays a pivotal role in all major diseases including cancer, heart disease, and so much more. As such, achieving and maintaining an optimal immune system is key to good health. An optimal immune system supplement should go well beyond symptom relief. While a quality multi-vitamin/mineral (such as the Core Science Ultimate Health Packs or Daily Wellness Packs) will always help to maintain your immune system, when your system is weak or needs boosting then Immune Boost Max should be added.

- It is produced by one of only four labs that received a five-star rating and is a Gold Medal ribbon winner (Douglas Labs).
- Its quality, source of raw materials, processing methods, and expertise are second to none.
- Core Science has the unique ability to change its formulas should new advances in science dictate it.
- Dissolution times meet or exceed the highest standards.
- It contains high levels of anti-oxidants including vitamin C and bioflavinoids.
- It contains numerous botanicals shown to boost the immune system.
- It contains Reishi mushrooms, which are scientifically shown to boost immune function.
- It contains North American ginseng and garlic.
- It contains antiviral zinc and other minerals.

In addition to the above, for those who are solely looking for symptomatic relief, the following natural health products are superior alternatives to the over the counter drugs used by many;

Natural Nasal Spray

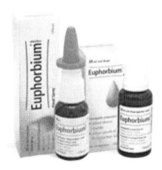

Euphorbium comp. is a homeopathic preparation to treat rhinitis of various origins (viral, bacterial or allergic) and sinusitis (chronic and acute). Benefits include:

- An effective alternative to conventional nasal sprays.
- Scientifically proven antiviral properties.
- Clinically demonstrated efficacy.
- May be combined with other natural or conventional medication.
- Extremely well tolerated.
- May be used in acute as well as in chronic conditions.
- Appropriate for long-term use.
- Neither habit-forming nor addictive.
- Suitable and effective for the entire family (children 2 years and up).

Natural Cough Syrup

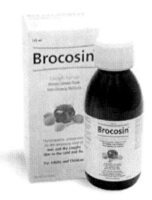

Brocosin is a homeopathic preparation used to provide relief of wet and dry coughs due to the cold and flu. It has a great honey-lemon taste and is suitable for the whole family. Benefits include:

- May be used for a wide variety of coughs.
- Gentle, well tolerated and highly effective.
- Suitable for the whole family.
- Soothes the respiratory tract.
- No known side effects or medicinal interactions.
- May be used by diabetics.

Sore Throat Remedy

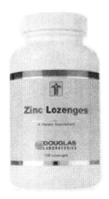

Why pop sugary cough drops into you when you can use anti-viral zinc?

35

CHOLESTEROL –
CHOL REDUCE 1000

This particular product is so new that this book will be available before the product is. I have designed it due to the great need for a natural alternative to fight high cholesterol, the overwhelming scientific evidence that shows it is beneficial and the terrible side effects that come from the grossly over-prescribed cholesterol lowering drugs. The following information sheet is blunt and to the point. This product should be available at www.yourhealthstore.ca by the end of February 2012.

Core Science Chol Reduce 1000
Data Sheet

Directions:

Take 2 to 4 packs per day with meals or as recommended by your healthcare professional.

Ingredients per pack:

> **Commiphora mukul Weighi (gum)**.. 1,000 mg
> **(standardized to 2.5% Guggulsterones Z & E)**
> **Plant Sterols (Phytosterols)** .... 400 mg
> **Sytrinol™** .... 150 mg
> **(proprietary blend of polymethoxylated flavones and**
> **tocotrienols from citrus and palm fruits)**
> **Standardized Pomegranate Extract (Fruit)** .... 50 mg
> **(Standardized to 40% ellagic acid)**
> **Niacin**.. 100 mg

Other ingredients: cellulose, gelatin, vegetable stearate

This product does not contain yeast, wheat gluten, soy protein, milk/dairy, corn, sodium, sugar, starch, artificial colouring, preservatives or flavouring. If seal around cap is broken, do not use. For optimal storage conditions, store in a cool, dry place. (15-20C/59-68F)

Manufactured in USA by Douglas Laboratories, Pittsburgh PA 15205 U.S.A.
Distributed by Core Science, Ottawa ON www.corescience.ca

36

OSTEOARTHRITIS – ARTHRI-JOINT MAX

Contrary to the belief of many, you should not accept it when your medical doctor tells you "you're getting older – it's natural that you're getting arthritic". There are many steps one can take to ensure they have the proper nutrients in their body with supplementation that is supported by science.

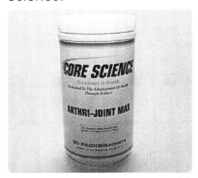

For those who still believe that they can get everything they need from food, they're wrong. Between ages 40 to 45, your body stops producing some of the key nutrients necessary for proper joint and cartilage health. Therefore, you could choose to accept this as age or you could supplement with key nutrients to not only live a long active life, but to help prevent degeneration in the first place.

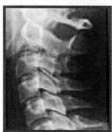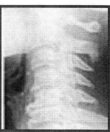

CORE SCIENCE ARTHRI-JOINT MAX – 30 PACKS

EACH PACK CONTAINS:
- 1 Glucosamine Plus Extra Strength capsule AND
- 1 Uni-Joint Formula capsule AND
- 1 Glucosamine + MSM Forte capsule

Suggested Usage: Take 1-2 packs daily with meals, or as directed by your health practitioner. Since this product provides nutrients that may help re-build degenerated discs and joints it is meant to be used on a long term basis. Years of degeneration takes the appropriate care over time for maximum results.

Use in conjunction with the Core Science Ultimate Men's or Women's Health Packs for a total Wellness program.

Glucosamine Plus Extra Strength TM
Each capsule contains: Natural vegetable capsule containing an off-white powder
2-Amino-2-deoxy-beta-D-glucopyranose (Glucosamine Sulfate.2KCl) 500mg
Chondroitin Sulfate 400mg
Non-medicinal ingredients: Cellulose, vegetable stearate and silica.

Uni-Joint Formula TM
Each capsule contains: Natural gelatin capsule containing grey powder
Glucosamine Sulfate 250mg
Sea cucumber (powder) 150mg
Shark cartilage powder 150mg
Bromelain (stem, pineapple plant) 150mcu.
Bovine cartilage (mucopolysaccharides) 50mg
In a base of Yucca powder (leaf) and Bilberry extract (fruit)
Non-medicinal ingredients: Gelatin (capsule), cellulose, vegetable stearate and silica.

Glucosamine + MSM Forte TM
Each capsule contains: Natural gelatin capsule containing off white powder w/purple specks
2-Amino-2-deoxy-beta-D-glucopyranose (Glucosamine Sulfate) 500mg
Methylsulfonylmethane (MSM) 250mg
Red Wine Proanthocyanidins 10mg
Bromelain 10mg
In a base of Vitamin C
Non-medicinal ingredients: Gelatin (capsule), vegetable stearate and silica.

Warning: If you have an allergy to shellfish, (including crab and shrimp) you should not use this product.

This product does not contain yeast, wheat gluten, soy protein, milk/dairy, corn, sodium, sugar, starch, artificial colouring, preservatives or flavouring.

If seal around cap is broken, do not use.

For optimal storage conditions, store in a cool, dry place. (15-25C)

Manufactured in USA by Douglas Laboratories, Pittsburgh PA 15205 U.S.A.
Distributed by Core Science, Ottawa ON www.corescience.ca

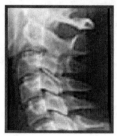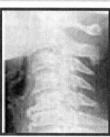

CORE SCIENCE ARTHRI-JOINT SUPREME – 30 PACKS

EACH PACK CONTAINS:
- 3 Glucosamine + MSM Forte capsule AND
- 1 Flex HA (hyaluronic acid)

Suggested Usage: Take 1-2 packs daily with meals, or as directed by your health practitioner. Since this product provides nutrients that may help re-build degenerated discs and joints it is meant to be used on a long term basis. Years of degeneration takes the appropriate care over time for maximum results.

Use in conjunction with the Core Science Ultimate Men's or Women's Health Packs for a total Wellness program.

Glucosamine + MSM Forte™

Each capsule contains: Natural gelatin capsule containing off white powder w/purple specks
2-Amino-2-deoxy-beta-D-glucopyranose (Glucosamine Sulfate) 500mg
Methylsulfonylmethane (MSM) 250mg
Red Wine Proanthocyanidins 10mg
Bromelain 10mg
Vitamin C (ascorbic acid) 50mg

Non-medicinal ingredients: Gelatin (capsule), vegetable stearate and silica.

Warning: If you have a significant allergy to shellfish, (including crab and shrimp) you should not use this product.

Flex HA™

Each capsule contains: Hyaluronic Acid 30 mg (non-animal source)

Therefore, each pack contains:
1500 mg glucosamine sulphate +
750 mg MSM +
150 mg vitamin C +
30 mg bromelain+
30 mg procyandins+
30 mg hyaluronic acid

This product does not contain yeast, wheat gluten, soy protein, milk/dairy, corn, sodium, sugar, starch, artificial colouring, preservatives or flavouring.

If seal around cap is broken, do not use.

For optimal storage conditions, store in a cool, dry place. (15-25C)

Manufactured in USA by Douglas Laboratories, Pittsburgh PA 15205 U.S.A. Distributed by Core Science, Ottawa ON www.corescience.ca

- They are produced by one of only four labs that received a five-star rating and is a Gold Medal ribbon winner (Douglas Labs).
- Its quality , source of raw materials, processing methods, and expertise are second to none.
- Core Science has the unique ability to change its formulas should new advances in science dictate it.
- Dissolution times meet or exceed the highest standards.
- It contains optimal levels of glucosamine sulphate. Glucosamine sulphate has been studied in over 200 clinical trials worldwide and is approved for use in over 70 countries.
- It contains MSM, scientifically shown to rebuild cartilage.
- Arthri-Joint Max contains chondroitin sulphate. While some research shows this molecule may be too large to be properly absorbed, other research shows that it may be beneficial in a small percentage of people without any side effects.
- New Arthri-Joint Supreme contains hyaluronic acid which has been shown beneficial to "lubricating" your joints.
- Bromelain papain has been added as a natural anti-inflammatory, which doubles as a digestive aid. Hence, it actually benefits your stomach.
- Powerful anti-oxidants are also present.

For a better understanding of osteoarthritis, I have included the following article, which was previously published in past books of mine.

37

SPINAL DEGENERATION IS NOT INEVITABLE

What you can do today to prevent your spine from aging

"You're getting older – what did you expect?" is the common response given by many doctors to explain the degeneration of your spine as you age. The problem is that this belief is a self-fulfilling prophecy as it absolves self-responsibility and results in inaction, allowing your spine to continue to degenerate.

If age were the sole factor in the degeneration of your spine, then please explain why some sixty-year-olds have no degeneration while some thirty-year-olds have advanced spinal degeneration. Or better yet, explain why your L_5 vertebra is degenerating while your L_3 isn't – they're obviously both the same age. It's not age or time that causes degeneration – it's what we do (or don't do) over that time. It may be common to degenerate over time, but there's nothing normal about it.

**Spinal Degeneration = Spinal Deterioration =
Spinal Decay = Degenerative Joint Disease =
Degenerative Disc Disease = Osteoarthritis**

The most common arthritis

There are over 100 different types of arthritis, of which osteoarthritis (OA) is the most common. Contrary to common belief OA is due to lifestyle factors and **not** genetics (unlike rheumatoid arthritis). It is essentially a "wear and tear" of the discs and the joints. There are two factors that cause this degeneration:

1) Damage

Quite simply, if you damage something, it will "wear and tear" faster. If your car gets in an accident, guess which part of your car will rust first. This damage can be what I call "fast damage" or "slow damage". Fast damage would include things such as car accidents (whiplash) or other types of injuries. Slow damage would include a much smaller amount of pressure but over a prolonged period of time. This would include chronic work posture, poor posture or uncorrected spinal subluxations (spinal misalignments).

2) Lack of movement

I'm sure you've heard the old adage "if you don't use it, you lose it". The reason it applies here is that while most of the body receives its nutrients via the blood stream, there are no blood vessels that go directly into the disc. Hence, a disc receives its nutrients through a process called imbibition, which means the more movement **specific** to each individual disc, the more nutrients that will be pumped into that disc. A lack of nutrients would obviously be likely to result in more degeneration.

Phase 1   Thinning of the disc and/or a loss of the normal spinal curve.

Phase 2   Advanced degeneration – significant thinning of the disc and/or bone spurs (osteophytes).

Phase 3   Severe degeneration – large bone spurs and/or partial or total fusion.

The natural approach

It is important to appreciate that spinal degeneration is an ***ongoing process***, not a static condition. In other words, if you do nothing to change your ways, it is likely to progress. To have a normal spine (and not a common one), steps must be taken to a) undo the damage, b) increase spinal range of motion and c) restock the disc with the proper nutrients. This would include;

1) Chiropractic adjustments

Chiropractic is an ideal form of treatment for spinal degeneration (osteoarthritis) as it can help undo fast damage, re-align slow damage and increase range of motion specific to the individual joint. (Simple stretching cannot replace chiropractic as it cannot correctly "unlock" or realign a subluxated vertebrae.)

2) Spinal stabilization exercises

This does not mean bigger pecs, biceps or running. In fact, running on a misaligned spine (just like driving your car on misaligned wheels) is likely to increase its wear and tear. Rather, these exercises must be prescribed by someone who has seen your x-rays and are specific to stabilizing the core muscles and ligaments that support your spine as well as helping to restore your normal curve.

3) Specific nutritional supplementation

The nutrients (and amounts) necessary to help you rebuild your discs cannot be achieved through diet. By supplying the proper nutrients (combined with chiropractic to help ensure they enter the disc), degeneration can be slowed, stopped and in some cases even reversed. The scientific research shows that glucosamine and MSN as well as the pre-cursors to chondroitin sulphate have shown positive benefits to the spine. Other nutrients such as shark cartilage, sea cucumber and bromelain-papain have also shown positive benefits. My highest recommendation goes to Core Science's Arthri-Joint Max as it includes all of the above.

How long should it take?

Most people have unknowingly spent years allowing their spine to degenerate when in fact they should spend a lifetime keeping it healthy. Spinal correction (chiropractic), spinal stabilization and nutritional support for a degenerated spine require a minimum of a year (and often more) for maximum improvement, just like a dentist putting braces on your teeth. Remember, you're not looking to mask the pain but rather help restore and rebuild your spine. By taking a comprehensive natural approach and addressing all three factors, your spine can last a lifetime.

38

MUSCLE REPAIR
MUSCLE REPAIR MAX

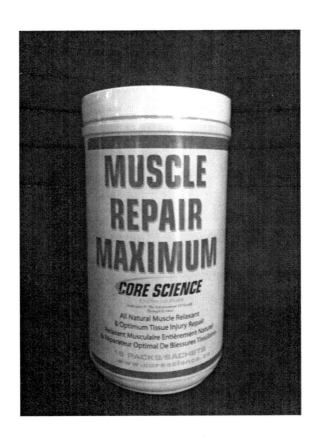

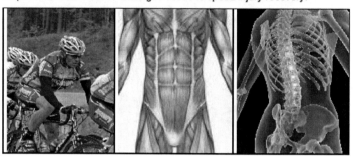

CORE SCIENCE MUSCLE REPAIR MAXIMUM – All Natural Optimum Muscle Injury Repair & Relaxant

Each Core Science Muscle Repair Maximum pack contains
1 Proteoenzyme Forte TM tablet,
2 Wobenzym N tablet,
1 Relora-Plex capsule and
1 Mag 2: Cal 1: tablet.

Each bottle contains 15 packs.

Proteozyme Forte TM:
Each tablet contains: Coated, oblong, yellow tablet with specks

Vitamin A (Palmitate) 500 I.U.	Folic Acid 100mcg
Vitamin B1 (Thiamin Hydrochloride) 5mg	Calcium (Proteinate±) 75mg
Vitamin B2 (Riboflavin) 5mg	Magnesium (Proteinate±) 37.5mg
Niacinamide 5mg	Zinc (Proteinate±) 37.5mg
Pantothenic Acid (Calcium Pantothenate) 25mg	Manganese (Sulphate) 75mg
Vitamin B6 (Pyridoxine Hydrochloride) 25mg	Potassium (Proteinate±) 37.5mg
Vitamin B12 25mcg	Papain 50mg
Vitamin C (Calcium Ascorbate) 250mg	Pepsin (1:3000) 30mg

Non-medicinal ingredients: Bromelain, Hesperidin complex, Rutin, Bioflavonoids, Valerian root, Passiflora (aerial parts), Bovine cartilage. Trypsin, Chymotrypsin, Glucosamine Sulfate, dried pineapple juice, shave grass (aerial parts) *HVP hydrolyzed vegetable protein

Wobenzym N:
Each tablet contains: Coated, yellowish white tablet

Pancreatin (Pancreas) 200mg
Papain (Fruit) 120mg
Bromelain (Pineapple stem) 90mg
Trypsin (Pancreas) 48mg
Chymotrypsin (Pancreas) 2mg
Rutoside Trihydrate (Rutin) 100mg

Non-medicinal ingredients: Calcium phosphate, Corn polysaccharides, Micro crystalline cellulose, Crospovidone, Polyethylene glycol, Vegetable stearate, Silica, pH resistant enteric coating, Magnesium silicate, Triethyl citrate, natural vanilla flavouring, Purified water.

Relora-Plex:
Each capsule contains: Natural vegetarian capsule containing brown powder with specks.

Thiamine 5mg
Riboflavin 5mg
Niacinamide 5mg
Vitamin B-6 5mg
Folic Acid 100mcg
Vitamin B-12 50mcg
Relora 250mcg (a proprietary blend of patent-pending plant extracts from Magnolia Phellodendron)

Non-medicinal ingredients: Cellulose and vegetable stearate.

Mag 2: Cal 1:
Each tablet contains: Cellulose coated, white, oblong tablet

Vitamin C 75mg
Vitamin D3 12.5 I.U.
Calcium (citrate, carbonate, ascorbate) 125mg
Magnesium (oxide, aspartate, ascorbate) 250mg
Boron (citrate, aspartate) 1.5mg
Glutamic Acid (from 50mg Glutamic Acid HCl) 20mg

Non-medicinal ingredients: Cellulose, vegetable stearate and silica.

Warning:

If you have an allergy to shellfish, (including crab and shrimp) you should not use this product.

If you are pregnant or breastfeeding, suffer from bleeding disorders or liver damage, or if you are taking any prescription medication (such as warfarin), consult a physician prior to use. Excessive consumption may impair ability to drive or operate heavy machinery. Not recommended for consumption with alcoholic beverages.

Suggested Usage: Take one pack at a time on an empty stomach at least 1 hour before each meal for a total of 3 packs per day or as prescribed by your healthcare practitioner. This product does not contain yeast, wheat gluten, soy protein, milk/dairy, sodium, sugar, artificial colouring, preservatives or flavouring. If seal around cap is broken, do not use. For optimal storage conditions, store in a cool, dry place. (15-25C)

Imported in Canada by Douglas Laboratories Canada, London ON
Distributed by Core Science, Ottawa ON www.corescience.ca

Muscle Repair Max goes well beyond an optimal natural muscle relaxant in that it also repairs muscle tissue and clears muscle tissue debris due to trauma. It is great for athletes and also good post workout, post deep massage, and post active release technique (A.R.T.) sessions.

- It is produced by one of only four labs that received a five-star rating and is a Gold Medal ribbon winner (Douglas Labs).
- Its quality , source of raw materials, processing methods, and expertise are second to none.
- Core Science has the unique ability to change its formulas should new advances in science dictate it.
- Dissolution times meet or exceed the highest standards.
- It contains a wide range of vitamins, minerals, anti-oxidants, and enzymes.
- It contains plant extracts.
- It contains calcium and magnesium.
- It contains Wobenzym that has been used in Germany and other advanced health countries for decades for muscle repair, immune system function, cardiovascular health, neurological function, and more.

39

NATURAL ANTI-INFLAMMATORIES ACUTE INJURY PLUS

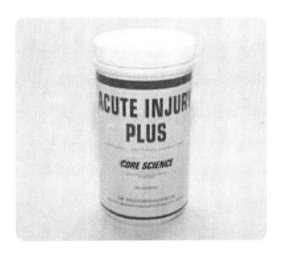

Quite simply I consider this to be the best natural anti-inflammatory on the market.

* It contains optimal levels of bromelain, boswellia, and tumeric (curcumin), all scientifically shown to naturally reduce inflammation.

- It also contains a wide variety of vitamins, minerals, and enzymes.
- It is produced by one of only four labs that received a five-star rating and is a Gold Medal ribbon winner (Douglas Labs).
- Its quality , source of raw materials, processing methods, and expertise are second to none.
- Core Science has the unique ability to change its formulas should new advances in science dictate it.
- Dissolution times meet or exceed the highest standards.

Injured? In pain? Inflamed?

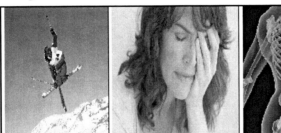

Whether a car accident, sports injury, fall, or any other type of acute injury, use what many consider to be the world's best and most effective all natural anti-inflammatory from Core Science.

ACUTE INJURY PLUS

This all natural anti-inflammatory, with specialized joint and tissue nutrients to maximize your injury recovery, is your best choice to quickly recover from acute injury and reduce inflammation and pain without delay. Based on the latest science, avoid the adverse side effects of prescription and over the counter drugs. Great for elite athletes, car accidents and everyday injuries.

SUPER MULTIPLYING FACTOR

Acute Injury Plus from Core Science utilizes its exclusive super multiplying factor. Each pack contains 4 tablets, each of which has been shown to be beneficial in treating acute injury. Combined, the effects are synergistic and unlike most other anti-inflammatories, it actually doubles as a digestive aid which is easy and beneficial to your stomach. Far beyond an anti-inflammatory its specialized joint and tissue nutrients including proteoenzymes also help repair and speed recovery of your injury safely and effectively.

Available from the OCNHC,
World Exchange Plaza, 111 Albert Street, Ground Floor, Ottawa
(613) 688-1036
or www.excellenceinhealth.com or www.corescience.ca

CORE SCIENCE
Dedicated to the Advancement of Health Through Science

CORE SCIENCE ACUTE INJURY PLUS – Natural Anti-Inflammatory – 15 packs

Suggested Usage:	Adults take one pack with each meal 3 to 5 times per day immediately after injury for the first 3 to 5 days or as recommended by your healthcare practitioner.

EACH PACK CONTAINS ONE OF EACH OF THE FOLLOWING

Bromelain 5000
Each capsule contains: Natural gelatine capsule containing white powder
Bromelain 5000 m.c.u.
Non-medicinal ingredients: Cellulose, gelatin (capsule), vegetable stearate

Ayur-Boswellia serrata
Each Capsule contains: Natural gelatine capsule containing an off-white powder
Boswellia 200mg (standardized to 65% Boswellic Acids)
Non-medicinal ingredients: Cellulose, gelatin (capsule), vegetable stearate

Ayur-Curcumin
(Turmeric) Natural vegetable capsule containing orange-yellow powder
Each capsule contains: **Turmeric (root) 300mg (standardized to provide 90% curcumin)**
Non-medicinal ingredients: Cellulose, gelatin (capsule), vegetable stearate

Proteozyme Forte TM
Each tablet contains: Coated, oblong, yellow tablet with specks
Vitamin A (Palmitate) 500 I.U.
Vitamin B1 (Thiamin Hydrochloride) 5mg
Vitamin B2 (Riboflavin) 5mg
Niacinamide 5mg
Pantothenic Acid (Calcium Pantothenate) 25mg
Vitamin B6 (Pyridoxine Hydrochloride) 25mg
Vitamin B12 25mcg
Vitamin C (Calcium Ascorbate) 250mg
Folic Acid 100mcg
Calcium (Proteinate*) 75mg
Magnesium (Proteinate*) 37.5mg
Zinc (Proteinate*) 37.5mg
Manganese (Sulphate) 75mg
Potassium (Proteinate*) 37.5mg
Papain 50mg
Pepsin (1:3000) 30mg

Non-medicinal ingredients: Bromelain, Hesperidin complex, Rutin, Bioflavonoids, Valerian root, Passiflora (aerial parts), Bovine cartilage, Trypsin, Chymotrypsin, Glucosamine Sulfate, dried pineapple juice, shave grass (aerial parts).
*HVP hydrolyzed vegetable protein

Warning: **If you have an allergy to shellfish, (including crab and shrimp) you should not use this product.**

This product does not contain yeast, wheat gluten, soy protein, milk/dairy, corn, sodium, sugar, starch, artificial colouring, preservatives or flavouring.

If seal around cap is broken, do not use.

For optimal storage conditions, store in a cool, dry place. (15-25C)

Manufactured in USA by Douglas Laboratories, Pittsburgh PA 15205 U.S.A.
Distributed by Core Science, Ottawa ON www.corescience.ca

40

ANTI-INFLAMMATORIES -
Their Side-Effects Could Be
More Serious Than You Think

If you think that people are insane when it comes to nutrition, they're even more insane when it comes to drugs. Consider this:

You're in pain. It could be low back pain, a headache, a fall, sports injury, car accident or even your arthritis. And you do what millions of Canadians and U.S. residents do every day. You reach for a pill. You're looking for the quick fix and what's wrong with just a pill or two, especially if it's going to make you feel better? After all, if millions are doing it and they're all approved by the FDA and Health Canada, what could possibly go wrong? The truth? The truth is that plenty could go wrong. And not just to the rare person but to thousands. Let's look at the facts, but first a little background.

Three types of drugs - Drugs for pain basically fall into three different categories: pain killers, muscle relaxants and anti-inflammatories.

- **Pain killers** – These include common over-the-counter drugs such as Tylenol. Why am I generally anti-Tylenol? Because it does absolutely nothing to fix the underlying cause of the problem and simply masks the pain. Why is masking the pain a problem? Because pain is your body's warning system that something is wrong. By masking the pain, not only are you short-circuiting this system, but you may actually go out and aggravate your condition even more. Not to be blunt, but no one ever died from pain. Furthermore, they do have their side-effects, especially so in children as much as we feel the need to do something for our kids. I only recommend pain killers in cases where they would allow for sleep, which is necessary for proper recovery and health.

- **Muscle relaxants** – As much as I don't like pain killers, I like muscle relaxants such as Robaxacet even less. Again, think **underlying cause**. People want quick fixes and think symptoms. In most cases, the muscle is not the underlying cause but rather has reacted to the irritated nerve or dysfunctional joint. This is especially true in seriously impinged nerves that result in an antalgic posture where the body's self-defense mechanism is literally pulling you off to one side off the nerve. Why would you want to try to defeat the body's self-defense mechanism and put pressure right back on the nerve?

- **Anti-inflammatories** – This is the one type of drug that makes sense as we do want to bring down inflammation as quickly as possible. Inflammation after an injury is one of the rare times when the body's innate wisdom messes up. It treats injury the same way it does infection and long- term inflammation is actually adverse to our health. This is why we should ice an injury immediately. Anti-inflammatories include over the counter drugs such as Advil, Ibuprofen and Motrin as well as prescription drugs such as Naprosyn, Voltaren, Arthrotec and Celebrex. So what's the problem with anti-inflammatories? There are many.

The side effects of anti-inflammatories

While you may believe that drugs are "safe" because they've been approved by Health Canada or the FDA, you'd have to be living under a rock not to be aware of the multiple drug recalls from supposedly "safe and approved" drugs. It is fairly common knowledge that anti-inflammatories can be tough on your stomach but do you know to what extent? Last year, 76,000 people went to hospital emergency rooms in the U.S. due to the "side-effects" of anti-inflammatories, many suffering from serious stomach bleeding and even death. Last year in Canada alone, 1,900 Canadians *died* from anti-inflammatory use.

The new death rate

Think it can't happen to you? We all know that studies can contradict one another. However, a few years ago, two scientists looked at every study that had ever been completed on the "chronic" use of anti-inflammatories and came up with a new *death rate*. How did they define "chronic"? Chronic was defined as anyone who had been using anti-inflammatories for two months or longer. This would include anyone with chronic headaches, arthritis, menstrual problems, chronic injuries and so much more. Please note that anti-inflammatories were only ever meant to be used in the short-term, meaning two weeks or less. If you still have inflammation two months later, obviously you're not correcting the underlying cause of the problem.

So what was the death rate? What are your chances of dying from taking anti-inflammatories for two months or longer? Is it one in a million? One in a hundred thousand? The new death rate is **1 in 1,200**. (This is not a misprint.)

The natural alternative

Aside from using ice, (read "Ice or Heat? ~ Applying common sense to your injury" in *"Healthellaneous"* or download the article from my website) there are many natural alternatives that are not only effective but extremely safe. My highest recommendation goes to Core Science's Acute Injury Plus. Based on the latest science and research, not only is it highly effective and of unparalleled quality, but it even has components that double as a digestive aid. Hence, instead of harming the stomach, it actually benefits the stomach. For best results it should be taken immediately after discovering the inflammation and continued until the inflammation is gone, while also addressing the underlying cause of the injury.

41

PROBIOTICS and PREBIOTICS

As previously discussed, probiotics are essential for optimal health. One of the problems however, is that tests have shown that some drug and nutrition store probiotics that claimed to have millions of bacteria in fact had zero by the time you popped that capsule in your mouth.

WHAT'S THE DIFFERENCE BETWEEN PROBIOTICS AND PREBIOTICS?

Probiotics are bacteria essential for good health. Prebiotics are substances such as fructooligosaccharides that allow probiotics to grow and flourish – essentially think of them as food for your probiotics. Remember, it's estimated that 70% of your immune system starts with your gut.

Finally, most commercial brands of yogurt are very poor sources of good probiotics, contrary to their marketing hype, and come with excessive amounts of sugar.

Both probiotics and prebiotics are contained in the Core Science Ultimate Health Packs but for those wishing for optimal levels or to supplement separately, my highest recommendation goes to either of the following;

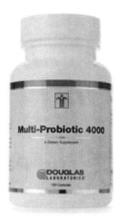

Each Multi-Probiotic 4000 capsule contains over 4 billion (4000 x 1 million) organisms in the following potencies:

Lactobacillus. acidophilus (DDS-1☐).............1.15 Billion
L. Rhamnosus...1.15 Billion
L. Rhamnosus (Type B, Bifidus) ....775 Million
Bifidobacterium lactis....................................275 Million
Bifidobacterium longum ....275 Million
B. Bifidum...275 Million
Streptococcus thermophilus..........................150 Million
In a base of FOS (fructooligosaccharides), special carbohydrates, enzymes and ulmus fulva.

I also recommend;

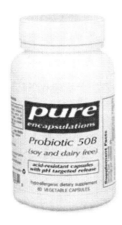

Probiotic 50B (soy and dairy free)

Each vegetable capsule contains a probiotic blend of50 billion CFU providing:

Lactobacillus plantarum (Lp-115)
Lactobacillus acidophilus (DDS-1)
Lactobacillus rhamnosus (Lr-32)
Bifidobacterium lactis (Bl-04)
Bifidobacterium longum (Bl-05)
with rice starch, vegetable capsule and gellan gum.

WHY I RECOMMEND THEM

- They are produced by two of the finest labs in the world. Their quality, source of raw materials, processing methods, and expertise are second to none.
- Dissolution times meet or exceed the highest standards.
- It contains billions of bacteria, far beyond most supplements.
- It contains a wide range of bacteria necessary for human health.
- Multiprobiotic 4000 also contains prebiotics in the form of fructooligosaccharides.

42

VITAMIN D

There is no need to reiterate the need for or science behind vitamin D supplementation. It is obviously present in the Core Science Ultimate Health Packs and Core Science Daily Wellness Packs but for those wishing to supplement additionally (Health Canada limits the amount in a daily vitamin to 1000 I.U.), my recommendation goes to:

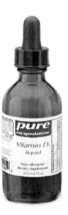

Vitamin D3 liquid
1 drop contains 1,000 IU Vitamin D3 with medium chain triglycerides

For individuals with greater short-term needs, this product allows for achieving 25,000-50,000 IU Vitamin D3 per week without having to take multiple capsules. For the elderly, Vitamin D3 liquid is an easy to use form. Vitamin D3 liquid, in a base of medium chain triglycerides, does not require emulsification for absorption. Vitamin D3 liquid is also free of preservatives, artificial colors, flavors and sugars. Not to be taken by pregnant and lactating women. It is recommended that individuals taking more than 2,000 i.u. vitamin D per day have their blood levels monitored. WARNING: Accidental overdose of liquid vitamin D products can lead to serious adverse side effects in infants. This product is not intended for infants. The recommended daily dose of vitamin D for infants is 400 I.U. whereas this product provides 1,000 IU per drop.

WHY I RECOMMEND IT
- It is produced by one of only four labs that received a five-star rating and is a Gold Medal ribbon winner (Douglas Labs).
- Its quality , source of raw materials, processing methods, and expertise are second to none.
- Dissolution times meet or exceed the highest standards.
- A single drop contains 1000 I.U. of vitamin D3 (cholecalciferol). As such, supplementation at 1000 I.U. to 2000 I.U. per day means your three-inch bottle would still last six months to a year.
- It also contains medium chain triglycerides for better absorption.

43

ESSENTIAL FATTY ACIDS

Again, as previously discussed, there is no question of the need for essential fatty acids in today's diet, nor any question about the science clearly supporting this need.

It is obviously present in the Core Science Ultimate Health Packs but for those wishing to supplement additionally my recommendation goes to either of the following;

Opti EPA™ Liquid
Ultra-Refined, Molecularly Distilled Liquid Fish Oil
1 teaspoon (5 ml) contains Ultra Pure Fish Oil Concentrate providing:
EPA (eicosapentaenoic acid) .... 1,331 mg
DHA (docosahexaenoic acid) .... 888 mg
with Rosemary extract, Ascorbyl palmitate, natural vitamin E and natural flavors.

And

QÜELL FISH OIL™
EPA+DHA with Vitamin D3
Supercritical CO2 Triglyceride

"QÜELL Fish Oil is Supercritical CO2 extracted oil in triglyceride form, manufactured in Germany exclusively for Douglas Laboratories. QÜELL Fish Oil is unique among other fish oils for its' critical extraction, purity, bioavailability and concentrations. Critical Extraction Supercritical CO2 advanced technology is the superior protection against oxidation. The extraction method of fish oil uses less heat and no chemical solvents when compared to molecular distillation, resulting in fewer unwanted isomer formations and "cleaner" oil.

Critical Purity Supercritical fluid extraction uses CO2 (carbon dioxide) instead of oxygen to gently extract the fatty acids, which also protects them from microorganisms that can't survive without oxygen. No chemical preservatives, solvents, or undesirable compounds are found in QÜELL Fish Oils. Heavy metal and contaminant levels measure significantly lower than the standard. Critical Bioavailability Recent scientific data shows the triglyceride form of fish oil is better absorbed when compared to ethyl esters. Recent data have demonstrated that omega-3 fatty acids delivered in a triglyceride form may result in greater plasma levels and a higher omega-3 index compared with omega-3 fatty acids delivered in the form of ethyl esters.

Critical Concentration: Many fish oils contain only about 30% omega-3 fatty acids, of which roughly 18% is EPA and 12% DHA. The remaining 70% is a varying mixture of other components. In other words, regular fish oil contains less than a third of the desired active ingredients and more than two thirds of "other" components. These other components may include cholesterol, omega-6 fatty acids, saturated fatty acids, oxidation products and contaminants. Highly concentrated fish oil, like QÜELL, provide at least 75% active ingredients, leaving less room for nonessential compounds."

WHY I RECOMMEND IT
- They are produced by one of only four labs that received a five-star rating and is a Gold Medal ribbon winner (Douglas Labs).
- Their quality, source of raw materials, processing methods, and expertise are second to none.
- Absorption/dissolution times meet or exceed the highest standards.
- Both are ultra pure refined fish oils.
- Both contain high levels of EPA and DHA.
- Both contain anti-oxidants to maintain stability.

44

DETOXIFICATION PROGRAMS

Contrary to the occasional newspaper headline or unqualified so called expert, metabolic detoxification programs are essential aspects of your health. (Please see chapter 45.)

I'm not talking of internet or infomercial hype, rather, good quality detox programs are backed by decades of high quality scientific research.

My highest recommendation goes to both of the following programs:

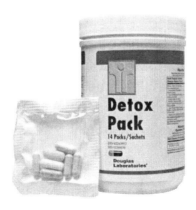

This detoxification program is intended to support liver detoxification pathways with various nutrients to assist in PHASE I (cytochrome P450 enzymes), antioxidant support to manage intermediary metabolites, and NAC for conjugation pathways of PHASE II detoxification. Additional fibre has been included to assist the excretory pathways.

Combined with

Metabolic Cleanse™
Delicious Natural Vanilla Flavored Protein Beverage

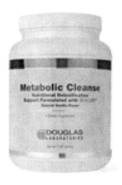

Metabolic Cleanse™ is a unique dietary supplement featuring beneficial amounts of rice, pea and fish proteins synergistically blended with essential amounts of vitamins, minerals, antioxidants and other nutrients important for the healthy maintenance of the entire gastrointestinal tract. It is designed to be a complete gastrointestinal support formula, perfect for detoxification, and now in a delicious, natural vanilla flavored powder naturally sweetened with organic coconut palm sugar. It provides beneficial amounts of LGlutamine and FOS (fructooligosaccharides) for their important roles in proper gastrointestinal maintenance. Increased N-acetyl L-cysteine and grape seed extracts have been added for the valuable antioxidant roles they perform in the body. Metabolic Cleanse™ contains no artificial colors or preservatives and is lactose, gluten, heavy metal and pesticide-free.

Or

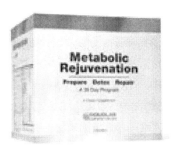

"Metabolic Rejuvenation by Douglas Laboratories is a comprehensive 28-day, 3 phase detoxification support program with nutrients specifically chosen to prepare the body through elimination, support phase 1 and 2 liver detoxification, and repair the body and intestinal tract. One Metabolic Rejuvenation box includes 4 bottles (one for each week) with convenience packs and a patient guidebook."

Douglas Labs describes Metabolic Rejuvenations as follows:

FUNCTIONS Week 1- Prepare
"The goal of the first week is to open pathways for elimination and prepare the body to properly detoxify in the next phase. The proprietary blend supplies a significant amount of detoxifying herbs, fibers, minerals, probiotics and vitamin C for proper bowel elimination and intestinal support. Fiber from citrus pectin and psyllium seed husks can naturally stimulate the bowel. Bentonite powder has

properties that tightly bind and immobilize toxic compounds in the gastrointestinal tract. Vitamin C acts as a free radical scavenger to cells. Magnesium may support infrequent bowel movements."

Week 2 and 3- Detox

"The goal of week 2 and 3 is to support phase 1 and phase 2 detoxification of the liver. As the body's main detoxification organ, the liver is responsible for removing all potentially detrimental molecules. This detoxification process occurs in 2 phases. The supplements in week 2 and 3convenience packs help to maintain liver structure and function in response to environmental toxins. Choline, betaine, and methionine are involved in methyl group metabolism, which is essential for normal liver function. Isothiocyanates (ITCs) found in Wasabia japonica are naturally occurring compounds that have the ability to stimulate detoxification pathways, and are 10-25 times more potent than ITCs found in cruciferous vegetables. Sulforaphanes in broccoli powder have been found to significantly increase the activity of Phase II enzymes. For efficient Phase two detoxification, the liver cells require sulphur-containing amino acids such as taurine, methionine and cysteine. N-Acetyl-L-cysteine is a biologically active precursor for glutathione synthesis, therefore raising intracellular glutathione levels. L-Glutathione scavenges toxic free radicals and inhibits peroxidation by slowing down free-radical catalyzed chain reactions. Glutathione is involved in DNA synthesis and repair, protein and prostaglandin synthesis, amino acid transport, metabolism of toxins and carcinogens, immune system function, prevention of oxidative cell damage, and enzyme activation. Dietary sulfur assumes a major role in detoxification as part of the hepatic sulfur conjugation pathways. Glutathione, sulfur and NAC support mercury detoxification. High mercury in the body can inhibit antioxidant enzymes and deplete intracellular glutathione. B vitamins, vitamin C and lipoic acid perform as antioxidants to scavenge free radicals. Garlic appears to prevent endothelial cell depletion of glutathione, which may be responsible for its antioxidant effects."

Week 4- Repair

"The goal of week 4 is to replenish lost nutrients through the detoxification phase and provide specific nutrients to repair the gut. A multivitamin/mineral with an organic fruit and vegetable blend provides adequate amounts of vitamins, minerals, and antioxidants to nutritionally replenish the body. Omega-3 fatty acids from fish oil support normal inflammatory processes. Glutamine helps maintain normal intestinal permeability, mucosal cell regeneration and structure, especially during periods of physiological stress. Glutamine also carries potentially toxic ammonia to the kidneys for excretion, which helps maintain normal acid-base balance. Healthy bacteria in the intestinal tract can be removed during extensive or frequent bowel elimination, thereby making supplementation with probiotic bacteria cultures necessary after a detoxification regimen. A normal intestinal microflora rich in lactobacilli creates acidic conditions that are unfavorable for the settlement of pathogenic microorganisms."

WHY I RECOMMEND THEM
- They're backed by decades of scientific research.
- They're produced by the top lab in North America.
- They contain all of the necessary nutrients as described in the next chapter.

45

Metabolic Detoxification and Intestinal Cleansing - How to Clean Yourself From the Inside Out

My late favourite aunt was a nutritionist extraordinaire, who always used to say that if she could do only one thing to improve a person's health it would be to turn them inside out and brush them off. She was absolutely right. Proper nutrition is one of the five Keys to Health, of which metabolic detoxification and intestinal cleansing is a key component.

Think of your body like a blast furnace. On a daily basis you consume a number of different foods and substances voluntarily as well as a number of other substances involuntarily. Now consider that these substances contain pesticides, pollutants, toxins, second-hand smoke, chemicals, preservatives, drugs, antibiotics, carcinogens, poor quality nutrients and a number of other undesirable components. No matter how hard you try (assuming that you do) what will the inside of your blast furnace look like over time? Now consider that this same blast furnace, essentially covered in years of "crusty black soot", is still responsible for effectively absorbing the proper nutrients and excreting the toxins from your body. It is little wonder then that this malfunctioning system can lead to fatigue, headaches, lack of mental clarity, bloating, weight gain, digestive troubles, irritable bowel, muscle and joint pain and a variety of significant diseases. This dysfunction occurs whether you feel its effects or not as your body's systems are over-stressed and forced to work overtime with less than optimal results. Times have changed in this over-polluted world. This is why regardless of your beliefs, a proper detox program is essential for everyone who desires optimum health.

A proper detox program

Not surprisingly, there are many different products of varying quality on the market. A proper program requires each of the following components:

1. The proper nutrients

A proper detox program appreciates that you have likely caused damage to your system. Hence, specific nutrients are necessary to repair this damage. As such, a proper detox program will contain the "**4 Rs**":

a) **Repair** – Specific nutrients are needed to repair the damage that you have done to your intestinal lining. This prevents the proper nutrients from escaping where they shouldn't, as well as allowing for the toxins to be excreted where they should.
b) **Remove** - Other specific nutrients are then needed to kill off the bad bacteria.
c) **Replace** – Good bacteria and other probiotics must be added to your system to allow for proper function.

d) **Rejuvenate** – The liver must then be detoxified, which again requires specific nutrients to help restore it to normal function.

2. The right foods

During your detox program, your health care professional should provide you with a list of specific foods you should eat as well as those to avoid. Quite simply, you do not want to eat the same toxin-filled foods while trying to detoxify. This can lead to the introduction of new healthier foods as well as being able to go on a counter rotation diet after your detox which will often allow you to identify foods that you may crave but are actually bad for you.

3. Proper supervision

While benefits may certainly be seen from doing such a program on your own, a proper detox program is best when under the supervision of a qualified health care professional who can anticipate and be prepared for how your body may react. Will a "die off" period occur (where your symptoms may originally increase as toxins exit the body)? Will there be some interaction with any prescription drugs that you are taking? (Always consult your medical doctor if this is the case.) What should you do if bloating occurs? These are all questions that a qualified health care professional can answer.

Just who is a qualified health care professional?

Anyone who has advanced nutritional training. This may include your chiropractor, naturopath, homeopath, advanced nutritionist and maybe your dietician, nurse or medical doctor. Please note, however, that many MDs and some dieticians may not necessarily get much training in advanced nutrition and in fact many "health consultants" may sometimes understand this topic much better.

Can't I just fast?

In a word, no. While many people fast for religious reasons, this is the equivalent of putting less in the blast furnace. Weight loss may occur and you may be giving your system "a rest" but you will never achieve proper detoxification and repair as this requires very specific nutrients.

What are the best detox programs?

In my office I utilize four different programs depending on the patient's needs and their health goals. The programs are provided by different labs, all of which are considered to be the best in the world. The majority of these programs are not available in nutrition stores or drug stores so that they may be properly supervised with professional support.

i) **Comprehensive Detox Cleansing Program** - This program typically lasts 3 to 4 weeks (longer for cases of fibromyalgia and other serious conditions) and may cost in the $300 to $500 range. Suppliers may include Douglas Laboratories or the Ultra Clear program. While this may initially seem expensive it will replace some meals which some people break down to $5 to $10 per meal. Also consider its value. It is a small price to pay for a properly functioning liver and digestive system.

ii) **Starter Detox Program** - This type of program lasts 7 to 10 days and costs in the $150 to $250 range. Suppliers include Core Science, Douglas Labs and Isagenix.

iii) **Easy Man's Detox -** Don't let the name fool you. While the other two programs are more comprehensive, this super convenient program from Core Science or Douglas Labs in the $75 to $100 range has significant benefits.

iv) **Metabolic Rejuvenation by Douglas Labs** – This program is fairly new and easy to take but still meets all of the requirements for the 4R program. It typically runs in the $150 - $200 range and is an all-pill based very easy to take program over a 4-week period. It may also be supplemented with a metabolic cleanse powder, which both increases your required effort and its cost.

The best programs (as described above) are backed by decades of well researched scientific evidence versus what you are likely to find in a drug store or on the internet. Given that new research shows that years of poor nutrition is just as bad for the liver as years of alcohol abuse, it is all the more essential that you consult a qualified health care professional. They can also guide you during the process and properly instruct you about things such as a "die off" period where you may actually see symptoms increase as toxins escape.

Who Should Detox and When?

Again, everyone should detox and in fact, given today's society, should do so on a regular basis. I personally detox 3 to 4 times per year to help ensure that my liver and intestinal system function at an optimal level year-round. Some of my patients find that timing is the bigger problem where they don't want to detoxify around holidays, birthdays, vacations, social events and travel. Unfortunately, it is exactly this lifestyle that results in your current less-than-optimal status.

A good detox program is not hard but does require some discipline. The benefits, however, can be amazing. This may include increased energy, fat loss, better mental clarity and concentration, better organ function, less bloating and much better overall health.

46

DIABETIC SUPPORT
GLYCEMIX

If I were to veer away from science for a second I would tell you that both my grandmother-in-law and my father live on this stuff. It's also backed by a wealth of science and is excellent for diabetes.

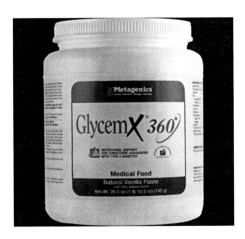

GlycemX 360° is a science-based, low-glycemic-index, delicious medical food formulated to provide specialized nutritional support for patients with type 2 diabetes. It features selective kinase response modulators (SKRMs) designed to improve fasting insulin and lipid parameters.

This product is to be used under the direct supervision of a physician or other licensed healthcare practitioner. In order to ensure proper use of their high-quality nutritional supplements, Metagenics only sells to licensed healthcare practitioners.

47

Where Do I Buy My Vitamin Supplements?

If you weren't aware already, by now you must fully appreciate just how much drug companies market to you and the sneaky, if not devious, ways in which they do so. Unfortunately, this dishonestly has had a huge impact on the health and wellness of society as a whole. But guess what? Nutritional companies also market to you, with some companies bending the truth. So whom do you trust? Please consider all of the following:

1. <u>Choose the Right Health Care Professional</u>

Often the best place to get your vitamin supplements is from a health care professional whom you trust. Health care professionals typically have access to supplements that you will not find in drug or nutrition stores and are produced by some of the world's top laboratories. These labs want their products distributed by professionals who know what they're talking about and have the academic expertise to do so.

The problem, however, is that many health care professionals, including most medical doctors, are perceived as experts but actually have very little training in nutritional supplements. Armed with the knowledge you now have from this book, don't hesitate to ask questions. Any good health care professional will have this information readily available or will certainly get it to you in a timely manner. Ask questions such as:

- What lab produces these supplements?
- What independent rating (out of 5 stars) did the lab receive?
- What certifications does the lab possess? See chapter 19
- Ask yourself how the product compares to the 18 criteria described in chapter 17 if it is a multivitamin and if there are significant discrepancies, ask your health care professional to explain why. Unless there's a very good reason, and even if there is, it may be time to purchase your vitamins elsewhere.

2. <u>Choose the Right Internet Site</u>

If you can't find the right health care professional and the best supplements aren't available in stores, that leaves the internet. There are actually a handful of good sites and obviously many poor sites. Again, ask these questions:

- Is the product produced by one of the 4 labs that received a 5 star rating?
- Is it easy to get the data on the ingredients of what the product actually contains? You would think that this would be a no-brainer but recently I went to mercola.com where Dr. Mercola is generally considered to be a very reputable health care professional. After 15 minutes of searching I am still unable to find out the dosage/potency of his Vitamin K capsules.

- Is the site run by a reputable health care professional? Obviously Dr. Mercola runs his and I run both www.corescience.ca and www.yourhealthstore.ca but most are sites that for all you know could be run by your plumber (with all due respect to plumbers). Just as important is what are the health care professional's qualifications? We discussed just how little training medical doctors get in nutrition and supplementation but did you know that 3 of the top 5 companies/labs are owned and/or run by chiropractors who typically have more knowledge of nutrition?
- Is there a physical location to the site? More credibility is typically given to an actual physical location that one could walk into and actually buy their supplements if they wanted to than an internet entity that could disappear overnight. My sites operate on the ground floor of the best known building complex in the heart of downtown Ottawa, our nation's capital.
- Everyone says they're the best. Can they back it up? Utilize the information in this book and look for obvious flaws. Let me give you a perfect example:

I recently did a search on natural supplementation for lowering cholesterol. The first site that came up (in Google Ads) was a site that was very specific in every ingredient that, according to them, one should look for in a cholesterol supplement. It also stated that it only contained substances that were based on the science and how you should avoid any product that had substances not based on the science. So what was the problem? It contains policosanol. As we discussed, almost all of the studies on policosanol are now considered fraudulent by many health care professionals as they were all done in Cuba by the company holding the patent for policosanol. Hence this particular site is not following its own rules and not keeping up on the science.

A second site, claiming to be a "nutritional supplement bible" specifies the benefits of gum guggul in lowering cholesterol and links to another site as the best product that they recommend. So what's the problem? Gum guggul is effective in lowering cholesterol – it's just that their linked product contains none.

- Is the deal too good? It is common practice to offer a better deal if one purchases in 3s or on some automatic recurring basis and there's nothing wrong with that. However, if the discount is too high (one of the above mentioned sites offers an 80% discount) then the product was obviously very inexpensive to produce in the first place. Quality products are expensive to produce and one usually, but not always, gets what they pay for.
- Does the site involve multi-level marketing? Guess what? There are many people who have seen significant benefits from supplements sold through some multi-level marketers and if you had to sell something there's nothing better than selling health. But be aware that since a significant amount of money goes to the various levels of marketing, the cost to make the actual product may be a factor in its quality. To be fair, a product sold in any store also usually has a significant mark-up. Just be aware that the person selling it to you obviously has a vested interest and again, can they back it up using the criteria discussed in this book?
- Is the site too heavy on testimonials? There is nothing wrong with testimonials provided that they're true and accurate. The problem occurs where there is nothing but glitz and testimonials and very little if any information on actual product data.

- Is the site selling you on fact or emotion? Unfortunately, most people, including those who are science-based contrary to their beliefs, still make most decisions based on emotion. When it comes to vitamins, try more fact and less emotion. Your health will thank you for it.

Of all the things to be sure about when it comes to quality, anything that you're going to put into your body for the sake of your health should be at the top of the list. Not all vitamins are created equally. Please invest the time to make sure you've made the right decision and choose someone you feel you can trust.

48

SPECIFIC HEALTH and DISEASE PROTOCOLS

The following are specific recommendations for lifetime optimal health and/or any specific sickness condition (why do we call these "health conditions"?) that you may have.

Please note that these recommendations may vary on a host of factors including:

1. Age
2. Gender
3. Past Health History
4. Other concurrent health problems, e.g. Diabetes
5. Contra- indications for each nutrient prescribed (e.g. In Wilson's Disease no copper supplementation is permissible even from a Multiple Vitamin)
6. Drug-nutrient interactions

Before beginning any of the following, it is recommended that you consult with your health care professional who is well versed with your specific health status, especially if you are currently taking prescription drugs. It is also highly recommended that you have a health care professional who is well versed in the need for natural supplementation as well as how this essential supplementation works in the body and its interaction with any other prescribed or non-prescribed drugs.

<u>LIFETIME OPTIMAL HEALTH</u>

As discussed in chapter 3, all human beings require the following essential vitamin supplementation throughout their lifetime:

High potency comprehensive multi-vitamin/mineral
Vitamin D
Essential Fatty Acids
Probiotics
Phytonutrients

Therefore, the one product that contains all of the above is:

- **Core Science Ultimate Health Pack**

  One could also obtain this with:
- **Core Science Ultimate Liquid Vitamin plus** or **Core Science Daily Wellness Pack**
- **High potency Essential Fatty Acids** (i.e. Opti-EPA Liquid)
- **Probiotics**
- **Phytonutrients**

Since I'm often asked, I personally take the Core Science Ultimate Health Packs twice per day plus I supplement with the following:

Vitamin D liquid – One to two drops (1,000 I.U. to 2,000 I.U.) twice per day. Why do I take this in addition if the Core Science Ultimate Health Packs are so good? Because the research shows fantastic benefits with Vitamin D and Health Canada limits the amount of Vitamin D in a daily supplement to 1,000 I.U.

Opti-EPA Liquid – One teaspoon twice per day (with my drops of vitamin D in it) again because the research on essential fatty acids is so overwhelmingly positive.

Multi-probiotic 4000 or 50 Billion – One extra capsule so that I can be obtaining probiotics at each meal in addition to the 2 meals at which I take the Ultimate Health Packs.

OTHER SICKNESS CONDITIONS

The following sickness conditions all require a high potency comprehensive multi-vitamin/mineral in addition to very specific nutrients. One might then ask why for instance a "brain formula" wouldn't just also include this multi-vitamin in the formula. The answer is that one needs to make the reasonable assumption that you may already be on a multi-vitamin. If it was included again in a specific condition formula you would essentially be doubling up and possibly overdoing your core vitamins. This would also be applicable if you had multiple sickness conditions, for instance, memory loss plus high cholesterol plus chronic pain. If each condition- specific formula had your core multi-vitamin in it, you would essentially be taking triple your core vitamin needs.

ACNE

High Potency Multi Vitamin and Mineral such as Core
Science Ultimate Health Packs, Core Science Daily
Wellness Packs or Core Science Ultimate Liquid Vitamin
plus
Vitamin A 10,000 IU twice daily
(for two months maximum and not if pregnant)
Essential Fatty Acids 2,000 to 4,000 mg daily
Oil of Oregano 250 to 450 mg, twice daily (kills skin bacteria)

AIDS/HIV

High Potency Multi Vitamin and Mineral such as Core
Science Ultimate Health Packs, Core Science Daily
Wellness Packs or Core Science Ultimate Liquid Vitamin
plus
Essential Fatty Acids 2,000 to 4,000 mg daily
Vitamin D 2,000 I.U. 2 to 3X daily
Core Science Immune Boost Max 1 to 3 packs daily

ALLERGIES

High Potency Multi Vitamin and Mineral such as Core
Science Ultimate Health Packs, Core Science Daily
Wellness Packs or Core Science Ultimate Liquid Vitamin
plus
Essential Fatty Acids 1,000 to 2,000 mg daily
Vitamin D 1,000 I.U. 2 to 3X daily
Quercetin 200-400 mg 3X daily
Grape seed extract 75 mg 3X daily
Vitamin C 1000 mg 3X daily
Probiotics and Prebiotics

ATHLETIC PERFORMANCE SUPPLEMENTS

High Potency Multi Vitamin and Mineral such as Core Science Ultimate Health Packs, Core Science Daily Wellness Packs or Core Science Ultimate Liquid Vitamin plus
Essential Fatty Acids 2,000 to 4,000 mg daily
Vitamin D 1,000 to 2,000 I.U. 2X daily
Creatine 5,000 to 25,000 grams per day
(depending on your level – drink plenty of fluids)
L- Glutamine 2,000 to 5,000 mg daily
Chromium 200-600 mcg daily
D - Ribose

ALZHEIMER'S DISEASE/ DEMENTIA

High Potency Multi Vitamin and Mineral such as Core Science Ultimate Health Packs, Core Science Daily Wellness Packs or Core Science Ultimate Liquid Vitamin plus
Essential Fatty Acids 1,000 to 2,000 mg daily
Vitamin D 1,000 I.U. 2 to 3X daily
Vitamin E 400 to 1600 I.U. daily
Phosphatidylserine
Bacopa (Bacopa monnieri)
Huperzine A
Choline
L-acetyl-carnitine

ANGINA

High Potency Multi Vitamin and Mineral such as Core
Science Ultimate Health Packs, Core Science Daily
Wellness Packs or Core Science Ultimate Liquid Vitamin
plus
Essential Fatty Acids 1,000 to 2,000 mg daily
Vitamin D 1,000 I.U. 2 to 3X daily
Vitamin E 200 to 1600 I.U. daily
Coenzyme Q10 50mg 1 to 2X daily
L-carnitine

ARTHRITIS (Osteoarthritis)

High Potency Multi Vitamin and Mineral such as Core
Science Ultimate Health Packs, Core Science Daily
Wellness Packs or Core Science Ultimate Liquid Vitamin
plus
Essential Fatty Acids 1,000 to 2,000 mg daily
Vitamin D 1,000 I.U. 2 to 3X daily
Core Science Arthri-Joint Max 1 to 2 packs daily or
Arthri-Joint Supreme 1 to 2 packs daily
or the following below:
Glucosamine sulfate 1,000 to 1,500 mg 1 to 2X daily
Methylsulfonyl sulfate (MSM)
Hyaluronic Acid
Bromelain
Boswellia
Curcumin (Turmeric)
Quercetin
Ginger

ARTHRITIS (Rheumatoid)

High Potency Multi Vitamin and Mineral such as Core
Science Ultimate Health Packs, Core Science Daily
Wellness Packs or Core Science Ultimate Liquid Vitamin
plus
Essential Fatty Acids 1,000 to 2,000 mg daily
Vitamin D 1,000 I.U. 2 to 3X daily
White Willow Bark
Curcumin (Turmeric)
Ginger
Boswellia
Devil's Claw
MSM
Digestive Enzymes
Probiotics and/or Prebiotics

ASTHMA

High Potency Multi Vitamin and Mineral such as Core
Science Ultimate Health Packs, Core Science Daily
Wellness Packs or Core Science Ultimate Liquid Vitamin
plus
Essential Fatty Acids 1,000 to 2,000 mg daily
Vitamin D 1,000 I.U. 2 to 3X daily
Quercetin 200 to 400 mg 3X daily
Grape seed extract 75 mg 3X daily

ATTENTION DEFICIT DISORDER (ADD AND ADHD)

High Potency Multi Vitamin and Mineral such as Core
Science Ultimate Health Packs, Core Science Daily
Wellness Packs or Core Science Ultimate Liquid Vitamin
plus

Essential Fatty Acids 1,000 to 3,000 mg daily
Vitamin D 1,000 I.U. 2 to 3X daily
Choline
Bacopa (Bacopa monnieri)

BRONCHITIS

High Potency Multi Vitamin and Mineral such as Core
Science Ultimate Health Packs, Core Science Daily
Wellness Packs or Core Science Ultimate Liquid Vitamin
plus
Essential Fatty Acids 1,000 to 2,000 mg daily
Vitamin D 1,000 I.U. 2 to 3X daily
Vitamin A 10,000 IU twice daily
(for two months maximum and not if pregnant)
Beta-carotene 25,000 to 75,000 I.U.
(watch skin colour – not if pregnant)
Bromelain
Oil of Oregano 250 to 450 mg 2X daily
Reishi Mushroom extract or
Core Science Immune Boost Max

CANCER TREATMENT SUPPORT

High Potency Multi Vitamin and Mineral such as Core
Science Ultimate Health Packs, Core Science Daily
Wellness Packs or Core Science Ultimate Liquid Vitamin
plus
Core Science Immune Boost Max 2 to 3 packs per day
Essential Fatty Acids 2,000 to 4,000 mg daily
Vitamin D 2,000 to 3,000 I.U. 2 to 3X daily
Vitamin C 1,000 to 4000 mg daily
Vitamin E 1,000 to 2,000 I.U. daily
Beta-carotene 50,000 to 100,000 I.U. daily

Selenium 200 to 800 mcg daily
Coenzyme Q10 100 to 200 mg 2X daily

CATARACTS
High Potency multi Vitamin and Mineral such as Core Science Ultimate Health Packs, Core Science Daily Wellness Packs or Core Science Ultimate Liquid Vitamin plus
Essential Fatty Acids 1,000 to 2,000 mg daily
Vitamin D 1,000 I.U. 2 to 3X daily
Vitamin C 1,000 to 2,000 mg daily
Vitamin E 200 to 400 I.U. daily
Beta-carotene 25,000 to 50,000 I.U. daily
Quercetin
Bilberry
Procyandins
Astaxanthin

CARPAL TUNNEL SYNDROME

High Potency Multi Vitamin and Mineral such as Core Science Ultimate Health Packs, Core Science Daily Wellness Packs or Core Science Ultimate Liquid Vitamin plus
Essential Fatty Acids 1,000 to 2,000 mg daily
Vitamin D 1,000 I.U. 2 to 3X daily
Vitamin B6 50 mg 1 to 3X daily
Curcumin (turmeric)
Boswellia

CHRONIC FATIGUE SYNDROME

High Potency Multi Vitamin and Mineral such as Core Science Ultimate Health Packs, Core Science Daily

Wellness Packs or Core Science Ultimate Liquid Vitamin
plus
Essential Fatty Acids 1,000 to 2,000 mg daily
Vitamin D 1,000 I.U. 2 to 3X daily
Magnesium
Malic Acid
D-Ribose
Creatine 2 to 5 grams daily

COLDS AND FLU

High Potency Multi Vitamin and Mineral such as Core
Science Ultimate Health Packs, Core Science Daily
Wellness Packs or Core Science Ultimate Liquid Vitamin
plus
Core Science Immune Boost Max 3 to 5 packs daily
or
Essential Fatty Acids 1,000 to 2,000 mg daily
Vitamin D 1,000 I.U. 2 to 3X daily
Oil of Oregano 250 to 450 mg 2 capsules every 4 hours
for up to 5 days
Vitamin C 1,000 to 2,000 mg 2 to 4X daily
Echinacea
Reishi mushroom extract
Zinc lozenges

CONGESTIVE HEART FAILURE

High Potency Multi Vitamin and Mineral such as Core
Science Ultimate Health Packs, Core Science Daily
Wellness Packs or Core Science Ultimate Liquid Vitamin
plus
Essential Fatty Acids 1,000 to 2,000 mg daily
Vitamin D 1,000 I.U. 2 to 3X daily

Coenzyme Q10 30 to 50 mg 2X daily
Hawthorn
L-carnitine
Taurine

CROHN'S DISEASE

High Potency Multi Vitamin and Mineral such as Core
Science Ultimate Health Packs, Core Science Daily
Wellness Packs or Core Science Ultimate Liquid Vitamin
plus
Essential Fatty Acids 1,000 to 2,000 mg daily
Vitamin D 1,000 I.U. 2 to 3X daily
Vitamin C 1000 to 2000 mg daily
Zinc 10 to 20 mg daily
Digestive enzymes
Probiotics and/or Prebiotics
L-Glutamine 500 mg 3X daily
Metabolic Detoxification Program

DEGENERATIVE DISK DISEASE
See Arthritis (Osteoarthritis)

DEPRESSION

High Potency Multi Vitamin and Mineral such as Core
Science Ultimate Health Packs, Core Science Daily
Wellness Packs or Core Science Ultimate Liquid Vitamin
plus
Essential Fatty Acids 1,000 to 2,000 mg daily
Vitamin D 1,000 I.U. 2 to 3X daily
St John's Wort or 5-Hydroxytryptophan (5-HTP) or
S-Adenosylmethionine (SAMe)

DIABETES TYPE I INSULIN- DEPENDENT

High Potency Multi Vitamin and Mineral such as Core
Science Ultimate Health Packs, Core Science Daily
Wellness Packs or Core Science Ultimate Liquid Vitamin
plus
Essential Fatty Acids 2,000 to 4,000 mg daily
Vitamin D 1,000 I.U. 2 to 3X daily
Bilberry extract
Grape seed extract
Vitamin E 400 to 900 I.U. daily to increase insulin sensitivity

DIABETES ADULT ONSET TYPE II

High Potency Multi Vitamin and Mineral such as Core
Science Ultimate Health Packs, Core Science Daily
Wellness Packs or Core Science Ultimate Liquid Vitamin
plus
Essential fatty Acids 1,000 to 2,000 mg daily
Vitamin D 1,000 I.U. 2 to 3X daily
Chromium 200 to 900 mcg daily
Bilberry extract
Grape seed extract
Vitamin E 400 to 900 I.U. daily to increase insulin sensitivity

DIARRHEA

Probiotic and prebiotics

ECZEMA

High Potency Multi Vitamin and Mineral such as Core
Science Ultimate Health Packs, Core Science Daily

Wellness Packs or Core Science Ultimate Liquid Vitamin plus
Essential fatty Acids 2,000 to 4,000 mg daily
Vitamin D 1,000 I.U. 2 to 3X daily
Selenium 100 to 200 mcg daily
Zinc 25 to 35 mg daily
Probiotics and Prebiotics
Digestive Enzymes
Milk Thistle
Indole-3-Carbinol
Reishi mushroom extract
Astragalus
Metabolic Detoxification Program

FIBROMYALGIA

High Potency Multi Vitamin and Mineral such as Core Science Ultimate Health Packs, Core Science Daily Wellness Packs or Core Science Ultimate Liquid Vitamin plus
Essential fatty Acids 1,000 to 2,000 mg daily
Vitamin D 1,000 I.U. 2 to 3X daily
D – Ribose
5-HTPor St John's Wort or Melatonin or SAMe
Malic acid 600 mg 2X daily
Magnesium 100 to 200 mg 1 to 2X daily
Curcumin (Turmeric)
Bowellia
Creatine 5,000 mg 2 times daily

HEART BURN AND INDIGESTION

High Potency Multi Vitamin and Mineral such as Core Science Ultimate Health Packs, Core Science Daily

Wellness Packs or Core Science Ultimate Liquid Vitamin
plus
Digestive Enzymes
Hydrochloric acid
Probiotics and Prebiotics

HEMORRHOIDS

High Potency Multi Vitamin and Mineral such as Core
Science Ultimate Health Packs, Core Science Daily
Wellness Packs or Core Science Ultimate Liquid Vitamin
plus
Essential fatty Acids 1,000 – 2,000 mg daily
Vitamin D 1,000 I.U. 2 to 3X daily
Grape seed extract
Bilberry extract
Dietary Fiber
Horse Chestnut 200 mg 2 to 3X daily
(standardized to 40% aescin content)

HEPATITIS (CHRONIC)

High Potency Multi Vitamin and Mineral such as Core
Science Ultimate Health Packs, Core Science Daily
Wellness Packs or Core Science Ultimate Liquid Vitamin
plus
Essential fatty Acids 2,000 to 4,000 mg daily
Vitamin D 1,000 I.U. 2 to 3X daily
Vitamin C 1,000 to 2,000 mg daily
Milk Thistle
Indole-3 Carbinol
Reishi Mushroom extract
Astragalus
Trimethylglycine 1,000 to 2,000 mg 3X daily

N-Acetylcysteine 1000 - 1800 mg
L-Glutamine 500 mg 3X daily
Alpha-Lipoic acid
Metabolic Detoxification Program

HIGH BLOOD PRESSURE

High Potency Multi Vitamin and Mineral such as Core
Science Ultimate Health Packs, Core Science Daily
Wellness Packs or Core Science Ultimate Liquid Vitamin
plus
Essential fatty Acids 2,000 to 4,000 mg daily
Vitamin D 1,000 I.U. 2 to 3X daily
Coenzyme Q10
Hawthorn
Calcium 500 to1500 mg daily
Magnesium 200 to 400 mg daily

HIGH CHOLESTEROL

High Potency Multi Vitamin and Mineral such as Core
Science Ultimate Health Packs, Core Science Daily
Wellness Packs or Core Science Ultimate Liquid Vitamin
plus
Core Science Chol Reduce 1000 3 to 4 packs daily
or
Essential fatty Acids 2,000 to 4,000 mg daily
Vitamin D 1,000 I.U. 2 to 3X daily
Gum Guggul
Chromium 200 to 600 mcg daily
Plant Sterols
Green Tea Extract
Niacin

HYPOGLYCEMIA

High Potency Multi Vitamin and Mineral such as Core
Science Ultimate Health Packs, Core Science Daily
Wellness Packs or Core Science Ultimate Liquid Vitamin
plus
Essential fatty Acids 1,000 to 2,000 mg daily
Vitamin D 1,000 I.U. 2 to 3X daily
Chromium 200 to 900 mcg daily
Soluble Fiber (Psyllium, Flaxseed powder, Fruits,
Vegetables, Beans and Peas)

INSOMNIA

High Potency Multi Vitamin and Mineral such as Core
Science Ultimate Health Packs, Core Science Daily
Wellness Packs or Core Science Ultimate Liquid Vitamin
plus
Melatonin

IRRITABLE BOWEL SYNDROME

Probiotics and Prebiotics
Digestive enzymes
Psyllium Husk Fiber

LIVER DISEASES (CIRRHOSIS, DRUG-INDUCED TOXICITIES
and CHRONIC HEPATITIS)

High Potency Multi Vitamin and Mineral such as Core
Science Ultimate Health Packs, Core Science Daily
Wellness Packs or Core Science Ultimate Liquid Vitamin
plus

Essential fatty Acids 1,000 to 2,000 mg daily
Vitamin D 1,000 I.U. 2 to 3X daily
Milk Thistle
Vitamin C 2000 to 3000 mg daily
Indole-3-Carbinol
Reishi Mushroom extract
Astragalus
Trimethylglycine 1,000 to 2,000 mg daily
N-Acetylcysteine
L Glutamine
Alpha-Lipoic acid
Metabolic Detoxification Program

MACULAR DEGENERATION

High Potency Multi vitamin and Mineral such as Core
Science Ultimate Health Packs, Core Science Daily
Wellness Packs or Core Science Ultimate Liquid Vitamin
plus
Essential fatty Acids 1,000 to 2,000 mg daily
Vitamin D 1,000 I.U. 2 to 3X daily
Lutein and zeaxanthin
Vitamin E 400 to 800 I.U. daily
Vitamin C 1,000 to 2,000 mg daily
Selenium 100 to 200 mcg daily
Zinc 25 to 50 mg daily
Bilberry
Grape seed extract

MENOPAUSE

High Potency Multi Vitamin and Mineral such as Core
Science Ultimate Health Packs, Core Science Daily

Wellness Packs or Core Science Ultimate Liquid Vitamin
plus
Essential fatty Acids 1,000 to 2,000 mg daily
Vitamin D 1,000 I.U. 2 to 3X daily
Black Cohosh
Genestein (Isoflavones)
Gamma Oryzanol
Calcium 500 to 1000 mg daily (500 mg at a time)
Magnesium 200 to 300 mg daily

MENSTRUAL DYSFUNCTION

High Potency Multi Vitamin and Mineral such as Core
Science Ultimate Health Packs, Core Science Daily
Wellness Packs or Core Science Ultimate Liquid Vitamin
plus
Essential fatty Acids 2,000 to 4,000 mg daily
Vitamin D 1,000 I.U. 2 to 3X daily
Vitamin E 200 to 400 I.U. daily
Magnesium 100 to 200 mg daily
Calcium 500 to 1,000 mg daily (500 mg at a time)
Vitamin B6 50 mg daily
Black Cohosh

MULTIPLE SCLEROSIS

High Potency Multi Vitamin and Mineral such as Core
Science Ultimate Health Packs, Core Science Daily
Wellness Packs or Core Science Ultimate Liquid Vitamin
plus
Essential fatty Acids 1,000 to 2,000 mg daily
Vitamin D 1,000 I.U. 2 to 3X daily
Vitamin E 200 to 600 I.U. daily
Vitamin B12 up to 60 mg daily under supervision

Selenium 100 to 200 mcg daily

MUSCLE CRAMPS (Spasm, cramps, repair)

High Potency Multi Vitamin and Mineral such as Core
Science Ultimate Health Packs, Core Science Daily
Wellness Packs or Core Science Ultimate Liquid Vitamin
plus
Essential fatty Acids 1,000 to 2,000 mg daily
Vitamin D 1,000 I.U. 2 to 3X daily
Core Science Muscle Repair

OSTEOARTHRITIS
See Arthritis

OSTEOPOROSIS AND OSTEOPENIA

High Potency Multi Vitamin and Mineral such as Core
Science Ultimate Health Packs, Core Science Daily
Wellness Packs or Core Science Ultimate Liquid Vitamin
plus
Core Science Bone Health Extreme
or
Essential fatty Acids 1,000 to 2,000 mg daily
Vitamin D 1,000 to 3,000 I.U. 2 to 3X daily
Calcium 500 to1,000 mg daily (500 mg at a time)
Magnesium 100 to 300 mg daily
Boron 1 to 3 mg daily
Genestein (Isoflavones)

PARKINSON'S DISEASE

High Potency Multi Vitamin and Mineral such as Core
Science Ultimate Health Packs, Core Science Daily

Wellness Packs or Core Science Ultimate Liquid Vitamin
plus
Essential fatty Acids 1,000 to 2,000 mg daily
Vitamin D 1,000 I.U. 2 to 3X daily
Vitamin E 400 to 600 I.U. daily
Vitamin C 1,000 to 2,000 mg daily
NADH 10 to 20 mg daily
Coenzyme Q10 50 to 100 mg 3X daily

PERIPHERAL VASCULAR DISEASE

High Potency Multi Vitamin and Mineral such as Core
Science Ultimate Health Packs, Core Science Daily
Wellness Packs or Core Science Ultimate Liquid Vitamin
plus
Essential fatty Acids 2,000 to 4,000 mg daily
Vitamin D 1,000 I.U. 2 to 3X daily
Vitamin E 200 to 1,600 I.U. daily

PREMENSTRUAL SYNDROME

High Potency Multi Vitamin and Mineral such as Core
Science Ultimate Health Packs, Core Science Daily
Wellness Packs or Core Science Ultimate Liquid Vitamin
plus
Essential fatty Acids 2,000 to 4,000 mg daily
Vitamin D 1,000 I.U. 2 to 3X daily
Black Cohosh
Genestein (Isoflavones)
Magnesium 100 to 300 mg daily
Vitamin B6 50 to 100 mg daily
Probiotics and Prebiotics

PROSTATE ENLARGEMENT

High Potency Multi Vitamin and Mineral such as Core Science Ultimate Health Packs, Core Science Daily Wellness Packs or Core Science Ultimate Liquid Vitamin
plus
Essential fatty Acids 1,000 to 2,000 mg daily
Vitamin D 1,000 I.U. 2 to 3X daily
Saw Palmetto
Pygeum Africanum
Beta-sitosterol
Stinging Nettle
Genestein (Isoflavones)
Pumpkinseed extract
Zinc 25 mg 1 to 2X daily

RAYNAUD'S DISEASE

High Potency Multi Vitamin and Mineral such as Core Science Ultimate Health Packs, Core Science Daily Wellness Packs or Core Science Ultimate Liquid Vitamin
plus
Essential fatty Acids 1,000 to 2,000 mg daily
Vitamin D 1,000 I.U. 2 to 3X daily
Hawthorn

RESTLESS LEG SYNDROME

High Potency Multi Vitamin and Mineral such as Core Science Ultimate Health Packs, Core Science Daily Wellness Packs or Core Science Ultimate Liquid Vitamin
plus
Essential fatty Acids 1,000 to 2,000 mg daily
Vitamin D 1,000 I.U. 2 to 3X daily

Magnesium 100 to 300 mg daily
Vitamin E 200 to 800 I.U. daily

RHEUMATOID ARTHRITIS
See Arthritis

TENDONITIS AND BURSITIS

High Potency Multi Vitamin and Mineral such as Core
Science Ultimate Health Packs, Core Science Daily
Wellness Packs or Core Science Ultimate Liquid Vitamin
plus
Essential fatty Acids 2,000 to 4,000 mg daily
Vitamin D 1,000 I.U. 2 to 3X daily
plus
Core Science Acute Injury Plus 3 to 5 packs daily
or
Curcumin (turmeric)
White Willow Bark extract
Ginger
Boswellia
MSM

ULCERATIVE COLITIS

High Potency Multi Vitamin and Mineral such as Core
Science Ultimate Health Packs, Core Science Daily
Wellness Packs or Core Science Ultimate Liquid Vitamin
plus
Essential Fatty Acids 1,000 to 2,000 mg daily
Vitamin D 1,000 I.U. 2 to 3X daily
L-Glutamine 500 mg 3X daily
Probiotics and Prebiotics
Curcumin (turmeric)

Ginger
Grape seed extract
Digestive Enzymes

URINARY TRACT INFECTIONS

High Potency Multi Vitamin and Mineral such as Core
Science Ultimate Health Packs, Core Science Daily
Wellness Packs or Core Science Ultimate Liquid Vitamin
plus
Essential Fatty Acids 1,000 to 2,000 mg daily
Vitamin D 1,000 I.U. 2 to 3X daily
Cranberry - For prevention of urinary tract infections
300 to 400 mg of concentrated
Cranberry juice capsules 2X per day
– **not** Cranberry Juice Cocktail

VARICOSE VEINS

High Potency Multi Vitamin and Mineral such as Core
Science Ultimate Health Packs, Core Science Daily
Wellness Packs or Core Science Ultimate Liquid Vitamin
plus
Essential Fatty Acids 1,000 to 2,000 mg daily
Vitamin D 1,000 I.U. 2 to 3X daily
Grape seed extract
Vitamin C 1000 to 2000 mg daily
Horse Chestnut 200 mg 2 to 3X daily
(standardized to 40% Aescin)

49

THE CHOICE IS YOURS

There have been numerous times throughout the writing of this book that I have come to the same conclusion. I can show you all of the science, but it still comes down to what I wrote about in one of my very first books, *"Healthy Beliefs Deadly Choices"*. The most important factor in determining your health is your belief system – what goes on in your head.

My hope was that by showing you the science of vitamins and the gross inaccuracies in the sick-care model, your belief system would either be reaffirmed towards taking the appropriate steps to optimal health or changed to accomplish that same goal.

Let's be blunt. There is no question and no ambiguity. The science, to any rational person applying common sense and from an optimal health paradigm, is abundantly clear. All you have to do now is act upon it. In today's day and age, everyone should take comprehensive vitamin supplementation in the right quantity and quality throughout the course of their lifetime. Any other belief is factually wrong. It is a need that is essential for everyone. Don't waste more time defending your false excuses for not being healthy than you do actually investing time in becoming and staying healthy.

I started this book with a quote, and I'd like to end it with a quote.

**"Only two things are infinite,
the universe and human stupidity,
and I'm not sure about the former"**
Albert Einstein

Einstein was recently proven wrong when he said that nothing could exceed the speed of light. Let's prove him wrong again and show him that the above quote doesn't need to be true if we take action now and for the rest of our lives. Take your vitamins.

About Dr. John Zielonka

Dr. Zielonka is one of Ottawa's best known and trusted health and wellness experts. His unique approach enables people to make informed choices and take an active role in their health. Only by looking at all of the factors related to one's health can they maximize their true health potential.

Dr. Zielonka is a Doctor of Chiropractic, holds a Bachelor of Science in Chemistry, has a Fellowship in Natural Supplementation and Anti-Aging, is a certified rehabilitation doctor, a certified occupational health consultant and is the Director of Health and Wellness Canada. He is the author of *"Healthellaneous"*, *"Nutrition Insanity"*, *"Healthy Beliefs Deadly Choices"* and co-author of the *"World's Best Kept Health Secret Revealed, Volume 3"* which pre-sold over 70,000 copies. His latest book, *"The Science of Vitamins Meets Optimum Health and Common Sense"* hit bookstores in February 2012. His Human Performance Lecture Series is the most comprehensive one of its kind in Canada with 63 different health topics of which some are now available on DVD. He has made numerous television and radio appearances including being a regular contributor to CTV Morning Live and he is the founder of National Health Day in Canada. He is the owner of the Ottawa Chiropractic & Natural Health Centre in Canada's capital, considered by many to be the premier centre for health in Ottawa.

His patients have included everyone from the world's fastest man, gold medal Olympic athletes, NHL, NFL and CFL players to past prime ministers, major corporations and newborn babies – yes, right there with them in the delivery room.

Dr. Zielonka, along with his wife Katherine, super-healthy daughter Breana, energy-filled twin boys Tyler and Ryan, dog Jack, cats Haley, Dexter and Darth and horses Billy and Tommy strive to make the world a healthier place.

Dr. Zielonka's websites:

www.drzonline.com

www.excellenceinhealth.com

www.yourhealthstore.ca

www.corescience.ca

www.facebook.com/excellenceinhealth
Please click the "like" button

Other books by Dr. Zielonka

Healthellaneous
This Book Could Save Your Life
2010

Nutrition Insanity
A Serious Look at Nutrition…and our lack of it.
2009

Healthy Beliefs Deadly Choices
2008

The World's Best Kept Health Secret Revealed Vol. 3
2006

Dr. Zielonka's books are available at www.drzonline.com as well as Amazon and all fine retail outlets.

They are also available at his health centre in the World Exchange Plaza in downtown Ottawa, Canada.

What People Are Saying About
"Healthy Beliefs Deadly Choices"

"Thank you for your timely book. I loved it! (Read it twice). Our society needs to be reminded that our health and well being are in our own hands. Even more – it's the beliefs we have about it which makes a difference. I choose to believe that my body is capable of healing itself as long as I give it proper nutrition, enough sleep, regular exercise and keep positive! That's why it was such a treat to read your "Healthy Beliefs, Deadly Choices". Those who are going to follow your advice will enjoy a healthy and happy life, abundance of energy and overall joy. Hope many more readers will decide to be responsible for their health! Looking forward to many more of your books!"

-R. Zitikiene, Carleton University

"In his book, "Healthy Beliefs, Deadly Choices", Dr. Zielonka brings to light the many discrepancies in our so called "health care" system, and makes us really look at how we take care of ourselves, not only as individuals, but as a society. Dr. Zielonka makes it perfectly clear that we must first take responsibility for our own health, first and foremost, by thinking clearly about what our choices are and then acting on what makes sense."

-Dr. Astrid Trim, President,
Momentum Healing Arts

Healthy Beliefs

Deadly Choices

How Your Beliefs Are Killing You

Dr. John Zielonka

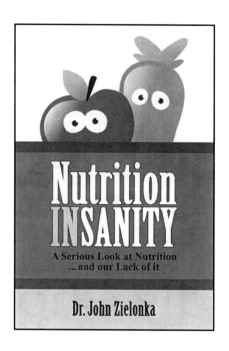

Nutrition Insanity
A Serious Look at Nutrition
...and our Lack of it

Dr. John Zielonka

"**Nutrition Insanity** brings a little common sense to the often perplexing and myth filled world of nutritional health. As health care practitioners we are frequently questioned by our patients about whether the latest fad diet or miracle exercise program will work to help "lose weight". Dr. Zielonka's latest book provides clear, concise and well researched insights that not only break weight loss myths, but more importantly, provide straightforward answers to questions of eating for Health. This book is written in no nonsense language that will be appreciated by patients and practitioners alike. From osteoarthritis to cardiovascular disease, Dr. Zielonka provides simple strategies that will help you regain control over your body and make you feel and look great!"

-Dr. Robert Fera B.Sc., H.K., D.C.
Integrated Wellness Concepts

DR. JOHN ZIELONKA

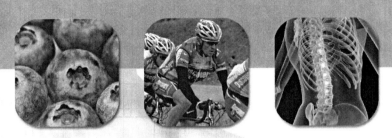

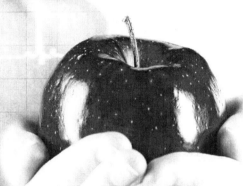

Healthellaneous
This Book Could Save Your Life

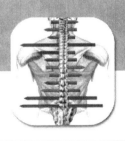
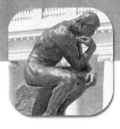
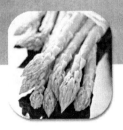

HEALTHELLANEOUS
THIS BOOK COULD SAVE YOUR LIFE

1. What do scientists say is the best form of treatment for headaches?
2. Can you safely lose 23 pounds of **fat** in 30 days?
3. What is the best way to slow, prevent and reverse arthritis?
4. How can improper backpack use have your child end up in the hospital?
5. Can a blind man climb and reach the peak of Mount Everest?
6. What daily activity is the # 1 cause of acute liver failure?
7. Do you really have all the facts when considering the Swine Flu vaccine?
8. What 3 things must everyone know about their spine and nervous system?
9. What common problem often caused by sitting can mimic a heart attack?

Dr. Zielonka's highly acclaimed health articles have benefited hundreds of his patients and thousands in the community to achieve a better way of life. Now in one collection, with the addition of numerous new, never before seen topics, whether you are a business executive, super mom, or both, you will discover answers to the above and so much more.

Dr. Zielonka has motivated and inspired me on my journey toward a healthier lifestyle. I have had the opportunity to re-think, re-evaluate and re-connect with all of the truly important things life has to offer, none of which are possible without optimal health. Dr. Zielonka's knowledge, enthusiasm and positive attitude is what makes every chapter interesting.

-Judy Grodsworth RN, BScN, (C)ONC
Medical Oncology Unit of the Ottawa Hospital

"Managing your health and wellness is an important part of building leadership resiliency and creating long-term business success. In his newest book, Healthellaneous, Dr. John Zielonka, shares many of his best insights and ideas, and provides concrete suggestions to help sustain your health and wellness and, in turn, enhance your leadership resiliency."

-Terrence B. Kulka, Ph.D., Director, Executive MBA
Telfer School of Management, University of Ottawa

#1 Best Seller

The World's Best Kept

Health Secret

REVEALED

VOLUME III

Dr. John Zielonka

and Leading Wellness Doctors

Book 3 of the Best Selling
Health Secret Series

CPSIA information can be obtained at www.ICGtesting.com
Printed in the USA
LVOW090935040212

266984LV00004B/5/P